Rheumatic Diseases and Syndromes Induced by Cancer Immunotherapy

Maria E. Suarez-Almazor
Leonard H. Calabrese
Editors

Rheumatic Diseases and Syndromes Induced by Cancer Immunotherapy

A Handbook for Diagnosis and Management

Springer

Editors
Maria E. Suarez-Almazor
Department of Health Services Research
University of Texas MD Anderson Cancer Center
Houston, TX
USA

Leonard H. Calabrese
Department of Rheumatic and Immunologic Diseases
Cleveland Clinic Lerner College of Medicine of Case Western Reserve University
Cleveland, OH
USA

ISBN 978-3-030-56823-8 ISBN 978-3-030-56824-5 (eBook)
https://doi.org/10.1007/978-3-030-56824-5

This Springer imprint is published by the registered company Springer Nature Switzerland AG
The registered company address is: Gewerbestrasse 11, 6330 Cham, Switzerland

Introduction

Immunotherapy has revolutionized the treatment of cancer. Although the concept of using one's immune system to attack tumor cells is not novel, it is the recent therapeutic use of immune checkpoint inhibition that has changed the landscape of cancer treatment. The discoveries leading to the development of immune checkpoint inhibitors were the basis for awarding the Noble Prize in Medicine in 2018 to James P. Allison, PhD, and Tasuku Honjo, MD, PhD. Immune checkpoint inhibitors are monoclonal antibodies that block physiologic and tumor-derived inhibitory immune responses, thus resulting in a broad upregulation of the immune system, enhancing antitumor immunity. These agents were initially approved for use in patients with metastatic melanoma, but in the past 5 years their use has exponentially increased to many other cancers, and they are also being used as adjuvant therapy in patients with extended local disease after surgery. Despite their benefits, immune checkpoint inhibitors are associated with important toxicity derived from the unrestrained upregulation of the immune system. They can cause inflammatory and autoimmune manifestations, termed immune-related adverse event (irAE). These adverse events can affect almost any organ or system and can result in severe morbidity and death. Often, the immune checkpoint inhibitor needs to be discontinued, and patients require immunosuppression to control the effects of irAE. Several rheumatic irAE have been described in cancer patients receiving immune checkpoint inhibitors, the most common being inflammatory arthritis, polymyalgia-like syndromes, myositis, and sicca syndromes. While the care of cancer patients receiving immunotherapy who develop immune toxicity must be multidisciplinary, rheumatologists play an important role in managing rheumatic irAE, given our experience in treating similar primary autoimmune diseases with immunosuppressive drugs.

The overall goal of the book is to provide clinicians with a handbook on the management of rheumatic irAE that develops from cancer immunotherapy. We address more comprehensively the irAE seen with immune checkpoint inhibitors, as these are the most frequently used agents. The first chapters of the handbook describe the origins of cancer immunotherapy, current therapies, and the pathogenesis of resulting irAE. The next chapters provide an overview of the various rheumatic inflammatory and autoimmune syndromes described in cancer patients who receive immune checkpoint inhibitors. Clinical cases are included in each chapter. Two additional chapters provide an overview of non-rheumatic immune-related adverse events, and adverse events that occur with cancer immunotherapies other than immune checkpoint inhibitors. The management of cancer patients with concomitant rheumatic autoimmune diseases who are eligible to receive immune checkpoint blockade is complex, as these patients may flare or be at higher risk for de novo irAE. Clinical trials have typically excluded patients with preexisting autoimmune disease, so current evidence is primarily from small case series. We provide a comprehensive review of the literature on this topic. Finally, the last three chapters discuss the general principles of management including how to choose the right therapy, risk-benefit considerations, and how to approach shared decision-making in clinical settings.

The handbook targets primarily clinicians: rheumatologists and clinical immunologists, including fellows in training programs, and also general oncologists and internists who may practice in underserved areas with a little access to rheumatology services. Our intent is to provide a concise review of current clinical knowledge on rheumatic irAE, with guidance for diagnosis and management. We have strived to include the latest clinical evidence in the field, incorporating current guidelines and professional societies' recommendations. Yet, knowledge in this area is continuously advancing, and best management practices are likely to evolve as new data on the pathogenesis and treatment of irAE becomes available. We hope clinicians find the handbook to be a practical, useful guide in the complex management of cancer patients who develop inflammatory and autoimmune adverse events as a consequence of cancer immunotherapy.

Contents

Contributors

Noha Abdel-Wahab, MD, PhD The University of Texas MD Anderson Cancer Center, Houston, TX, USA

Assiut University Hospital, Faculty of Medicine, Assiut, Egypt

Alan N. Baer, MD, FACP Sjögren's Syndrome Clinic, National Institute of Dental and Craniofacial Research, Bethesda, MD, USA

Division of Rheumatology, Johns Hopkins University School of Medicine, Baltimore, MD, USA

Aanika Balaji, MPH Johns Hopkins University School of Medicine, Baltimore, MD, USA

Clifton O. Bingham III, MD Division of Rheumatology, Johns Hopkins School of Medicine, Baltimore, MD, USA

Sebastian Bruera, MD Department of Medicine, Section of Immunology, Allergy, and Rheumatology, Baylor College of Medicine, Houston, TX, USA

Cassandra Calabrese, DO Department of Rheumatologic and Immunologic Diseases, Cleveland Clinic Foundation, Cleveland, OH, USA

Leonard H. Calabrese, DO Department of Rheumatic and Immunologic Diseases, Cleveland Clinic Lerner College of Medicine of Case Western Reserve University, Cleveland, OH, USA

Laura C. Cappelli, MD MHS Division of Rheumatology, Johns Hopkins School of Medicine, Baltimore, MD, USA

Adi Diab Department of Melanoma Medical Oncology, Division of Cancer Medicine, University of Texas MD Anderson Cancer Center, Houston, TX, USA

Margarita Divenko, MS Department of Immunology, The University of Texas MD Anderson Cancer Center, Houston, TX, USA

Faisal Fa'ak, MD Department of Graduate Medical Education, Piedmont Athens Regional Medical Center, Athens, GA, USA

Tamiko R. Katsumoto, MD Division of Immunology and Rheumatology, Stanford University, Palo Alto, CA, USA

Sang Kim, MD, PhD Section of Rheumatology, Department of General Internal Medicine, The University of Texas MD Anderson Cancer Center, Houston, TX, USA

Marie Kostine, MD, PhD Department of Rheumatology, Bordeaux University Hospital, Bordeaux, France

Olivier Lambotte, MD, PhD AP-HP-Paris Saclay, Médecine Interne/Immunologie Clinique, Hôpital Bicêtre, Paris, France

Université-Paris-Saclay; INSERM; CEA, Immunology of Viral Infections and Autoimmune Diseases Centre, IDMIT Department, Le Kremlin-Bicêtre, France

Cerena K. Leung, MD Department of General Internal Medicine, The University of Texas MD Anderson Cancer Center, Houston, TX, USA

Maria A. Lopez-Olivo, MD, PhD Department of Health Services Research, The University of Texas, MD Anderson Cancer Center, Houston, TX, USA

Andrew L. Mammen, MD, PhD Laboratory of Muscle Stem Cells and Gene Expression, National Institute of Arthritis and Musculoskeletal and Skin Diseases, National Institutes of Health, Bethesda, MD, USA

Xavier Mariette, MD, PhD Rhumatologie, Université Paris-Saclay, Assistance Publique – Hôpitaux de Paris, Hôpital Bicêtre, Le Kremlin Bicêtre, France

Alexa Simon Meara, MD MS The Ohio State University Wexner Medical Center, Division of Immunology and Rheumatology, Columbus, OH, USA

Jarushka Naidoo, MBBCh MHS Department of Oncology, Sidney Kimmel Comprehensive Cancer Center Johns Hopkins University, Baltimore, MD, USA

Bloomberg-Kimmel Institute for Cancer Immunotherapy at Johns Hopkins University, Baltimore, MD, USA

Roza Nurieva, PhD Department of Immunology, The University of Texas MD Anderson Cancer Center, Houston, TX, USA

Xerxes Pundole, MD, PhD Department of Health Services Research, The University of Texas MD Anderson Cancer Center, Houston, TX, USA

Manuel Ramos-Casals, MD Department of Autoimmune Diseases, ICMiD, Barcelona, Spain

Sjögren Syndrome Research Group (AGAUR), Laboratory of Autoimmune Diseases Josep Font, IDIBAPS-CELLEX, Barcelona, Spain

Department of Medicine, University of Barcelona, Hospital Clínic, Barcelona, Spain

Bairavi Shankar, BA Johns Hopkins University School of Medicine, Baltimore, MD, USA

Maria E. Suarez-Almazor, MD, PhD Department of Health Services Research, University of Texas MD Anderson Cancer Center, Houston, TX, USA

Uma Thanarajasingam, MD, PhD Mayo Clinic, Rochester, MN, USA

Alice Tison, MD Department of Rheumatology, Brest University Hospital, Brest, France

Blake M. Warner, DDS, PhD, MPH Salivary Disorders Unit, National Institute of Dental and Craniofacial Research, Bethesda, MD, USA

Sjögren's Syndrome Clinic, National Institute of Dental and Craniofacial Research, Bethesda, MD, USA

Part I
Introduction

Chapter 1
Cancer Immunology and the Evolution of Immunotherapy

Roza Nurieva, Margarita Divenko, and Sang Kim

Cancer Immunology: Immunoediting Hypothesis

More than a century ago, Virchow detected immune cells within tumors and suggested crosstalk between host immune system and tumors [1]. Several decades later, experiments utilizing murine models with either carcinogen-induced or spontaneous developed tumors revealed that tumor cells are antigenic and that host immune systems sense and eradicate them [2]. These experiments generated the immunosurveillance hypothesis postulating that the immune system identifies and eradicates nascent transformed cells to prevent

---

R. Nurieva (✉) · M. Divenko
Department of Immunology, The University of Texas MD Anderson Cancer Center, Houston, TX, USA
e-mail: RNurieva@mdanderson.org; MADivenko@mdanderson.org

S. Kim
Section of Rheumatology, Department of General Internal Medicine, The University of Texas MD Anderson Cancer Center, Houston, TX, USA
e-mail: STKim@mdanderson.org

M. E. Suarez-Almazor, L. H. Calabrese (eds.), *Rheumatic Diseases and Syndromes Induced by Cancer Immunotherapy*,
https://doi.org/10.1007/978-3-030-56824-5_1

development and growth of tumors [3]. The immunosurveillance hypothesis was later challenged as tumors, either induced by carcinogens or developing spontaneously, grew in both wild-type and athymic mice [4]. This hypothesis was revived in the 1990s with the development of murine models of immunodeficiency with pure genetic backgrounds [3]. Indeed, the immunosurveillance hypothesis was further expanded to the more comprehensive cancer immunoediting theory postulating that the immune system does not only protect from cancer but also shapes tumor cell immunogenicity. The immunoediting process comprises of three E phases: "elimination," "equilibrium," and "escape" [3].

Elimination

In the elimination phase, both the innate and adaptive immune systems cooperate to identify and eliminate transformed cells before they develop into a tumor. Initially, immune cells recognize the transformed cells through classical danger signals including type I interferon (IFN), damage-associated molecular patterns, and transformed cell-specific molecules such as H60, MICA/B, and RAE-1 [5]. Subsequently, immune cells including tumor-specific $CD4^+$ and $CD8^+$ T cells, natural killer (NK) cells, $\gamma\delta$ T cells, and M1 macrophages eliminate transformed cells via direct phagocytosis as well as through cytotoxic molecules including IFNγ, tumor necrosis factor alpha (TNFα), perforin, granzyme, NK cell receptor group 2D, and TNF-related apoptosis-inducing ligand [3].

Equilibrium

Some transformed cells evade elimination and enter the equilibrium phase. During this phase, tumors do not grow but are not completely eradicated by immune cells. In some transplantable tumor models, mice do not develop visible tumors for a long period of time even though tumor cells are microscopically detected at the injection site of tumor cells; however, when T cells or IFNγ are depleted, tumors begin to grow rapidly [6]. Equilibrium appears to be the longest of the three phases, lasting decades in some cancers [5]. During equilibrium, the host immune system shapes the immunogenicity of tumors by providing continuous selection pressure.

Escape

In the escape phase, tumor cells gradually lose antigenicity and finally escape immune cell recognition and elimination. Both intrinsic and extrinsic mechanisms contribute to tumor cell escape [7]. Intrinsically, tumor cells (1) express less tumor-specific antigens as well as surface major histocompatibility (MHC) class I molecules, (2) down-modulate the formation of self-peptide-MHC class I complex, (3) decrease expression of co-stimulatory molecules while increasing expression of co-inhibitory molecules, and (4) secrete immunosuppressive mediators. Extrinsically, suppressive immune cells including regulatory T cells, myeloid-derived suppressor cells, and M2 macrophages emerge and suppress anti-tumor immunity, helping tumor cells escape.

Cancer Immunotherapy

Major milestones in the history of cancer immunotherapy are shown in Fig. 1.1. Various immune-based cancer therapies have been approved by the Food and Drug Administration (FDA) and European Medicines Agency (EMA) or are being studied in clinical trials (Table 1.1). Here, we will briefly review each therapy.

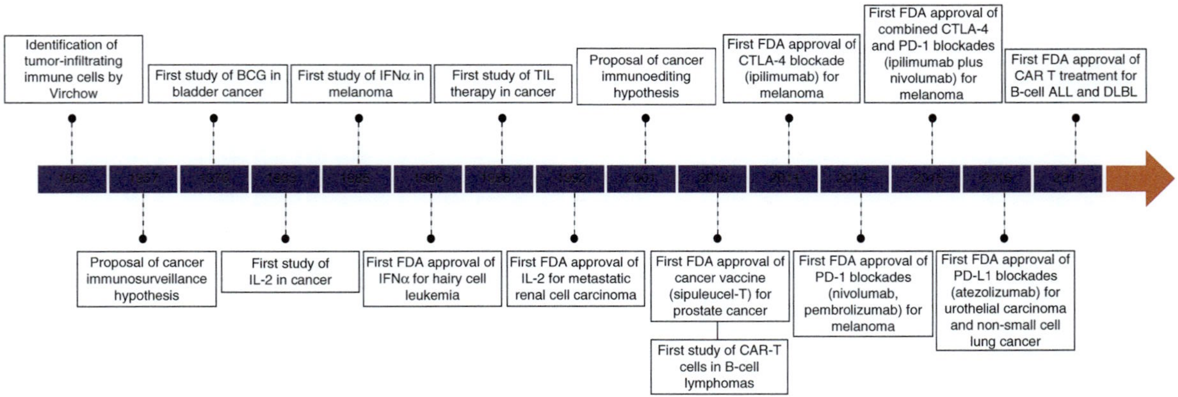

BCG, Bacilli Calmettee-Guerin; IFN, interferon; TIL, tumor-infiltrating lymphocyte; CAR, Chimeric antigen receptor; CTLA-4, Cytotoxic T-lymphocyte-associated antigen-4; PD-1, programmed cell death 1; PD-L1, programmed cell death ligand 1; IL-2 interleukin 2; All Acute lymphoblastic leukemia; DLBL, diffuse large B-cell lymphoma

FIGURE 1.1 Timeline in cancer immunotherapy

TABLE 1.1 Major immune-based cancer therapies

Modality	Target(s)	Current status
Immune checkpoint inhibitors	CTLA-4	FDA approved for treatment of multiple cancers
	PD-1	FDA approved for treatment of multiple cancers
	PD-L1	FDA approved for treatment of multiple cancers
	Multiple[a]	Phase I–III
Exogenous cytokines	n/a	IL-2: FDA approved for treatment of melanoma
		IFNα: FDA approved for treatment of multiple cancers
		IL-12, 15, 21, and GM-CSF: Phase I–III
Tumor vaccines	n/a	HPV vaccines: FDA approved for prevention of HPV-related malignancies HBV vaccine: FDA approved for prevention of HBV-related malignancies DC vaccine: FDA approved for treatment of prostate cancer
Adoptive cell therapy	n/a	CAR-T-cell therapy: FDA approved for treatment of B-cell ALL and DLBL TIL therapy, NK cell therapy, engineered T-cell receptor therapy: Phase I–III
Epigenetic drugs	HDAC	FDA approved for treatment of cutaneous/peripheral T-cell lymphoma and multiple myeloma
	DNMT	FDA approved for treatment of myelodysplastic syndrome and acute myeloid leukemia

(continued)

TABLE 1.1 (continued)

CLL chronic lymphocytic leukemia, *ALL* acute lymphocytic leukemia, *IFN* interferon, *GM-CSF* granulocyte-macrophage colony-stimulating factor, *HPV* human papilloma virus, *HBV* hepatitis B virus, *DC* dendritic cells, *CAR* chimeric antigen receptor, *TIL* tumor-infiltrating lymphocytes, *DLBL* diffuse large B-cell lymphoma, *HDAC* histone deacetylase, *DNMT* DNA methyltransferase
[a]Described in the main text

Immune Checkpoint Inhibitors

Immune checkpoint inhibitors (ICIs) have revolutionized the treatment of multiple cancers by releasing the breaks on the immune system so it can destroy cancer cells [8]. Inhibitory immune checkpoint molecules, including cytotoxic T lymphocyte-associated antigen 4 (CTLA-4), programmed cell death-1 (PD-1), and programmed cell death ligand-1 (PD-L1), play a decisive role in the maintenance of peripheral tolerance and prevention of autoimmunity. Blocking antibodies to CTLA-4, PD-1, and PD-L1 have shown significant success by enhancing anti-tumor immunity with subsequent eradication of tumor cells in many patients.

In 2011, the FDA approved the first ICI, ipilimumab (a human IgG1 monoclonal antibody against CTLA-4), for the treatment of metastatic melanoma [9]. Ipilimumab was the first treatment to significantly extend survival in metastatic melanoma when compared with a peptide vaccine or with standard dacarbazine chemotherapy [10]. It is undergoing clinical trials for the treatment of renal cell carcinoma, non-small cell lung carcinoma, bladder cancer, and prostate cancer [11]. The mechanisms of action of CTLA-4 blockade lie on unrestrained CD28-mediated positive co-stimulation in T cells [12], depletion of immunosuppressive regulatory T cells [13], and remodeling and broadening of the peripheral T-cell receptor (TCR) repertoire [10]. In

2014, the FDA approved two additional ICIs, both of which target PD-1, pembrolizumab and nivolumab, for the treatment of refractory melanoma [13, 14]. Later, the FDA also approved them for advanced non-small cell lung cancer, renal cell carcinoma, Hodgkin's lymphoma, head and neck cancer, and urothelial cancer [10, 15]. Regarding PD-L1 blockade, the FDA approved atezolizumab in 2016 for urothelial cancer and non-small cell lung cancer [10] followed by durvalumab (bladder cancer) and avelumab (urothelial cancer and Merkel cell carcinoma) in 2017 [10]. Clinical trials on other cancer types are ongoing for many of these agents. Inhibition of PD-1/PD-L1 pathways mainly induces tumor rejection by preventing PD-L1 inhibitory signals from tumor and non-tumor cells, with resultant reinvigoration of exhausted $CD8^+$ T cells in the tumor microenvironment [16, 17]. Compared to the CTLA-4 blockade, PD-1/PD-L1 blockade is more efficacious and less toxic [10]. More recently, clinical trials have reported that the combination of CTLA-4 and PD-1 blockade can be highly effective and prolong patients' survival [18]; however, ICI combination therapy is associated with a higher frequency of immune-related adverse events when compared to therapy with a single ICI [19].

While CTLA-4 and PD-1/PD-L1 blockade has demonstrated durable clinical responses for various malignancies, not all patients benefit from these treatments. Expanding clinical benefit to the majority of patients and preventing cancer resistance require a better understanding of the mechanisms that lead to an effective anti-tumor response. Beyond CTLA-4 and PD-1/PD-L1, a number of co-stimulatory (OX40, ICOS, GITR, 4-1BB, CD27, and CD40) or co-inhibitory (LAG-3, TIM-3, TIGIT, VISTA, B7-H3 (CD274), B7S1 (B7-H4, B7x, or Vtcn1), B7-H6, and B7-H7 (HHLA2)) immune checkpoint pathways have emerged with key role in regulating T-cell responses, and their therapeutic exploitation has shown success in preclinical models and currently under investigation in clinical trials [12, 20–30].

Cytokines

Cytokines including IFNα, interleukin (IL)-2, granulocyte-macrophage colony-stimulating factor (GM-CSF), IL-12, IL-15, and IL-21 have shown to have anti-tumor efficacy in preclinical murine studies [31]; among them, only IL-2 and IFNα have demonstrated clinical benefit and received FDA approval for the treatment of several cancers [32]. IFNα-2a was the first approved cytokine for the treatment of hairy cell leukemia in 1986. Later, IFNα-2a and IFNα-2b were approved for patients with high-risk melanoma or renal cell carcinoma [33]. IFNα ligation is critical for the host immune response against tumor – for generation and survival of $CD4^+$ T helper 1 (Th1) cells, cytotoxic T lymphocytes (CTL), and memory $CD8^+$ T cells, cytotoxic function and survival of NK cells, and dendritic cell (DC) maturation [33]. However, adverse events of systemic long-term treatments and suboptimal anti-tumor efficacy have relegated IFNα to second-line therapy as an adjunctive agent [34]. IL-2 is a key cytokine in promoting the expansion and cytotoxic function of NK cells and T lymphocytes. High-dose IL-2 (aldesleukin) was approved by the FDA in 1992 for metastatic renal cell carcinoma and in 1998 for metastatic melanoma [33, 35, 36]. However, high-dose IL-2 monotherapy failed to improve patients' survival due to its functional properties on expansion of regulatory T cells and association with severe adverse events including vascular leak syndrome, pulmonary edema, hypotension, renal insufficiency, and myocarditis [33]. To enhance anti-tumor efficacy while lowering adverse events, newly engineered IL-2 mutants (IL-2 superkine) or chimeric antibody-IL-2 fusion protein (IL-2 immunokine) [33, 37–41], either alone or combined with other cancer immunotherapies such as cytokines, adoptive cell-based immunotherapy, antigen-specific vaccination, and ICIs, are being investigated. These therapies have shown survival benefits in patients with advanced cancers [42, 43].

Other cytokines including GM-CSF, IL-12, IL-21, and IL-15 showed promise in preclinical settings; however, their clinical utility has been modest due to severe dose-limiting toxicity and/or inadequate tumoral responses [33, 44–47]. To overcome these barriers, modified cytokines (superkines and immunokines) are being investigated alone or in combination with anticancer vaccines, and ICIs to sustain anticancer efficacy, while aiming to limit toxicity [33]. For example, since GM-CSF leads to immunosuppression through the dysfunction of T-cell responses by myeloid-derived suppressor cells, the combination of GM-CSF with chemotherapies (gemcitabine, 5-fluorouracil, and docetaxel) can reduce the number of myeloid-derived suppressor cells and overcome GM-CSF-mediated immunosuppression [44, 45, 48]. While IL-12 administration showed significant therapeutic activity and acceptable toxicity in primary and metastatic preclinical models [49, 50], systemic administration of IL-12 to cancer patients is associated with severe toxicity, limiting its clinical utilization [46, 51]. To overcome toxicities, various approaches to deliver IL-12 (gene transfer via viral vectors, and liposomes, or electroporation of IL-12-encoding plasmids) in accessible tumor lesions as a single agent or in combination with ICIs are currently being tested in mice and humans [49, 50]. Clinical trials utilizing IL-21, either alone (acute myeloid leukemia) or in combination with CTLA-4 blockade (metastatic melanoma) and PD-1 blockade (advanced solid tumors), are underway [52]. A number of clinical trials testing IL-15 solely or in conjunction with NK cell transfer or DC vaccination in hematologic and solid malignancies are ongoing [53].

Cytokines such as TNFα, transforming growth factor beta (TGFβ), IL-1β, and IL-6 are involved in cancer-related inflammation and are proposed as therapeutic targets to enhance anti-tumor immunity [54, 55]. A recent study showed that TNFα diminishes the efficacy of anti-PD-1 therapy in mouse and human cancers by inducing expression of T-cell immunoglobulin mucin-3 (TIM-3), one of co-inhibitory molecules, on tumor-infiltrating lymphocytes after PD-1 blockade treatment [56]. Currently, the combination of TNFα blockage (infliximab or certolizumab) with ICIs is being evaluated for patients with metastatic melanoma (NCT: 03293784 on ClinicalTrials.gov). TGFβ promotes tumorigenesis in the later stages of tumor development by recruiting regulatory T cells and myeloid-derived suppressor cells to tumor sites and by inhibiting $CD8^+$ T cell and NK cell cytotoxicity [57]. TGFβ blocking agents such as galunisertib (small molecule) and fresolimumab (antagonistic antibody) showed synergistic effects with ICIs in breast and colon cancer treatment [58]. IL-1β, one of the most potent proinflammatory cytokines, plays a key role in growth, invasion, and dissemination of nearly all types of cancer cells [54, 55]. Currently, the IL-1 receptor antagonist (anakinra) is being utilized in clinical trials of patients with melanoma [59]. The IL-6 signaling pathway is critical for proliferation, survival, differentiation, and dissemination of various types of cancer cells including multiple myeloma, lung cancer, renal cell carcinoma, breast cancer, colorectal cancer, cervical cancer, and ovarian cancer [54, 60, 61]. Agents targeting IL-6 (siltuximab, clazakizumab, mAb1339), IL-6 receptor (tocilizumab, SANT-7), and IL-6 trans-signaling (sgp130Fc) are actively being evaluated in preclinical and clinical studies of various cancers with promising results [54, 60, 61].

Cancer Vaccines

The main purpose of cancer vaccines is to expose the patient's immune system to molecules associated with cancer to enable the immune system to recognize and destroy cancer cells. Cancer vaccines can be classified into preventive or therapeutic [62]. Human papilloma virus (HPV) and hepatitis B virus (HBV) vaccines can prevent HPV (cervical, head and neck, penile, vulvar, and vaginal cancers) and HBV-related (liver cancer) cancers [63]. Other viruses causing cancer include the human T-cell leukemia-lymphoma virus (adult T-cell leukemia), human herpesvirus-8 (Kaposi's sarcoma), and Epstein-Barr virus (Burkitt's lymphoma, gastric adenocarcinoma, and nasopharyngeal carcinoma), which cause malignancies as indicated; however, no vaccines exist against these viruses as of now [64].

While preventive vaccines are administered to healthy individuals and designed to target oncogenic viruses, therapeutic cancer vaccines, including cell vaccines (tumor and immune cells), protein/peptide vaccines, and genetic (DNA, RNA, and viral) vaccines, aim to eradicate malignancies [65]. Autologous tumor vaccines, utilizing patient-derived tumor cells genetically modified ex vivo with heightened antigenicity, were one of the first types of vaccines successfully tested in various cancers; however, these vaccines require sufficient tumor specimen, limiting implementation to only certain tumor types and/or stages [65]. To overcome the challenge, allogeneic whole tumor cell vaccines containing established human tumor cell lines have been developed [66, 67], but to date, clinical trials have shown limited success due to interpatient heterogeneity [68]. DCs are an attractive biologic tool for therapeutic vaccines because the most critical step in vaccination is the effective presentation of cancer antigens to T cells. The first FDA-approved DC vaccine, Sipuleucel-T (Provenge®), containing patient-derived DCs activated with prostate cancer antigen (prostatic acid phosphatase) and GM-CSF, was utilized for the treatment of metastatic castrate-resistant prostate cancer [69]. Despite the safety and immunogenicity of Sipuleucel-T, its efficacy is suboptimal due to insufficient antigen presentation, cytokine secretion, and migratory capacity of DCs. Recent genetic approaches to enhance expression of co-stimulatory molecules (CD40, CD70, GITRL, 4-1BBL, and OX-40 L) and/or pro-inflammatory factors (IL-12p70, IL-2, IL-18, CCR7, and CXCL10) by DCs have shown improvement of potency of DC-based vaccines [70–76] .

Utilizing peptides derived from defined tumor-associated antigens including cancer-testis antigens (MAGE, BAGE, NY-ESO-1, and SSX-2), tissue differentiation antigens (gp100 and Melan-A/MART-1 for melanoma; PSA and PAP for prostate cancer; mammaglobin-A for breast cancer), mutational antigens (ras, B-raf, and p53), viral antigens (Merkel cell polyomavirus for Merkel cell carcinoma; HPV for cervical or oropharyngeal cancers), and oncofetal antigens (CFA and MUC-1) and recombinant vaccines are an attractive option as they are easily produced and administered with minimal toxicity in clinics [77–82]. Since tumor-associated antigens can be poorly immunogenic, immunostimulatory adjuvants are essential for generation of effective immune responses [83, 84]. The challenges of recombinant vaccines include identifying the best and/or combination of Tumor-Associated Antigens (TAAs), selecting the most effective adjuvant, and identifying concurrent immunotherapies with synergistic effects [65].

Genetic vaccines are one of the most promising methodologies. They utilize viral or plasmid DNA vectors to deliver an expression cassette carrying the DNA- or mRNA-encoding tumor antigens, which are taken up by antigen-presenting cells and presented to tumor-specific T cells [85]. Genetic vaccines are cost-effective, as they deliver multiple tumor antigens in one immunization and do not require adjuvants to activate anti-tumor immune system effectively [85]. However, due to low uptake efficacy, genetic vaccines cannot induce efficient anti-tumor immunity. Technologies such as electroporation, ultrasound, laser, gene gun, liposome, microparticles, and nanoparticles are being examined to improve the delivery of genetic vaccines effectively and found to improve the vaccine efficacy [86–88].

Tumor-specific antigens (neoantigens), originating from nonsynonymous mutations and other genetic alterations in cancer cells, are expressed on the surface of tumor cells but not on normal cells. They are highly immunogenic, and, thus, they are ideal targets for therapeutic cancer vaccine to effectively induce tumor-specific T cells without killing normal cells. Several clinical trials have demonstrated the safety and efficacy of neoantigen vaccines [89–91].

Adoptive Cell Therapy

Adoptive cell therapy (ACT) employing patient-derived lymphocytes is a novel class of therapy providing high efficiency in an antigen-specific manner [92–95]. ACTs can be classified into four different types: tumor-infiltrating lymphocyte (TIL) therapy, engineered T-cell receptor (TCR) gene therapy, chimeric antigen receptor (CAR)-T-cell therapy, and NK cell therapy [96].

In 1987, Rosenberg's team showed that ex vivo expanded TILs from murine malignancies have a potent in vivo anti-tumor capacity [97]. Preclinical models and initial human trials showed remarkable tumor responses in patients with metastatic melanoma. This approach is now being evaluated in other cancers [98].

In TCR gene therapy, peripheral blood T cells are isolated and genetically modified in vitro to express TCRs that sense tumor-associated antigens such as MART-1, gp100, Y-ESO-1, MAGE-family, SSX, and HPV [92, 99]. TCR-T cells recognize the antigens bound to MHC molecules on tumor cells and eradicate them after recognition [100]. While clinical trials demonstrate the therapeutic potential of TCR gene therapy [100], the tumor antigens that have been explored up until now are not solely expressed by the tumor cells; thus, the identification of antigens restricted to tumor cells is essential to improve efficacy and safety profiles of the TCR gene therapy [101]. Another obstacle of TCR gene therapy is that cancer cells can escape T cell-mediated immune responses by downregulation or loss of their MHC expression [102].

Chimeric antigen receptor (CAR)-T-cell therapy can circumvent the need for the presence of MHC on tumor cells for recognition by tumor-specific T cells. Different from TCR-T cells, CAR-T cells function independently of MHC expression [103–107]. The engineering of CARs has evolved over time and resulted in four generations of CAR molecules. Currently, CAR-T-cell therapies have shown therapeutic benefits, especially for CD19 expressing B-cell malignancies, and the FDA has recently approved two anti-CD19 CAR-T-cell therapies (axicabtagene ciloleucel and tisagenlecleucel) for diffuse B-cell lymphoma and acute lymphoblastic leukemia [108–111]. In addition to hematological malignancies, CAR-T-cell therapy is being explored in solid tumors [112–114]. Despite its efficacy, CAR-T-cell therapy can cause significant toxicity, including cytokine release syndrome and "on-target, off-tumor" effects, which are related to uncontrolled CAR-T-cell activity and/or cross-reactivity. To avoid such toxicity of CAR-T cells, incorporation of suicide genes into the engineered T cells is a safe and efficient way to abrogate the adverse effects through elimination of transferred T cells [115, 116].

NK cells are innate effector lymphocytes with potent anti-tumor activity [117]. NK cell-based therapy including autologous NK, allogenic NK, and CAR-NK are of great clinical interest for the following reasons: (i) allogeneic NK cells do not cause graft-versus-host disease [118–122]; (ii) their relatively short life span can allow an effective anti-tumor activity while reducing long-term adverse events such as cytopenia; and (iii) since CAR-NK cells recognize and target tumor cells through their native receptors, tumor escape with CAR-NK cells by downregulating the CAR target antigen is less likely to occur than with CAR-T cells [123]. Preclinical and clinical studies have demonstrated the safety and efficacy of NK cell-based therapies against various hematological and solid malignancies, and several clinical trials are currently ongoing [124]. Genetic manipulation to improve persistency and cytotoxicity of NK cells will further enhance the efficacy of NK cell-based therapies while preserving their outstanding safety profile.

Epigenetic Drugs

Epigenetic alterations are a critical element in generation, proliferation, and survival of tumor cells, and epigenetic modifiers can be potential druggable targets for anticancer therapy [125]. During tumorigenesis, the epigenome goes through multiple alterations, including genome-wide loss of DNA methylation and regional hypermethylation of promoter of tumor suppressor genes, global loss in histone modification marks, overexpression of histone deacetylases (HDACs), and deregulation of histone methyltransferases (HMTs) [125]. The most effective and commonly used epigenetic drugs are inhibitors of the key enzymes involved in DNA methylation, DNA Methyltransferase Inhibitors (iDNMTs), and histone deacetylation, Histone Deacetylase Inhibitors (iHDACs) [126, 127]. Four iHDACs and two iDNMTs have been approved by the FDA for the treatment of various hematologic malignancies [128–130]; these agents are not as effective in patients with solid tumors, possibly due to their more differentiated cell status and lesser gene reprogramming plasticity [125].

Future of Cancer Immunotherapy

With durable tumor responses, immunotherapy is becoming a frontline treatment for various malignancies. Recent clinical trials of immunotherapy combined with other cancer treatments such as surgery, chemotherapy, and radiation therapy demonstrate promising results [131–134]. Various cancer immunotherapeutic modalities are currently in the pipeline, targeting various other components of the immune system. Given its paradigm-shifting clinical success, immunotherapy is becoming a mainstream option in cancer therapeutics, either alone or in combination with other conventional cancer therapies.

References

1. Hanahan D, Weinberg RA. Hallmarks of cancer: the next generation. Cell. 2011;144(5):646–74.
2. Smith HJ. Antigenicity of carcinogen-induced and spontaneous tumours in inbred mice. Br J Cancer. 1966;20(4):831–7.
3. Dunn GP, Bruce AT, Ikeda H, Old LJ, Schreiber RD. Cancer immunoediting: from immunosurveillance to tumor escape. Nat Immunol. 2002;3(11):991–8.
4. Stutman O. Tumor development after 3-methylcholanthrene in immunologically deficient athymic-nude mice. Science. 1974;183(4124):534–6.
5. Schreiber RD, Old LJ, Smyth MJ. Cancer immunoediting: integrating immunity's roles in cancer suppression and promotion. Science. 2011;331(6024):1565–70.
6. Koebel CM, Vermi W, Swann JB, Zerafa N, Rodig SJ, Old LJ, et al. Adaptive immunity maintains occult cancer in an equilibrium state. Nature. 2007;450(7171):903–7.
7. Suarez-Almazor ME, Kim ST, Abdel-Wahab N, Diab A. Review: immune-related adverse events with use of checkpoint inhibitors for immunotherapy of Cancer. Arthritis Rheumatol. 2017;69(4):687–99.
8. Ribas A. Releasing the brakes on Cancer immunotherapy. N Engl J Med. 2015;373(16):1490–2.
9. Lipson EJ, Drake CG. Ipilimumab: an anti-CTLA-4 antibody for metastatic melanoma. Clin Cancer Res. 2011;17(22):6958–62.
10. Ribas A, Wolchok JD. Cancer immunotherapy using checkpoint blockade. Science. 2018;359(6382):1350–5.
11. Hargadon KM, Johnson CE, Williams CJ. Immune checkpoint blockade therapy for cancer: an overview of FDA-approved immune checkpoint inhibitors. Int Immunopharmacol. 2018;62:29–39.
12. Wei SC, Duffy CR, Allison JP. Fundamental mechanisms of immune checkpoint blockade therapy. Cancer Discov. 2018;8(9):1069–86.
13. Galluzzi L, Kroemer G, Eggermont A. Novel immune checkpoint blocker approved for the treatment of advanced melanoma. Onco Targets Ther. 2014;3(11):e967147.
14. Raedler LA. Opdivo (Nivolumab): second PD-1 inhibitor receives FDA approval for Unresectable or metastatic melanoma. Am Health Drug Benefits. 2015;8(Spec Feature):180–3.

15. Waqar SN, Morgensztern D. Immunotherapy for non-small cell lung cancer: are we on the cusp of a new era? Expert Rev Clin Immunol. 2015;11(8):871–3.
16. Baumeister SH, Freeman GJ, Dranoff G, Sharpe AH. Coinhibitory pathways in immunotherapy for Cancer. Annu Rev Immunol. 2016;34:539–73.
17. Yokosuka T, Takamatsu M, Kobayashi-Imanishi W, Hashimoto-Tane A, Azuma M, Saito T. Programmed cell death 1 forms negative costimulatory microclusters that directly inhibit T cell receptor signaling by recruiting phosphatase SHP2. J Exp Med. 2012;209(6):1201–17.
18. Wu K, Yi M, Qin S, Chu Q, Zheng X, Wu K. The efficacy and safety of combination of PD-1 and CTLA-4 inhibitors: a meta-analysis. Exp Hematol Oncol. 2019;8:26.
19. Almutairi AR, McBride A, Slack M, Erstad BL, Abraham I. Potential immune-related adverse events associated with monotherapy and combination therapy of Ipilimumab, Nivolumab, and Pembrolizumab for advanced melanoma: a systematic review and meta-analysis. Front Oncol. 2020;10:91.
20. Ni L, Dong C. New checkpoints in cancer immunotherapy. Immunol Rev. 2017;276(1):52–65.
21. Moran AE, Kovacsovics-Bankowski M, Weinberg AD. The TNFRs OX40, 4-1BB, and CD40 as targets for cancer immunotherapy. Curr Opin Immunol. 2013;25(2):230–7.
22. Vonderheide RH, Dutcher JP, Anderson JE, Eckhardt SG, Stephans KF, Razvillas B, et al. Phase I study of recombinant human CD40 ligand in cancer patients. J Clin Oncol. 2001;19(13):3280–7.
23. Dangaj D, Lanitis E, Zhao A, Joshi S, Cheng Y, Sandaltzopoulos R, et al. Novel recombinant human b7-h4 antibodies overcome tumoral immune escape to potentiate T-cell antitumor responses. Cancer Res. 2013;73(15):4820–9.
24. Janakiram M, Shah UA, Liu W, Zhao A, Schoenberg MP, Zang X. The third group of the B7-CD28 immune checkpoint family: HHLA2, TMIGD2, B7x, and B7-H3. Immunol Rev. 2017;276(1):26–39.
25. Lines JL, Sempere LF, Broughton T, Wang L, Noelle R. VISTA is a novel broad-spectrum negative checkpoint regulator for cancer immunotherapy. Cancer Immunol Res. 2014;2(6):510–7.
26. He Y, Cao J, Zhao C, Li X, Zhou C, Hirsch FR. TIM-3, a promising target for cancer immunotherapy. Onco Targets Ther. 2018;11:7005–9.

27. Ndhlovu LC, Lopez-Verges S, Barbour JD, Jones RB, Jha AR, Long BR, et al. Tim-3 marks human natural killer cell maturation and suppresses cell-mediated cytotoxicity. Blood. 2012;119(16):3734–43.
28. Du W, Yang M, Turner A, Xu C, Ferris RL, Huang J, et al. TIM-3 as a target for cancer immunotherapy and mechanisms of action. Int J Mol Sci. 2017;18(3):645.
29. Johnston RJ, Comps-Agrar L, Hackney J, Yu X, Huseni M, Yang Y, et al. The immunoreceptor TIGIT regulates antitumor and antiviral CD8(+) T cell effector function. Cancer Cell. 2014;26(6):923–37.
30. Andrews LP, Marciscano AE, Drake CG, Vignali DA. LAG3 (CD223) as a cancer immunotherapy target. Immunol Rev. 2017;276(1):80–96.
31. Waldmann TA. Cytokines in Cancer Immunotherapy. Cold Spring Harb Perspect Biol. 2018;10(12):a028472.
32. Rosenberg SA. IL-2: the first effective immunotherapy for human cancer. J Immunol. 2014;192(12):5451–8.
33. Conlon KC, Miljkovic MD, Waldmann TA. Cytokines in the treatment of Cancer. J Interf Cytokine Res. 2019;39(1):6–21.
34. Quesada JR, Hersh EM, Manning J, Reuben J, Keating M, Schnipper E, et al. Treatment of hairy cell leukemia with recombinant alpha-interferon. Blood. 1986;68(2):493–7.
35. Abrams DI, Volberding PA. Alpha interferon therapy of AIDS-associated Kaposi's sarcoma. Semin Oncol. 1986;13(3 Suppl 2):43–7.
36. Soiffer RJ, Murray C, Shapiro C, Collins H, Chartier S, Lazo S, et al. Expansion and manipulation of natural killer cells in patients with metastatic cancer by low-dose continuous infusion and intermittent bolus administration of interleukin 2. Clin Cancer Res. 1996;2(3):493–9.
37. Levin AM, Bates DL, Ring AM, Krieg C, Lin JT, Su L, et al. Exploiting a natural conformational switch to engineer an interleukin-2 'superkine'. Nature. 2012;484(7395):529–33.
38. Spangler JB, Moraga I, Mendoza JL, Garcia KC. Insights into cytokine-receptor interactions from cytokine engineering. Annu Rev Immunol. 2015;33:139–67.
39. Hu P, Mizokami M, Ruoff G, Khawli LA, Epstein AL. Generation of low-toxicity interleukin-2 fusion proteins devoid of vasopermeability activity. Blood. 2003;101(12):4853–61.
40. Charych D, Khalili S, Dixit V, Kirk P, Chang T, Langowski J, et al. Modeling the receptor pharmacology, pharmacokinetics,

and pharmacodynamics of NKTR-214, a kinetically-controlled interleukin-2 (IL2) receptor agonist for cancer immunotherapy. PLoS One. 2017;12(7):e0179431.
41. Klein C, Waldhauer I, Nicolini VG, Freimoser-Grundschober A, Nayak T, Vugts DJ, et al. Cergutuzumab amunaleukin (CEA-IL2v), a CEA-targeted IL-2 variant-based immunocytokine for combination cancer immunotherapy: overcoming limitations of aldesleukin and conventional IL-2-based immunocytokines. Onco Targets Ther. 2017;6(3):e1277306.
42. Fehniger TA, Cooper MA, Caligiuri MA. Interleukin-2 and interleukin-15: immunotherapy for cancer. Cytokine Growth Factor Rev. 2002;13(2):169–83.
43. Junghans RP, Ma Q, Rathore R, Gomes EM, Bais AJ, Lo AS, et al. Phase I trial of anti-PSMA designer CAR-T cells in prostate Cancer: possible role for interacting interleukin 2-T cell pharmacodynamics as a determinant of clinical response. Prostate. 2016;76(14):1257–70.
44. Mach N, Dranoff G. Cytokine-secreting tumor cell vaccines. Curr Opin Immunol. 2000;12(5):571–5.
45. Kaufman HL, Ruby CE, Hughes T, Slingluff CL Jr. Current status of granulocyte-macrophage colony-stimulating factor in the immunotherapy of melanoma. J Immunother Cancer. 2014;2:11.
46. Lasek W, Zagozdzon R, Jakobisiak M. Interleukin 12: still a promising candidate for tumor immunotherapy? Cancer Immunol Immunother. 2014;63(5):419–35.
47. Zaidi MR, Merlino G. The two faces of interferon-gamma in cancer. Clin Cancer Res. 2011;17(19):6118–24.
48. Jinushi M, Hodi FS, Dranoff G. Enhancing the clinical activity of granulocyte-macrophage colony-stimulating factor-secreting tumor cell vaccines. Immunol Rev. 2008;222:287–98.
49. Quetglas JI, Labiano S, Aznar MA, Bolanos E, Azpilikueta A, Rodriguez I, et al. Virotherapy with a Semliki Forest virus-based vector encoding IL12 synergizes with PD-1/PD-L1 blockade. Cancer Immunol Res. 2015;3(5):449–54.
50. Fallon J, Tighe R, Kradjian G, Guzman W, Bernhardt A, Neuteboom B, et al. The immunocytokine NHS-IL12 as a potential cancer therapeutic. Oncotarget. 2014;5(7):1869–84.
51. Leonard JP, Sherman ML, Fisher GL, Buchanan LJ, Larsen G, Atkins MB, et al. Effects of single-dose interleukin-12 exposure on interleukin-12-associated toxicity and interferon-gamma production. Blood. 1997;90(7):2541–8.

52. Floros T, Tarhini AA. Anticancer cytokines: biology and clinical effects of interferon-alpha2, interleukin (IL)-2, IL-15, IL-21, and IL-12. Semin Oncol. 2015;42(4):539–48.
53. Anguille S, Lion E, Van den Bergh J, Van Acker HH, Willemen Y, Smits EL, et al. Interleukin-15 dendritic cells as vaccine candidates for cancer immunotherapy. Hum Vaccin Immunother. 2013;9(9):1956–61.
54. Setrerrahmane S, Xu H. Tumor-related interleukins: old validated targets for new anti-cancer drug development. Mol Cancer. 2017;16(1):153.
55. Chen X, Lv Q, Hong Y, Chen X, Cheng B, Wu T. IL-1beta maintains the redox balance by regulating glutaredoxin 1 expression during oral carcinogenesis. J Oral Pathol Med. 2017;46(5):332–9.
56. Bertrand F, Montfort A, Marcheteau E, Imbert C, Gilhodes J, Filleron T, et al. TNFalpha blockade overcomes resistance to anti-PD-1 in experimental melanoma. Nat Commun. 2017;8(1):2256.
57. Berraondo P, Sanmamed MF, Ochoa MC, Etxeberria I, Aznar MA, Perez-Gracia JL, et al. Cytokines in clinical cancer immunotherapy. Br J Cancer. 2019;120(1):6–15.
58. Knudson KM, Hicks KC, Luo X, Chen JQ, Schlom J, Gameiro SR. M7824, a novel bifunctional anti-PD-L1/TGFbeta trap fusion protein, promotes anti-tumor efficacy as monotherapy and in combination with vaccine. Onco Targets Ther. 2018;7(5):e1426519.
59. Baker KJ, Houston A, Brint E. IL-1 family members in Cancer; two sides to every story. Front Immunol. 2019;10:1197.
60. Lauta VM. Interleukin-6 and the network of several cytokines in multiple myeloma: an overview of clinical and experimental data. Cytokine. 2001;16(3):79–86.
61. Bellone S, Watts K, Cane S, Palmieri M, Cannon MJ, Burnett A, et al. High serum levels of interleukin-6 in endometrial carcinoma are associated with uterine serous papillary histology, a highly aggressive and chemotherapy-resistant variant of endometrial cancer. Gynecol Oncol. 2005;98(1):92–8.
62. Cassarino DS, Miller WJ, Auerbach A, Yang A, Sherry R, Duray PH. The effects of gp100 and tyrosinase peptide vaccinations on nevi in melanoma patients. J Cutan Pathol. 2006;33(5):335–42.
63. Harper DM, DeMars LR. HPV vaccines - a review of the first decade. Gynecol Oncol. 2017;146(1):196–204.
64. Melief CJ, van Hall T, Arens R, Ossendorp F, van der Burg SH. Therapeutic cancer vaccines. J Clin Invest. 2015;125(9):3401–12.

65. Guo C, Manjili MH, Subjeck JR, Sarkar D, Fisher PB, Wang XY. Therapeutic cancer vaccines: past, present, and future. Adv Cancer Res. 2013;119:421–75.
66. Heicappell R, Schirrmacher V, von Hoegen P, Ahlert T, Appelhans B. Prevention of metastatic spread by postoperative immunotherapy with virally modified autologous tumor cells. I. Parameters for optimal therapeutic effects. Int J Cancer. 1986;37(4):569–77.
67. Plaksin D, Porgador A, Vadai E, Feldman M, Schirrmacher V, Eisenbach L. Effective anti-metastatic melanoma vaccination with tumor cells transfected with MHC genes and/or infected with Newcastle disease virus (NDV). Int J Cancer. 1994;59(6):796–801.
68. Dillman RO. Is there a role for therapeutic cancer vaccines in the age of checkpoint inhibitors? Hum Vaccin Immunother. 2017;13(3):528–32.
69. Longo DL. New therapies for castration-resistant prostate cancer. N Engl J Med. 2010;363(5):479–81.
70. Kikuchi T, Moore MA, Crystal RG. Dendritic cells modified to express CD40 ligand elicit therapeutic immunity against preexisting murine tumors. Blood. 2000;96(1):91–9.
71. Koya RC, Kasahara N, Favaro PM, Lau R, Ta HQ, Weber JS, et al. Potent maturation of monocyte-derived dendritic cells after CD40L lentiviral gene delivery. J Immunother. 2003;26(5):451–60.
72. Bonehill A, Van Nuffel AM, Corthals J, Tuyaerts S, Heirman C, Francois V, et al. Single-step antigen loading and activation of dendritic cells by mRNA electroporation for the purpose of therapeutic vaccination in melanoma patients. Clin Cancer Res. 2009;15(10):3366–75.
73. Bonehill A, Tuyaerts S, Van Nuffel AM, Heirman C, Bos TJ, Fostier K, et al. Enhancing the T-cell stimulatory capacity of human dendritic cells by co-electroporation with CD40L, CD70 and constitutively active TLR4 encoding mRNA. Mol Ther. 2008;16(6):1170–80.
74. Iinuma H, Okinaga K, Fukushima R, Inaba T, Iwasaki K, Okinaga A, et al. Superior protective and therapeutic effects of IL-12 and IL-18 gene-transduced dendritic neuroblastoma fusion cells on liver metastasis of murine neuroblastoma. J Immunol. 2006;176(6):3461–9.
75. Kang TH, Bae HC, Kim SH, Seo SH, Son SW, Choi EY, et al. Modification of dendritic cells with interferon-gamma-inducible

protein-10 gene to enhance vaccine potency. J Gene Med. 2009;11(10):889–98.
76. Minkis K, Kavanagh DG, Alter G, Bogunovic D, O'Neill D, Adams S, et al. Type 2 Bias of T cells expanded from the blood of melanoma patients switched to type 1 by IL-12p70 mRNA-transfected dendritic cells. Cancer Res. 2008;68(22):9441–50.
77. Slingluff CL Jr, Yamshchikov G, Neese P, Galavotti H, Eastham S, Engelhard VH, et al. Phase I trial of a melanoma vaccine with gp100(280-288) peptide and tetanus helper peptide in adjuvant: immunologic and clinical outcomes. Clin Cancer Res. 2001;7(10):3012–24.
78. Chen PL, Roh W, Reuben A, Cooper ZA, Spencer CN, Prieto PA, et al. Analysis of immune signatures in longitudinal tumor samples yields insight into biomarkers of response and mechanisms of resistance to immune checkpoint blockade. Cancer Discov. 2016;6(8):827–37.
79. Butts C, Maksymiuk A, Goss G, Soulieres D, Marshall E, Cormier Y, et al. Updated survival analysis in patients with stage IIIB or IV non-small-cell lung cancer receiving BLP25 liposome vaccine (L-BLP25): phase IIB randomized, multicenter, open-label trial. J Cancer Res Clin Oncol. 2011;137(9):1337–42.
80. Sienel W, Varwerk C, Linder A, Kaiser D, Teschner M, Delire M, et al. Melanoma associated antigen (MAGE)-A3 expression in stages I and II non-small cell lung cancer: results of a multi-center study. Eur J Cardiothorac Surg. 2004;25(1):131–4.
81. De Smet C, Lurquin C, van der Bruggen P, De Plaen E, Brasseur F, Boon T. Sequence and expression pattern of the human MAGE2 gene. Immunogenetics. 1994;39(2):121–9.
82. Azuma K, Shichijo S, Maeda Y, Nakatsura T, Nonaka Y, Fujii T, et al. Mutated p53 gene encodes a nonmutated epitope recognized by HLA-B*4601-restricted and tumor cell-reactive CTLs at tumor site. Cancer Res. 2003;63(4):854–8.
83. Heldwein KA, Liang MD, Andresen TK, Thomas KE, Marty AM, Cuesta N, et al. TLR2 and TLR4 serve distinct roles in the host immune response against Mycobacterium bovis BCG. J Leukoc Biol. 2003;74(2):277–86.
84. Todryk SM, Melcher AA, Dalgleish AG, Vile RG. Heat shock proteins refine the danger theory. Immunology. 2000;99(3):334–7.
85. Aurisicchio L, Ciliberto G. Genetic cancer vaccines: current status and perspectives. Expert Opin Biol Ther. 2012;12(8):1043–58.
86. Bins AD, Jorritsma A, Wolkers MC, Hung CF, Wu TC, Schumacher TN, et al. A rapid and potent DNA vaccination

strategy defined by in vivo monitoring of antigen expression. Nat Med. 2005;11(8):899–904.
87. Dupuis M, Denis-Mize K, Woo C, Goldbeck C, Selby MJ, Chen M, et al. Distribution of DNA vaccines determines their immunogenicity after intramuscular injection in mice. J Immunol. 2000;165(5):2850–8.
88. Greenland JR, Letvin NL. Chemical adjuvants for plasmid DNA vaccines. Vaccine. 2007;25(19):3731–41.
89. Gubin MM, Zhang X, Schuster H, Caron E, Ward JP, Noguchi T, et al. Checkpoint blockade cancer immunotherapy targets tumour-specific mutant antigens. Nature. 2014;515(7528):577–81.
90. Kreiter S, Castle JC, Tureci O, Sahin U. Targeting the tumor mutanome for personalized vaccination therapy. Onco Targets Ther. 2012;1(5):768–9.
91. Castle JC, Kreiter S, Diekmann J, Lower M, van de Roemer N, de Graaf J, et al. Exploiting the mutanome for tumor vaccination. Cancer Res. 2012;72(5):1081–91.
92. Johnson LA, Morgan RA, Dudley ME, Cassard L, Yang JC, Hughes MS, et al. Gene therapy with human and mouse T-cell receptors mediates cancer regression and targets normal tissues expressing cognate antigen. Blood. 2009;114(3):535–46.
93. Rosenberg SA, Spiess P, Lafreniere R. A new approach to the adoptive immunotherapy of cancer with tumor-infiltrating lymphocytes. Science. 1986;233(4770):1318–21.
94. Khalil DN, Smith EL, Brentjens RJ, Wolchok JD. The future of cancer treatment: immunomodulation, CARs and combination immunotherapy. Nat Rev Clin Oncol. 2016;13(6):394.
95. Foley KC, Nishimura MI, Moore TV. Combination immunotherapies implementing adoptive T-cell transfer for advanced-stage melanoma. Melanoma Res. 2018;28(3):171–84.
96. June CH, Riddell SR, Schumacher TN. Adoptive cellular therapy: a race to the finish line. Sci Transl Med. 2015;7(280):280ps7.
97. Spiess PJ, Yang JC, Rosenberg SA. In vivo antitumor activity of tumor-infiltrating lymphocytes expanded in recombinant interleukin-2. J Natl Cancer Inst. 1987;79(5):1067–75.
98. Muranski P, Boni A, Wrzesinski C, Citrin DE, Rosenberg SA, Childs R, et al. Increased intensity lymphodepletion and adoptive immunotherapy--how far can we go? Nat Clin Pract Oncol. 2006;3(12):668–81.
99. Morgan DA, Ruscetti FW, Gallo R. Selective in vitro growth of T lymphocytes from normal human bone marrows. Science. 1976;193(4257):1007–8.

100. He Q, Jiang X, Zhou X, Weng J. Targeting cancers through TCR-peptide/MHC interactions. J Hematol Oncol. 2019;12(1):139.
101. Rosenberg SA, Restifo NP. Adoptive cell transfer as personalized immunotherapy for human cancer. Science. 2015;348(6230):62–8.
102. Bubenik J. Tumour MHC class I downregulation and immunotherapy (review). Oncol Rep. 2003;10(6):2005–8.
103. Gross G, Waks T, Eshhar Z. Expression of immunoglobulin-T-cell receptor chimeric molecules as functional receptors with antibody-type specificity. Proc Natl Acad Sci U S A. 1989;86(24):10024–8.
104. Kershaw MH, Westwood JA, Parker LL, Wang G, Eshhar Z, Mavroukakis SA, et al. A phase I study on adoptive immunotherapy using gene-modified T cells for ovarian cancer. Clin Cancer Res. 2006;12(20 Pt 1):6106–15.
105. Lamers CH, Sleijfer S, Vulto AG, Kruit WH, Kliffen M, Debets R, et al. Treatment of metastatic renal cell carcinoma with autologous T-lymphocytes genetically retargeted against carbonic anhydrase IX: first clinical experience. J Clin Oncol. 2006;24(13):e20–2.
106. Park JR, Digiusto DL, Slovak M, Wright C, Naranjo A, Wagner J, et al. Adoptive transfer of chimeric antigen receptor re-directed cytolytic T lymphocyte clones in patients with neuroblastoma. Mol Ther. 2007;15(4):825–33.
107. Brentjens RJ, Latouche JB, Santos E, Marti F, Gong MC, Lyddane C, et al. Eradication of systemic B-cell tumors by genetically targeted human T lymphocytes co-stimulated by CD80 and interleukin-15. Nat Med. 2003;9(3):279–86.
108. Brentjens RJ, Santos E, Nikhamin Y, Yeh R, Matsushita M, La Perle K, et al. Genetically targeted T cells eradicate systemic acute lymphoblastic leukemia xenografts. Clin Cancer Res. 2007;13(18 Pt 1):5426–35.
109. Davila ML, Riviere I, Wang X, Bartido S, Park J, Curran K, et al. Efficacy and toxicity management of 19-28z CAR T cell therapy in B cell acute lymphoblastic leukemia. Sci Transl Med. 2014;6(224):224ra25.
110. Imai C, Mihara K, Andreansky M, Nicholson IC, Pui CH, Geiger TL, et al. Chimeric receptors with 4-1BB signaling capacity provoke potent cytotoxicity against acute lymphoblastic leukemia. Leukemia. 2004;18(4):676–84.

111. Maude SL, Frey N, Shaw PA, Aplenc R, Barrett DM, Bunin NJ, et al. Chimeric antigen receptor T cells for sustained remissions in leukemia. N Engl J Med. 2014;371(16):1507–17.
112. Adusumilli PS, Cherkassky L, Villena-Vargas J, Colovos C, Servais E, Plotkin J, et al. Regional delivery of mesothelin-targeted CAR T cell therapy generates potent and long-lasting CD4-dependent tumor immunity. Sci Transl Med. 2014;6(261):261ra151.
113. Beatty GL, Haas AR, Maus MV, Torigian DA, Soulen MC, Plesa G, et al. Mesothelin-specific chimeric antigen receptor mRNA-engineered T cells induce anti-tumor activity in solid malignancies. Cancer Immunol Res. 2014;2(2):112–20.
114. Jackson HJ, Rafiq S, Brentjens RJ. Driving CAR T-cells forward. Nat Rev Clin Oncol. 2016;13(6):370–83.
115. Hoyos V, Savoldo B, Quintarelli C, Mahendravada A, Zhang M, Vera J, et al. Engineering CD19-specific T lymphocytes with interleukin-15 and a suicide gene to enhance their anti-lymphoma/leukemia effects and safety. Leukemia. 2010;24(6):1160–70.
116. Miliotou AN, Papadopoulou LC. CAR T-cell therapy: a new era in Cancer immunotherapy. Curr Pharm Biotechnol. 2018;19(1):5–18.
117. Rezvani K. Adoptive cell therapy using engineered natural killer cells. Bone Marrow Transplant. 2019;54(Suppl 2):785–8.
118. Olson JA, Leveson-Gower DB, Gill S, Baker J, Beilhack A, Negrin RS. NK cells mediate reduction of GVHD by inhibiting activated, alloreactive T cells while retaining GVT effects. Blood. 2010;115(21):4293–301.
119. Ruggeri L, Capanni M, Urbani E, Perruccio K, Shlomchik WD, Tosti A, et al. Effectiveness of donor natural killer cell alloreactivity in mismatched hematopoietic transplants. Science. 2002;295(5562):2097–100.
120. Miller JS, Soignier Y, Panoskaltsis-Mortari A, McNearney SA, Yun GH, Fautsch SK, et al. Successful adoptive transfer and in vivo expansion of human haploidentical NK cells in patients with cancer. Blood. 2005;105(8):3051–7.
121. Curti A, Ruggeri L, D'Addio A, Bontadini A, Dan E, Motta MR, et al. Successful transfer of alloreactive haploidentical KIR ligand-mismatched natural killer cells after infusion in elderly high risk acute myeloid leukemia patients. Blood. 2011;118(12):3273–9.

122. Shah N, Li L, McCarty J, Kaur I, Yvon E, Shaim H, et al. Phase I study of cord blood-derived natural killer cells combined with autologous stem cell transplantation in multiple myeloma. Br J Haematol. 2017;177(3):457–66.
123. Sotillo E, Barrett DM, Black KL, Bagashev A, Oldridge D, Wu G, et al. Convergence of acquired mutations and alternative splicing of CD19 enables resistance to CART-19 immunotherapy. Cancer Discov. 2015;5(12):1282–95.
124. Lupo KB, Matosevic S. Natural Killer Cells as Allogeneic Effectors in Adoptive Cancer Immunotherapy. Cancers (Basel). 2019;11(6):769.
125. Roberti A, Valdes AF, Torrecillas R, Fraga MF, Fernandez AF. Epigenetics in cancer therapy and nanomedicine. Clin Epigenetics. 2019;11(1):81.
126. Morel D, Jeffery D, Aspeslagh S, Almouzni G, Postel-Vinay S. Combining epigenetic drugs with other therapies for solid tumours - past lessons and future promise. Nat Rev Clin Oncol. 2020;17(2):91–107.
127. Li B, Wang Z, Wu H, Xue M, Lin P, Wang S, et al. Epigenetic regulation of CXCL12 plays a critical role in mediating tumor progression and the immune response in osteosarcoma. Cancer Res. 2018;78(14):3938–53.
128. Shen L, Orillion A, Pili R. Histone deacetylase inhibitors as immunomodulators in cancer therapeutics. Epigenomics. 2016;8(3):415–28.
129. Raj K, Mufti GJ. Azacytidine (Vidaza(R)) in the treatment of myelodysplastic syndromes. Ther Clin Risk Manag. 2006;2(4):377–88.
130. Momparler RL. A perspective on the comparative Antileukemic activity of 5-Aza-2′-deoxycytidine (Decitabine) and 5-Azacytidine (Vidaza). Pharmaceuticals (Basel). 2012;5(8):875–81.
131. Ishihara D, Pop L, Takeshima T, Iyengar P, Hannan R. Rationale and evidence to combine radiation therapy and immunotherapy for cancer treatment. Cancer Immunol Immunother. 2017;66(3):281–98.
132. Cook AM, Lesterhuis WJ, Nowak AK, Lake RA. Chemotherapy and immunotherapy: mapping the road ahead. Curr Opin Immunol. 2016;39:23–9.

133. Hanoteau A, Moser M. Chemotherapy and immunotherapy: a close interplay to fight cancer? Onco Targets Ther. 2016;5(7):e1190061.
134. Herrscher H, Robert C. Immune checkpoint inhibitors in melanoma in the metastatic, neoadjuvant, and adjuvant setting. Curr Opin Oncol. 2020;32(2):106–13.

Chapter 2
Cancer Immunotherapy: Overview of Immune Checkpoint Inhibitors

Faisal Fa'ak and Adi Diab

Cancer treatment has been fully transformed with the development of cancer immunotherapies. Cancer immunotherapy manipulates the immune system to identify, target, and destroy cancer cells. It is classified into passive therapies such as tumor-specific antibodies, recombinant cytokines, and the transfer of ex vivo-activated immune cells and the active type such as cancer vaccines and antibodies against checkpoints of T-cell activation [1]. The resultant antitumor response is characterized by several properties, including constant surveillance, specificity against tumor antigen, and the presence of a long-lasting memory to protect against tumor relapse.

In a process called peripheral tolerance, the immune system uses several intrinsic T-cell immune checkpoint pathways

F. Fa'ak
Department of Graduate Medical Education, Piedmont Athens Regional Medical Center, Athens, GA, USA

A. Diab (✉)
Department of Melanoma Medical Oncology, Division of Cancer Medicine, University of Texas MD Anderson Cancer Center, Houston, TX, USA
e-mail: adiab@mdaderson.org

M. E. Suarez-Almazor, L. H. Calabrese (eds.), *Rheumatic Diseases and Syndromes Induced by Cancer Immunotherapy*,
https://doi.org/10.1007/978-3-030-56824-5_2

to regulate the immune response [2]. Tumor antigen-specific T cells attempt to attack cancer. However, tumor cells hijack the anti-inflammatory checkpoints to protect themselves from T-cell attacks, a process called adaptive immune resistance [3]. The progress in the understanding of the immune system has led to the development of monoclonal antibodies (mAbs) targeted against regulatory immune checkpoints, which control T-cell activation. The US Food and Drug Administration (FDA) has approved seven immune checkpoint inhibitors (ICIs) for the treatment of various malignancies, targeting two main signaling pathways, cytotoxic T-lymphocyte antigen 4 (CTLA-4) and programmed cell death 1 (PD-1)/programmed cell death ligand-1(PD-L1).

CTLA-4 Inhibitors

Tumor-specific effector T-cell activation, proliferation, and migration require two signals [4]. It starts with the interaction of the T-cell receptor (TCR) with antigen bound to major histocompatibility complex (MHC) molecules, complemented by the co-stimulatory signals mediated by CD28 on the T-cell surface binding to B7 proteins (CD80 or CD86) on antigen-presenting cells (APCs) [5]. CTLA-4 is a negative regulator expressed by the activated T effector and T regulatory cells that competes for binding to B7 to counteract the positive CD28-mediated signals [6, 7] (Fig. 2.1). This engagement leads to decreased T-cell proliferation and cytotoxicity. Under physiological conditions, this pathway controls inflammation and prevents autoimmunity. In cancer, it shuts down the antitumor immune response leading to T-cell exhaustion and downregulation of the antitumor response.

Ipilimumab is a fully human mAb (IgG1) that blocks CTLA-4 to reverse tumor-induced downregulation of T-cell function and, consequently, preserve and maintain T-cell activation within the tumor microenvironment. James Allison's group initially described in 1995 the potent inhibitory role of CTLA-4 in regulating T-cell responses [8]. They showed that anti-CTLA-4 antibodies enhanced the rejection of several types of established tumors in mice [8]. This preclinical research led to the first-in-human pilot study, which showed prolonged progression-free survival in a few cancer patients [9, 10]. Phase II and III randomized clinical trials showed significant improvements in overall survival, compared to the peptide vaccine or standard dacarbazine chemotherapy leading to FDA approval of ipilimumab for the treatment of

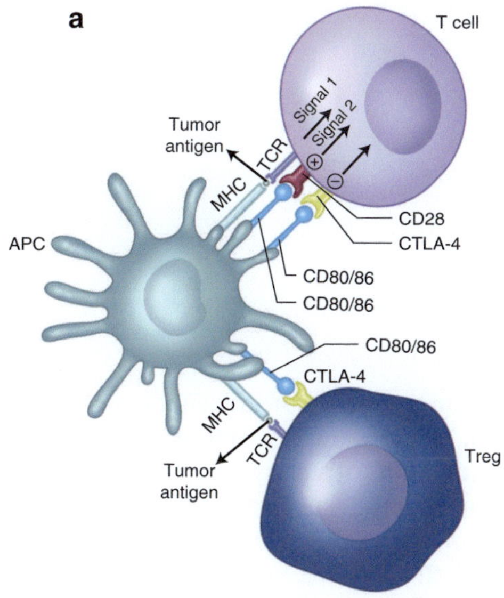

FIGURE 2.1 Mechanism of anti-CTLA-4 checkpoint inhibitors. (**a**) T-cell activation requires two signals. Signal 1 starts with the interaction of the T-cell receptor (TCR) with antigen bound to major histocompatibility complex (MHC) molecules, complemented by the co-stimulatory signal 2 mediated by CD28 on the T-cell surface binding to B7 proteins (CD80 or CD86) on antigen-presenting cells (APCs). CTLA-4 expressed by the activated T effector and T regulatory cells that compete for binding to B7 (CD80 or CD86) to counteract T-cell activation. (**b**) Anti-CTLA inhibitor blocks CTLA-4 engagement with B7 (CD80 or CD86) to reverse downregulation of T-cell function

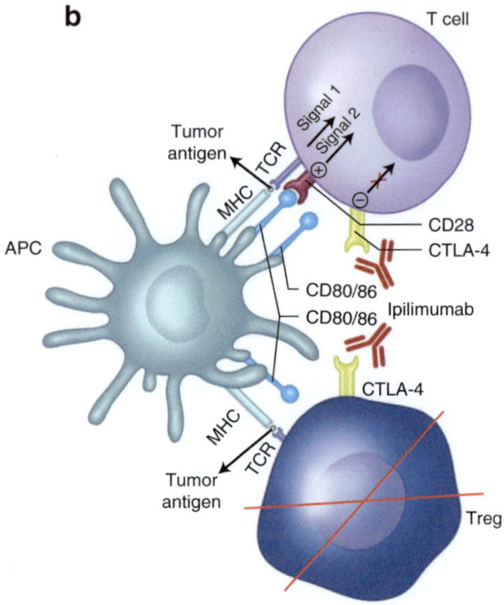

FIGURE 2.1 (continued)

patients with unresectable or metastatic melanoma in March 2011 [11–15]. A meta-analysis including 1861 patients with advanced melanoma treated with ipilimumab showed a pooled 3-year overall survival of 22%. A plateau in the pooled Kaplan–Meier curve began at approximately 3 years and extended through 10 years [16]. Ipilimumab was also approved in 2015 for use in the adjuvant setting for patients with high-risk stage III melanoma, after resection. Significant improvement in recurrence-free and overall survival was observed in patients treated with ipilimumab, compared to placebo [17, 18].

The use of ipilimumab as a monotherapy has only been approved for patients with melanoma. Ipilimumab monotherapy has also shown some benefits in patients with castration-resistant prostate cancer but is not approved for this indication [19, 20].

PD-1 and PD-L1 Inhibitors

Programmed cell death-1 is a transmembrane protein receptor that was initially described as a receptor inducing cell death of an activated T cell [21]. However, preclinical studies demonstrated that it is a negative regulator of T-cell effector function [22, 23]. PD-1 appears shortly after T-cell activation and decreases with the clearance of antigen [24]. T-cell identification of tumor antigens triggers the production of pro-inflammatory cytokines, such as interferon-γ (IFN-γ), which stimulate reactive PD-L1 expression on tumor cells. PDL-1 binding PD-1 results in inhibitory functions mediated through tyrosine phosphatase SH2 domain-containing protein tyrosine phosphatase-2 (SHP-2), which

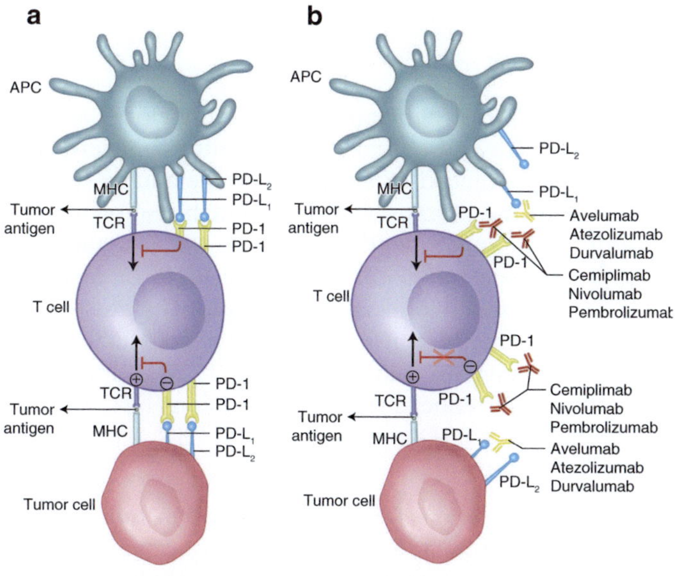

FIGURE 2.2 Mechanism of anti-programmed cell death 1 (anti-PD-1)/anti-PD ligand 1 (anti-PD-L1) checkpoint inhibitors. (**a**) After activation of T cells, PD-1 appears on the surface of T cells. PDL-1 binding PD-1 results in inhibitory signal mediated downstream of the TCR leading to T-cell exhaustion, inhibiting antitumor cytotoxic T-cell responses. (**b**) PD-1 and PD-L1 inhibitors reverse T-cells exhaustion

dephosphorylates signaling molecules downstream of the TCR (Fig. 2.2) leading to decreased T-cell activation and cytokine production [24]. Also, PD-1 signals induce T regulatory cells and promote the expression of proteins that impair T-cell proliferation, cytokine production, and survival [24]. Inflammation-induced PD-L1 expression in the tumor microenvironment results in PD-1-mediated T-cell exhaustion, inhibiting antitumor cytotoxic T-cell responses. These findings led to the development of PD-1 and PD-L1 inhibitors as immunotherapy agents. Six PD-1/PDL-1 inhibitors are approved by the FDA for the treatment of various cancers, controlling activation, exhaustion, tolerance, and resolution of inflammation.

PD-1 Inhibitors

Pembrolizumab

Pembrolizumab is a humanized IgG4 monoclonal antibody against PD-1. It was the first PD-1 inhibitor to receive FDA approval, for advanced or unresectable melanoma that progressed following therapy with ipilimumab and/or a BRAF inhibitor [25]. Subsequently, approval was expanded for use as a first-line treatment for unresectable or metastatic melanoma, irrespective of BRAF mutational status, given a significantly higher response rate of 32.9% in patients treated with pembrolizumab compared to 11.9% for ipilimumab ($P < 0.001$), with reduced risk of progression (HR, 0.58; 95% CI, 0.47–0.72, $p < .001$) and risk of death (HR, 0.69; 95% CI, 0.52–0.90, $p = .0036$).

Other major indications for pembrolizumab include [26]

- First-line treatment for metastatic non-squamous non-small cell lung cancer (NSCLC) with no epidermal growth factor receptor (EGFR) or anaplastic lymphoma kinase (ALK) genomic tumor aberrations, in combination with pemetrexed and platinum chemotherapy.

- First-line treatment for metastatic squamous NSCLC in combination with carboplatin and either paclitaxel or paclitaxel protein bound.
- Locally advanced/metastatic NSCLC expressing PD-L1 with no EGFR or ALK genomic tumor aberrations.
- Metastatic NSCLC whose tumors express PD-L with disease progression on or after platinum-containing chemotherapy.
- Patients with EGFR or ALK genomic tumor aberrations should have disease progression on FDA-approved therapy for these aberrations.
- Metastatic SCLC with disease progression on or after platinum-based chemotherapy and at least one other prior line of therapy.
- First-line treatment for metastatic, unresectable, or recurrent head and neck squamous cell carcinoma (HNSCC), in combination with platinum and FU.
- First-line treatment for metastatic, unresectable, or recurrent HNSCC whose tumors express PD-L1.
- Treatment for patients with recurrent or metastatic HNSCC with disease progression on or after platinum-containing chemotherapy.
- Treatment for patients with refractory classical hodgkin lymphoma (cHL) or who have relapsed after three or more prior lines of therapy.
- Treatment for patients with refractory primary mediastinal large B-cell lymphoma (PMBCL) or who have relapsed after two or more prior lines of therapy.
- Treatment for patients with locally advanced or metastatic disease who are not eligible for cisplatin-containing chemotherapy and whose tumors express PD-L1 or in patients who are not eligible for any platinum-containing chemotherapy regardless of PD-L1 status.
- Treatment for patients with locally advanced or metastatic disease who have disease progression during or following platinum-containing chemotherapy or within 12 months of

neoadjuvant or adjuvant treatment with platinum-containing chemotherapy.

- Treatment for patients with bacillus Calmette–Guerin-unresponsive, high-risk, non-muscle invasive bladder cancer with carcinoma in situ with or without papillary tumors who are ineligible for or have elected not to undergo cystectomy.
- Treatment for patients with unresectable or metastatic solid tumors with microsatellite instability-high (MSI-H) or mismatch repair deficient.
- Treatment for patients with recurrent locally advanced or metastatic gastric or gastroesophageal junction adenocarcinoma whose tumors express PD-L1, with disease progression on or after two or more prior lines of therapy including fluoropyrimidine- and platinum-containing chemotherapy and, if appropriate, human epidermal growth factor receptor 2 (HER2)/neu-targeted therapy.
- Treatment for patients with recurrent locally advanced or metastatic squamous cell carcinoma of the esophagus whose tumors express PD-L1 with disease progression after one or more prior lines of systemic therapy.
- Treatment for patients with recurrent or metastatic cancer with disease progression on or after chemotherapy whose tumors express PD-L1.
- Treatment for patients with hepatocellular carcinoma (HCC) who have been previously treated with sorafenib.
- Treatment for patients with recurrent locally advanced or metastatic Merkel cell carcinoma.
- First-line treatment for advanced renal cell carcinoma (RCC) in combination with axitinib.
- Treatment for axitinib advanced endometrial carcinoma that is not MSI-H or deficient mismatch repair (dMMR), who have disease progression following prior systemic therapy and are not candidates for curative surgery or radiation, in combination with lenvatinib.

Nivolumab

Nivolumab is a fully human IgG4 monoclonal antibody against PD-1. Similar to pembrolizumab, it was first approved in 2014 for stage IIIC/IV melanoma that progressed after treatment with ipilimumab, with an overall response rate of 31.7% compared to 10.6% with chemotherapy. Nivolumab has also shown significant benefits in 1-year progression-free survival in the adjuvant setting for patients with stage IIIB, IIIC, or IV who underwent complete resection of their melanoma, compared to ipilimumab (HR, 0.65; 97.56% CI, 0.51–0.83; $p < .001$) [27].

Other major indications include [28]
- Metastatic NSCLC and progressive on or after platinum-based chemotherapy or EGFR/ALK-targeted therapy
- Metastatic small cell lung cancer with progression after platinum-based chemotherapy and at least one other line of therapy
- Patients with advanced RCC who have received prior anti-angiogenic therapy
- Relapsed or progressive disease after autologous hematopoietic stem cell transplantation (HSCT) and brentuximab vedotin or three or more lines of systemic therapy that includes autologous HSCT
- Recurrent or metastatic squamous cell carcinoma of the head and neck with disease progression on or after a platinum-based therapy
- Patients with locally advanced or metastatic urothelial carcinoma who have disease progression during or following platinum-containing chemotherapy, within 12 months of neoadjuvant or adjuvant treatment with platinum-containing chemotherapy
- Patients with HCC who have been previously treated with sorafenib

Cemiplimab

Cemiplimab is the latest human IgG4 monoclonal antibody against PD-1. In 2018, the FDA approved cemiplimab for use in patients with metastatic cutaneous squamous cell carcinoma (CSCC) or locally advanced CSCC who are not candidates for curative surgery or curative radiation. The overall response rates exceeded 45% for both metastatic and locally advanced disease [29].

PDL-1 Inhibitors

Atezolizumab

Atezolizumab is a fully humanized IgG1 monoclonal antibody against PDL-1. It was the first PD-L1 inhibitor to be granted accelerated approval in 2016 for locally advanced or metastatic urothelial cancer following progression after chemotherapy [30]. In 2017, the FDA expanded the approved indications to include first-line treatment of locally advanced/metastatic disease among cisplatin-ineligible patients, based on an overall response rate of 23%, with a median overall survival of 15.9 months [31].

Other major indications include [32]

- Metastatic non-squamous NSCLC with no EGFR or ALK genomic tumor aberrations, in combination with bevacizumab, paclitaxel, and carboplatin.
- Metastatic non-squamous NSCLC with no EGFR or ALK genomic tumor aberrations, in combination with paclitaxel protein bound and carboplatin.
- Patients with metastatic NSCLC who have disease progression during or following platinum-containing chemotherapy.
- Patients with EGFR or ALK genomic tumor aberrations should have disease progression on FDA-approved therapy for NSCLC harboring these aberrations.

- Unresectable locally advanced or metastatic triple-negative breast cancer (TNBC) whose tumors express PD-L1, in combination with paclitaxel protein bound.
- First-line treatment for extensive-stage small cell lung cancer (ES-SCLC), in combination with carboplatin and etoposide.

Durvalumab

Durvalumab is a fully human IgG1 monoclonal antibody against PD-L1. It received FDA approval in 2017 to treat patients with platinum-refractory locally advanced/metastatic urothelial carcinoma, based on phase I/II open-label, dose-escalation trial (Study 1108) [27, 33, 34]. Overall response rate was 17.8%, with a median overall survival of 8.2 months; 55% of patients were alive at 12 months [34].

The FDA expanded durvalumab indication in 2018 to include stage III unresectable NSCLC, given its superior overall response rates compared to placebo (28.4% vs. 16.0%; $P < 0.001$) [35, 36].

Avelumab

Avelumab is a fully human IgG1 monoclonal antibody against PDL-1. In 2017, avelumab received FDA approval for metastatic Merkel cell carcinoma [27, 37] [38]. Avelumab has been also granted approval to treat patients with locally advanced or metastatic urothelial cancer refractory to chemotherapy and to be used in combination with axitinib for advanced renal cell carcinoma [39].

Combination Immunotherapy

Over the past decade, there has been a rapid proliferation in the use of ICI for the treatment of various malignancies. Despite this success, most cancer patients still do not respond to treatment or become resistant. This challenge has opened the door to find new strategies to overcome this resistance. Using a combination of immunotherapy agents with different mechanisms of action can target different immune pathways simultaneously and improve response [40]. Currently, the only FDA-approved immunotherapy combination regimen includes CTLA-4 and PD-1/PDL-1 blocking antibodies [41].

Ipilimumab and nivolumab in combination were approved by the FDA in 2016 as a first-line treatment for the untreated unresectable stage III or stage IV melanoma. Combination therapy showed an overall response rate of 57.6% (95% CI, 52.0–63.2), compared to 43.7% (95% CI, 38.1–49.3%) in the nivolumab, and 19.0% (95% CI, 14.9–23.8) in the ipilimumab monotherapy groups [41, 42]. The median overall survival was >60.0 months (median not reached) in the combination group compared to 36.9 months and 19.9 months in the nivolumab group and ipilimumab group, respectively [43].

Ipilimumab and nivolumab in combination significantly improve response rates in patients with untreated advanced RCC and those with metastatic colorectal cancer with microsatellite instability or mismatch repair protein deficiency and have received approval for these indications [44–46].

One of the most promising combinations is the use of nivolumab with bempegaldesleukin. Bempegaldesleukin is an IL-2 pathway agonist designed to provide prolonged signaling through heterodimeric IL-2-receptor beta/gamma leading to increased proliferation and activation of CD8+ T and NK cells rather than the T regulatory cells (Tregs) in the tumor microenvironment. This combination received FDA breakthrough therapy designation for previously untreated unresectable or metastatic melanoma following a high response rate of 53% [47].

References

1. Papaioannou NE, Beniata OV, Vitsos P, Tsitsilonis O, Samara P. Harnessing the immune system to improve cancer therapy. Ann Transl Med. 2016;4(14):261.
2. Fife BT, Bluestone JA. Control of peripheral T-cell tolerance and autoimmunity via the CTLA-4 and PD-1 pathways. Immunol Rev. 2008;224(1):166–82.
3. Ribas A. Adaptive immune resistance: how cancer protects from immune attack. Cancer Discov. 2015;5(9):915–9.
4. Sharma P, Wagner K, Wolchok JD, Allison JP. Novel cancer immunotherapy agents with survival benefit: recent successes and next steps. Nat Rev Cancer. 2011;11(11):805–12.
5. Lizée G, Overwijk WW, Radvanyi L, Gao J, Sharma P, Hwu P. Harnessing the power of the immune system to target cancer. Annu Rev Med. 2013;64(1):71–90.
6. Krummel MF, Allison JP. CD28 and CTLA-4 have opposing effects on the response of T cells to stimulation. J Exp Med. 1995;182(2):459–65.
7. Poschke I, Mougiakakos D, Kiessling R. Camouflage and sabotage: tumor escape from the immune system. - Abstract - Europe PMC [Internet]. [cited 2020 Feb 2]. Available from: https://europepmc.org/article/med/21626032
8. R. Leach D, F. Krummel M, P. Allison J. Enhancement of Antitumor Immunity by CTLA-4 Blockade. Science [Internet]. [cited 2020 Feb 2]. Available from: https://science.sciencemag.org/content/271/5256/1734
9. Weber J. Ipilimumab: controversies in its development, utility and autoimmune adverse events. Cancer Immunol Immunother. 2009;58(5):823–30.
10. Hodi FS, Mihm MC, Soiffer RJ, Haluska FG, Butler M, Seiden MV, et al. Biologic activity of cytotoxic T lymphocyte-associated antigen 4 antibody blockade in previously vaccinated metastatic melanoma and ovarian carcinoma patients. Proc Natl Acad Sci U S A. 2003;100(8):4712–7.
11. Weber JS, Hersh EM, Yellin M, Nichol GM, Urba W, Powderly JD, et al. The efficacy and safety of ipilimumab (MDX-010)

in patients with unresectable stage III or stage IV malignant melanoma. J Clin Oncol [Internet]. 2016;12. cited 2020 Feb 2]. Available from: https://ascopubs.org/doi/abs/10.1200/jco.2007.25.18_suppl.8523
12. Weber JS, Berman D, Siegel J, Minor D, Amin A, Thompson JA, et al. Safety and efficacy of ipilimumab with or without prophylactic budesonide in treatment-naive and previously treated patients with advanced melanoma. JCO. 2008;26(15_suppl):9010.
13. Hamid O, Chin K, Li J, Neyns B, Linette G, Negrier S, et al. Dose effect of ipilimumab in patients with advanced melanoma: results from a phase II, randomized, dose-ranging study. JCO. 2008;26(15_suppl):9025.
14. Hodi FS, O'Day SJ, McDermott DF, Weber RW, Sosman JA, Haanen JB, et al. Improved Survival with Ipilimumab in Patients with Metastatic Melanoma [Internet]. https://doi.org/10.1056/NEJMoa1003466. 2010 [cited 2020 Feb 2]. Available from: https://www.nejm.org/doi/10.1056/NEJMoa1003466?url_ver=Z39.88-2003&rfr_id=ori%3Arid%3Acrossref.org&rfr_dat=cr_pub%3Dwww.ncbi.nlm.nih.gov
15. Robert C, Thomas L, Igor B. Ipilimumab plus Dacarbazine for Previously Untreated Metastatic Melanoma | NEJM [Internet]. [cited 2020 Feb 2]. Available from: https://www.nejm.org/doi/10.1056/NEJMoa1104621?url_ver=Z39.88-2003&rfr_id=ori:rid:crossref.org&rfr_dat=cr_pub%3dwww.ncbi.nlm.nih.gov.
16. Schadendorf D, Hodi FS, Robert C, Weber JS, Margolin K, Hamid O, et al. Pooled analysis of long-term survival data from phase II and phase III trials of Ipilimumab in Unresectable or metastatic melanoma. J Clin Oncol. 2015;33(17):1889–94.
17. Eggermont AMM, Chiarion-Sileni V, Grob J-J, Dummer R, Wolchok JD, Schmidt H, et al. Adjuvant ipilimumab versus placebo after complete resection of high-risk stage III melanoma (EORTC 18071): a randomised, double-blind, phase 3 trial. Lancet Oncol. 2015;16(5):522–30.
18. Eggermont AMM, Chiario-Sileni V, Grob J-J, Dummer R, Wolchok JD, Schmidt H, et al. Prolonged survival in stage III melanoma with Ipilimumab adjuvant therapy. N Engl J Med. 2016;375(19):1845–55.
19. Kwon ED, Drake CG, Scher HI, Fizazi K, Bossi A, van den Eertwegh AJM, et al. Ipilimumab versus placebo after radiotherapy in patients with metastatic castration-resistant prostate cancer that had progressed after docetaxel chemotherapy

(CA184-043): a multicentre, randomised, double-blind, phase 3 trial. Lancet Oncol. 2014;15(7):700–12.
20. Beer TM, Kwon ED, Drake CG, Fizazi K, Logothetis C, Gravis G, et al. Randomized, double-blind, phase III trial of Ipilimumab versus placebo in asymptomatic or minimally symptomatic patients with metastatic chemotherapy-naive castration-resistant prostate Cancer. J Clin Oncol. 2017;35(1):40–7.
21. Ishida Y, Agata Y, Shibahara K, Honjo T. Induced expression of PD-1, a novel member of the immunoglobulin gene superfamily, upon programmed cell death. EMBO J. 1992;11(11):3887–95.
22. Dong H, Strome SE, Salomao DR, Tamura H, Hirano F, Flies DB, et al. Tumor-associated B7-H1 promotes T-cell apoptosis: a potential mechanism of immune evasion. Nat Med. 2002;8(8):793–800.
23. He J, Hu Y, Hu M, Li B. Development of PD-1/PD-L1 pathway in tumor immune microenvironment and treatment for non-small cell lung Cancer. Sci Rep. 2015;5:1):1–9.
24. Baumeister SH, Freeman GJ, Dranoff G, Sharpe AH. Coinhibitory pathways in immunotherapy for Cancer. Annu Rev Immunol. 2016;34:539–73.
25. Robert C, Ribas A, Wolchok JD, Hodi FS, Hamid O, Kefford R, et al. Anti-programmed-death-receptor-1 treatment with pembrolizumab in ipilimumab-refractory advanced melanoma: a randomised dose-comparison cohort of a phase 1 trial. Lancet. 2014;384(9948):1109–17.
26. Drugs@FDA: FDA-Approved Drugs [Internet]. [cited 2020 Feb 3]. Available from: https://www.accessdata.fda.gov/scripts/cder/daf/index.cfm?event=overview.process&ApplNo=125514
27. Gong J, Chehrazi-Raffle A, Reddi S, Salgia R. Development of PD-1 and PD-L1 inhibitors as a form of cancer immunotherapy: a comprehensive review of registration trials and future considerations. J Immunother Cancer. 2018;6(1):8.
28. Drugs@FDA: FDA-Approved Drugs [Internet]. [cited 2020 Feb 3]. Available from: https://www.accessdata.fda.gov/scripts/cder/daf/index.cfm?event=overview.process&ApplNo=125554.
29. Migden MR, Rischin D, Schmults CD, Guminski A, Hauschild A, Lewis KD, et al. PD-1 blockade with Cemiplimab in advanced cutaneous squamous-cell carcinoma. N Engl J Med [Internet]. 2018 [cited 2020 Feb 9]. Available from: https://www.nejm.org/doi/10.1056/NEJMoa1805131?url_ver=Z39.88-2003&rfr_id=ori%3Arid%3Acrossref.org&rfr_dat=cr_pub%3Dwww.ncbi.nlm.nih.gov.

30. Rosenberg JE, Hoffman-Censits J, Powles T, van der Heijden MS, Balar AV, Necchi A, et al. Atezolizumab in patients with locally advanced and metastatic urothelial carcinoma who have progressed following treatment with platinum-based chemotherapy: a single arm, phase 2 trial. Lancet. 2016;387(10031):1909–20.
31. Balar AV, Galsky MD, Rosenberg JE, Powles T, Petrylak DP, Bellmunt J, et al. Atezolizumab as first-line therapy in cisplatin-ineligible patients with locally advanced and metastatic urothelial carcinoma: a single-arm, multicentre, phase 2 trial. Lancet. 2017;389(10064):67–76.
32. Drugs@FDA: FDA-Approved Drugs [Internet]. [cited 2020 Feb 3]. Available from: https://www.accessdata.fda.gov/scripts/cder/daf/index.cfm?event=overview.process&ApplNo=761041.
33. Massard C, Gordon MS, Sharma S, Rafii S, Wainberg ZA, Luke J, et al. Safety and efficacy of Durvalumab (MEDI4736), an anti-programmed cell death Ligand-1 immune checkpoint inhibitor, in patients with advanced urothelial bladder Cancer. J Clin Oncol. 2016;34(26):3119–25.
34. Powles T, O'Donnell PH, Massard C, Arkenau H-T, Friedlander TW, Hoimes CJ, et al. Efficacy and safety of Durvalumab in locally advanced or metastatic urothelial carcinoma: updated results from a phase 1/2 open-label study. JAMA Oncol. 2017;3(9):e172411.
35. Antonia SJ, Villegas A, Daniel D, Vicente D, Murakami S, Hui R, et al. Durvalumab after Chemoradiotherapy in stage III non-small-cell lung Cancer. N Engl J Med. 2017;377(20):1919–29.
36. Gray JE, Villegas AE, Daniel DB, Vicente D, Murakami S, Hui R, et al. Three-year overall survival update from the PACIFIC trial. JCO. 2019;37(15_suppl):8526.
37. Kaufman HL, Russell J, Hamid O, Bhatia S, Terheyden P, D'Angelo SP, et al. Avelumab in patients with chemotherapy-refractory metastatic Merkel cell carcinoma: a multicentre, single-group, open-label, phase 2 trial. Lancet Oncol. 2016;17(10):1374–85.
38. Patel MR, Ellerton J, Infante JR, Agrawal M, Gordon M, Aljumaily R, et al. Avelumab in metastatic urothelial carcinoma after platinum failure (JAVELIN solid tumor): pooled results from two expansion cohorts of an open-label, phase 1 trial. Lancet Oncol. 2018;19(1):51–64.
39. Motzer RJ, Penkov K, Haanen J, Rini B, Albiges L, Campbell MT, et al. Avelumab plus Axitinib versus Sunitinib for advanced renal-cell carcinoma. N Engl J Med. 2019;380(12):1103–15.

40. Postow MA, Callahan MK, Wolchok JD. Immune checkpoint blockade in cancer therapy. J Clin Oncol. 2015;33(17):1974–82.
41. Larkin J, Chiarion-Sileni V, Gonzalez R, Grob JJ, Cowey CL, Lao CD, et al. Combined Nivolumab and Ipilimumab or monotherapy in untreated melanoma. N Engl J Med. 2015;373(1):23–34.
42. Larkin J, Chiarion-Sileni V, Gonzalez R, Grob JJ, Cowey CL, Lao CD, et al. 3303 Efficacy and safety in key patient subgroups of nivolumab (NIVO) alone or combined with ipilimumab (IPI) versus IPI alone in treatment-naïve patients with advanced melanoma (MEL) (CheckMate 067). Eur J Cancer. 2015;51:S664–5.
43. Larkin J, Chiarion-Sileni V, Gonzalez R, Grob J-J, Rutkowski P, Lao CD, et al. Five-year survival with combined Nivolumab and Ipilimumab in advanced melanoma. N Engl J Med. 2019;381(16):1535–46.
44. Motzer RJ, Tannir NM, McDermott DF, Arén Frontera O, Melichar B, Choueiri TK, et al. Nivolumab plus Ipilimumab versus Sunitinib in advanced renal-cell carcinoma. N Engl J Med. 2018;378(14):1277–90.
45. Overman MJ, Lonardi S, Wong KYM, Lenz H-J, Gelsomino F, Aglietta M, et al. Nivolumab (NIVO) + low-dose ipilimumab (IPI) in previously treated patients (pts) with microsatellite instability-high/mismatch repair-deficient (MSI-H/dMMR) metastatic colorectal cancer (mCRC): long-term follow-up. JCO. 2019;37(4_suppl):635.
46. Morse MA, Overman MJ, Hartman L, Khoukaz T, Brutcher E, Lenz H-J, et al. Safety of Nivolumab plus low-dose Ipilimumab in previously treated microsatellite instability-high/mismatch repair-deficient metastatic colorectal Cancer. Oncologist. 2019;24(11):1453–61.
47. Hurwitz ME, Cho DC, Balar AV, Curti BD, Siefker-Radtke AO, Sznol M, et al. Baseline tumor-immune signatures associated with response to bempegaldesleukin (NKTR-214) and nivolumab. JCO. 2019;37(15_suppl):2623.

Chapter 3
Immunopathogenesis of Immune-Related Adverse Events from Cancer Immunotherapy

Leonard H. Calabrese

The field of cancer therapy experienced a paradigm shift in 2011 with the introduction of the first checkpoint inhibitor (ICI), the anti-CTLA-4 molecule ipilimumab. Since then six more agents have been approved, all targeting either PD-1 or its cognate ligand PD-L1. ICI treatments now constitute a new pillar of cancer therapy but have also introduced a new array of complications known as immune-related adverse events (irAEs), which have been proffered as a possible Achilles heel of these therapeutics [1]. These irAEs can affect virtually any organ system, range from mild to severe, and can be fatal [2]. As the therapies employed to manage irAEs have been culled from the therapeutic armamentarium used to treat idiopathic forms of autoimmunity (i.e., glucocorticoids,

L. H. Calabrese (✉)
Department of Rheumatic and Immunologic Diseases,
Cleveland Clinic Lerner College of Medicine of Case Western Reserve University, Cleveland, OH, USA
e-mail: calabrl@ccf.org

M. E. Suarez-Almazor, L. H. Calabrese (eds.), *Rheumatic Diseases and Syndromes Induced by Cancer Immunotherapy*,
https://doi.org/10.1007/978-3-030-56824-5_3

anti-TNF agents, other targeted therapies, antimetabolites), it is reasonable to ask on just what scientific basis they are utilized. In fact, an even more fundamental question plaguing the field of irAEs is whether these complications represent similar but slightly different forms of idiopathic autoimmune conditions with shared immunopathogenic pathways (i.e., rheumatoid arthritis, Sjögren's syndrome, polymyalgia rheumatic, vasculitis, myositis) or whether they represent mere avatars of immune diseases with potentially unique immunopathogenic origins. Answering this question has profound implications in our search for therapies, which balance effective anti-inflammatory capacity with sparing of immune effector pathways involved in fighting cancer [3].

Autoimmunity or Autoinflammation?

Over the past 20 years, the fundamental concepts of immunopathogenesis surrounding the very nature of human autoimmune disease have been shifting, largely due to an increased understanding of the concept of autoinflammation [4]. Diseases labeled as classic autoimmune disorders (i.e., SLE, RA, Sjögren's) have long been believed to be largely polygenic in origin, involving breaches in immunologic tolerance with the generation of pathogenic autoreactive B cells and organ-specific autoantibodies as well as self-directed T cells. Autoinflammatory diseases, while also associated with chronic immune activation, largely involve innate immune dysregulation; they often display a strong propensity for distinct anatomic localization (i.e., skin, mucous membranes, eye) and were originally viewed as primarily monogenic in origin [3]. An evolution in the understanding of these concepts reveals they are more nuanced: in classic autoimmune disorders, there is also evidence of innate immune activation and involvement of the inflammasome [5]. Furthermore, there are also diseases that now appear to bridge these concepts such as Crohn's disease, which, while polygenic, has many features of autoinflammation as well as some elements characteristic of autoimmunity [5, 6]. Environmental factors (e.g., infection, microbiome, diet, toxin exposure) have been epidemiologically linked to both autoimmune and autoinflammatory disorders, but their relative contributions are far from clear.

With this background, it is reasonable to ask: where do irAEs fit within this theoretical framework? A simple examination of the spectrum of irAEs reveals remarkable clinical, anatomic, and pathologic diversity, making it unlikely that these diseases are homogeneous in their immunopathogenesis. Indeed some irAEs do display features of classic autoimmunity such as select cases of type 1 diabetes and inflammatory arthritis with characteristics of rheumatoid arthritis [7]. Each of these disorders is accompanied by the documented presence of signature autoantibodies as well as background MHC genes as observed in the idiopathic forms of these diseases [7]. In reality, adverse events of this description represent a very small minority of all reported irAEs. Autoreactive T cells have been identified in several cases of myositis [8] and pneumonitis [9]; however, detailed studies of large numbers of patients, which include screening for the evolution of autoreactive T cells in the wake of ICI therapy, have not been reported.

Factors hindering an increased understanding of immunopathogenesis are multiple. First, the vast majority of reports of irAEs are clinical and descriptive; there is a paucity of in-depth immunopathogenic and translational studies. Second, irAEs are diverse by nature, and some are relatively rare making comprehensive pathophysiologic studies difficult when done at single institutions. Finally, there is also a paucity of preclinical investigations into the mechanisms of irAEs in comparison to the massive quantity of studies on efficacy of immune-based therapies for cancer. Further limiting our understanding of irAEs are some technical limitations of preclinical investigations, including the use of animals traditionally used to study cancer immunotherapies such as B6 and BLAB/c strains which are generally resistant to autoimmunity [9], imposing a barrier for the development of immune toxicities. Efforts to adopt models that mimic both efficacy and toxicity of immune-based therapeutics are urgently needed. Perhaps the greatest resource that is lacking is a comprehensive study of irAEs analogous to the multicenter AIDS cohort study (MACS), which has categorized, curated, and investigated the natural history of HIV disease for over three decades at multiple sites throughout the United States. A similar effort is urgently needed to effectively and comprehensively track and study irAEs.

Putative Mechanisms of Immunopathogenesis

Preclinical Models

It has been known for over two decades that CTLA-4 knockout mice suffer rapidly progressive lymphoproliferation and fatal multi-organ inflammatory disease [10]; therefore, the fact that interfering with classical immune checkpoints such as the CTLA-4 and PD-1 pathways can result in immune disease should come as no surprise. Genetic models inducing PD-1 deficiency result in spontaneous autoimmunity and can induce or exacerbate autoimmune diseases such as diabetes and systemic lupus [11]. Furthermore, anti-PD-1 treatment can exacerbate diabetes in nonobese diabetic (NOD) mice as well as exacerbate disease in animal models of multiple sclerosis in the form of experimental autoimmune encephalitis [11]. Collectively, these data assert a central role of CTLA-4 and PD-1 pathways in terms of control of tolerance and autoimmunity.

Lessons from Primary Immunodeficiency States

Even more compelling for the role of the CTLA-4 pathway in maintaining control of autoimmunity has been the elucidation of several genetic diseases characterized by under-expression of CTLA-4 on the lymphocyte cell surface, resulting in multi-organ inflammation and autoimmunity [12]. Two disorders, CHAI (CTLA-4 haploinsufficiency) and LATAIE (LRBA deficiency with autoantibodies, Treg defects, autoimmune infiltration, and enteropathy), while genetically and mechanistically different, both result in under-expression and dysfunction of CTLA-4 signaling [13]. A detailed report of the phenotype, penetrance, and treatment of a large international cohort of CHAI patients has recently been published [14]. Immunologically, loss of CTLA-4 signaling results in T cell activation and hyperproliferation, a functional deficit of Treg cells, and expansion of CD21lo B cells. This latter finding of perturbed B cell populations also correlates with the development of irAEs in patients treated with combined anti-CTLA-4 and anti-PD-1 agents [15]. Clinical lessons from these two immune deficiency disorders include appreciation of the variety of immune-mediated diseases found in these patients (type 1 diabetes, arthritis, thyroiditis, hepatitis, and other end-organ manifestations) along with the presence of autoantibodies. The similarity of the clinical presentation and laboratory findings of CHAI and LATAIE patients when compared to irAE patients is striking [14]. One important difference between genetic forms of CLTA-4 deficiency and irAEs is that most patients with these primary immunodeficiencies also develop progressive hypogammaglobulinemia, a feature not observed in irAEs from ICIs. Further work to explore a more detailed understanding of these and other forms of human primary immunodeficiency states is likely to shed additional light on the immunopathogenesis of irAEs.

Drugs and Disease Effects

Within the class of ICIs, there are differential effects stemming from characteristics of the individual drugs as well as the dose of these agents in the development of irAEs. In general, irAEs are more common with anti-CTLA-4 agents versus those targeting PD-1/PD-L1 pathways; higher doses of all agents enhance toxicity, albeit with broad variation [16, 17]. In addition, there are also drug-irAE associations in which specific drugs are associated with trends for specific irAEs. For example, the vast majority of hypophysitis is linked to anti-CTLA-4 therapy, while the vast majority of inflammatory polyarthritis is linked to anti-PD-1/PD-L1 therapy [7]. Finally, certain tumors are linked to certain toxicities (e.g., lung cancer and pneumonitis; melanoma and vitiligo) suggesting that anatomic location may affect toxicity [18]. Such anatomic linking may be very important in the immunopathogenesis of irAEs of autoinflammatory mechanisms as discussed above.

Basic Mechanisms of Autoimmunity and Autoinflammation for Checkpoint Inhibitors

Experimental Construct for the Evolution of Autoimmune Diseases

A theoretical construct had been proposed interrelating a variety of risk factors, which, over time, can ultimately lead to clinical autoimmune disease [19]. This construct is useful for modeling our understanding of irAEs (Fig. 3.1). In this model, individuals are placed at some degree of risk by their genetic composition, which, for most, is insufficient alone to cause clinical autoimmunity. Over time, numerous environmental factors (e.g., diet, stress, tobacco, microbiome composition, pollution) may contribute to further breaches of tolerance leading to increasing self-reactivity [19]. In the absence of clinical disease or other immune-mediated disease manifestations, this stage is referred to as asymptomatic autoimmunity. Beyond this, additional environmental factors may contribute to the ultimate development of clinical disease in either an insidious or fulminant fashion. Accepting this construct and applying it to our understanding of irAEs, we may then postulate that the introduction of ICI therapy

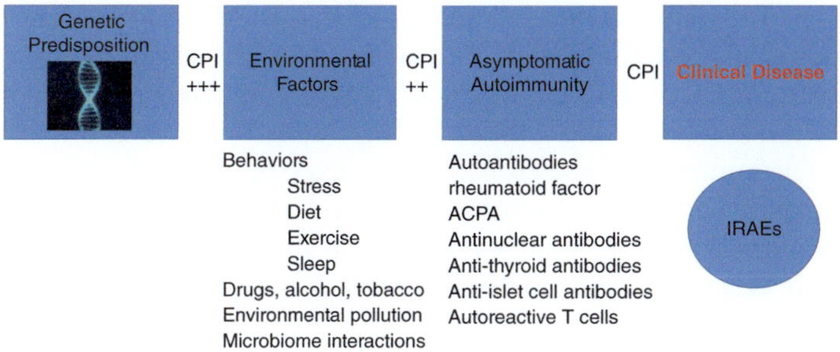

Figure 3.1 Timeline of the theoretic evolution of autoimmunity examining the influence of genes, environmental factors, and exposure to checkpoint inhibitors (CPIs) in the development of autoreactivity and autoimmune disease. At the left is the patient with some genetic risks for autoimmunity but no additional environmental risks for autoimmunity and free of any evidence of autoreactivity (i.e., autoreactive T cells or autoantibodies). At this stage of the balance between autoreactivity and tolerance, the hurdles needed to overcome to develop autoimmune disease are high, and thus there are barriers and resistance for CPIs to ultimately drive the evolution of autoimmune disease. As the stages to autoimmunity progress facilitated by environmental risks (i.e., tobacco exposure, others) such exposure may already be driving the subject to overcome tolerance, and then exposure to CPIs may be more likely to drive the generation of autoantibodies and/or autoimmune diseases. Finally if the genetically predisposed individual has already developed the stage autoreactivity (i.e., asymptomatic autoimmunity with laboratory evidence of autoantibodies or autoreactive T cells), then exposure to CPIs may be the final step in a more rapid evolution or the development of particularly fulminate autoimmune disease. *CPI* checkpoint inhibitor, *ACPA* anti-citrullinated antibodies, *IRAEs* immune-related adverse events

can be viewed as a profound environmental factor which could potentially drive the expression of autoimmunity/autoinflammation in patients with some degree of genetic predisposition. Implicit in this theory is that higher genetic risk will enable irAE induction more than in those with lower risk propensity. In some individuals with minimal underlying genetic/environmental proclivity for autoimmunity, higher doses or combined ICI therapy may be required to drive immune-mediated toxicities; in others with high risks, such as those with strong genetic backgrounds or more abundant environmental risk factors, far less exposure to ICIs may be needed to express immune toxicities. Such a model could account for the dramatic variation in incidence and severity of irAEs in patients undergoing ICI therapy.

Proposed Immunologic Pathways Contributing to irAEs

As noted above, our understanding of the immunologic underpinnings of most irAEs is far from complete, and much more work at the preclinical, translational, and clinical levels is needed. For now, however, it is useful to segregate putative immunopathogenesis into a number of discreet pathways, each of which may contribute to various irAEs, singly or in combination (Fig. 3.2). Consider these mechanistic theories as building blocks for our understanding of how irAEs may come about, recognizing that linking them to individual complications is problematic given our lack of immunopathogenic data for most.

Generalized Immune Activation

Generalized immune activation following interdiction of the CTLA-4 or the PD-1 pathways by ICIs has been well documented [20], though the extent of the relative contributions of both innate and adaptive immune pathways is not well understood. A fundamental question to address before gaining further understanding is whether generalized inflammation (i.e., autoinflammation) in an organ-nonspecific manner can explain some of the clinical spectrum of irAEs.

As previously discussed, many irAEs are devoid of meaningful evidence for organ-specific autoimmunity of either T or B cell origin; this may represent deficits in our current

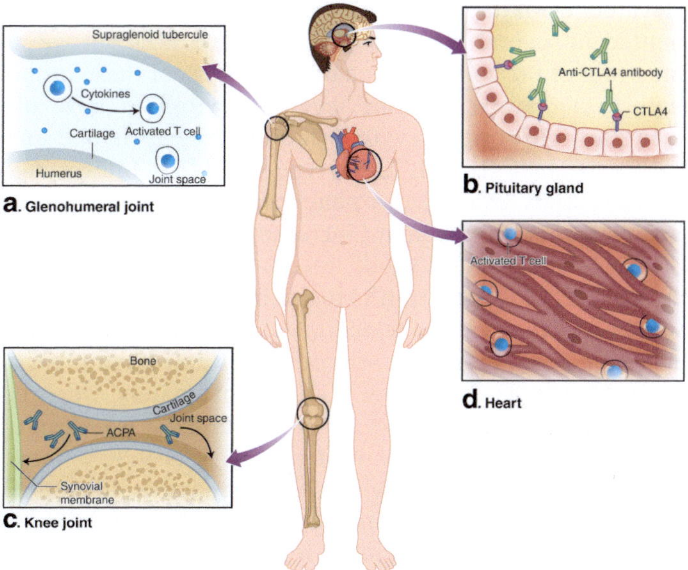

FIGURE 3.2 Immunopathogenic mechanisms of irAEs. (**a**) Generalized immune activation due to checkpoint neutralization, which could lead to conditions such as patient with polymyalgia rheumatic. (**b**) Direct off-target effects of CPIs such as anti-CTLA-4 antibodies binding to CTLA-4 expressed by hypothalamic tissues contributing to hypophysitis. (**c**) Preexisting asymptomatic autoimmunity showing the effects of ACPA that may be preexisting in an asymptomatic state prior to CPI exposure. (**d**) Off-target effects of T cell-mediated immunity, which can occur in multiple organs such as the muscle, heart, or joint

state of investigations rather than proof that they do not exist. It is possible that many irAEs may indeed be more autoinflammatory than autoimmune in the classic sense. Consider polymyalgia rheumatica (PMR), a condition that among rheumatic irAE complications is relatively common and for which we have only limited immunopathogenic understanding of to begin with. Similar to idiopathic PMR, the irAE form is highly inflammatory, but some are described as atypical (Fig. 3.1a) with only about 70% of PMR irAE patients meeting ACR/EULAR classification criteria [21].

Elevated cytokines, in particular, IL-17, have been documented in several irAEs, especially colitis [22], yet we are uncertain of the cellular or anatomic origins of these inflammatory mediators. Baseline levels of cytokines have also been shown to correlate with incidence of irAEs in one small study, especially IL-1, IL-2, and type 1 IFN [23]. Interestingly, a recent study examined a panel of 40 cytokines pre- and post- ICI therapy revealing increases in CXCL9, CXCL10, CXCL11, and CXCL13, but not IL-1 and IL6 [24]. These chemokines serve cell trafficking of innate and adaptive cell lines and have been implicated in autoimmune diseases such as multiple sclerosis and scleroderma. Other cytokines of interest such as TNF and IL-17 unfortunately were not assayed [24]. Finally, while our understanding is extremely limited as to how and to what degree ICIs induce innate immune activation, a study of skin immunohistology in the irAE of lichenoid dermatitis has been informative. In this study of irAE and spontaneous forms of lichenoid dermatitis, patients exposed to ICIs demonstrated an increase in CD14/TLR4 innate-mediated tissue damage suggesting a prominent role of innate immune response in this clinical subtype [25]. More work is urgently needed to better understand the interrelationship between ICIs and innate immune effector mechanisms.

Direct Off-Target Effects of ICIs

Another potential mechanism for immune-mediated toxicity is that of off-target effects of ICIs, which could induce tissue damage on non-hematopoietic cell lines bearing the target ligand (Fig. 3.1b). Some evidence of this has been demonstrated for hypophysitis secondary to anti-CTLA-4 agents, as CTLA-4 has been demonstrated to be expressed on hypothalamic and pituitary tissues and thus can readily serve as a target for antibody-mediated injury [26, 27]. No other irAEs have shown similar cross-reaction between healthy host tissue and target antigens of ICIs.

Preexisting Asymptomatic Autoimmunity

There are now numerous reports of ICIs leading to rapid onset of autoimmunity in what appear to be examples of patients with preexisting autoimmune states. In the currently embraced model depicted in Fig. 3.1, some classic autoimmune disorders may originate in a milieu of genetic predisposition followed by encounters with unknown environmental triggers that may lead to states of asymptomatic autoimmunity. In this state, patients may display characteristic autoantibodies, such as ACPA, but remain asymptomatic. What happens to individuals with asymptomatic autoimmunity is variable, with perhaps the majority remaining asymptomatic while others progress to clinical disease.

Although most reports of ICI-associated inflammatory polyarthritis are seronegative for ACPA and RF, more recently several reports suggest that some patients are ACPA-positive before therapy and thus may represent examples of this putative mechanism for autoimmunity [7, 28, 29] (Fig. 3.1c). This scenario of an irAE with serologic features of RA has been reported exclusively, thus far, in the setting of anti-PD-1 therapeutics (36). Clinically these patients often present fulminantly with short incubation times following ICI administration. A similar scenario has been described for the irAE of type 1 diabetes presenting with acute ketoacidosis, in which some patients are positive for disease-associated antibodies such as anti-islet cell antibodies [30] in serum prior to treatment. Similar examples of other irAEs in which patients have documented disease-associated autoantibodies prior to developing organ-specific irAEs include rare examples of myasthenia gravis, autoimmune hemolytic anemia, and autoimmune thyroid disease [31–33]. Against this argument of preexisting asymptomatic autoimmunity is the fact that most patients with irAEs of rheumatic and non-rheumatic origin test negatively for serum autoantibodies; studies examining the value of clinically utilized autoantibodies as predictive biomarkers of irAEs have mixed results but are largely disappointing [34, 35]. There are now several studies which document that in patients with preexisting autoimmune conditions, only about 50% develop a flare of the underlying immune condition when treated with ICIs [7, 36, 37].

Off-Target Effects of T Cell-Mediated Immunity

Given that current ICIs affect regulatory pathways essential to maintaining T cell homeostasis, and that most irAEs are devoid of strong evidence of pathogenic autoantibodies, cell-mediated immunity has been considered central in their pathogenesis. Anti-CTLA-4 and anti-PD-1/anti-PD-L1 appear to have differential effects on T cell populations with CTLA-4 blocking antibodies primarily affecting CD4 cells, while drugs affecting PD-1/PD-L1 pathways appear to affect a subset of exhausted-like CD-8 cells [38]. A role for quantitative and functional compromise of Treg cells may also contribute to breaching T cell tolerance [1]. The generation of autoreactive T cells could further come about via two non-mutually exclusive pathways leading to loss of self-tolerance. The first involves the generation of autoreactive T cells within the tumor milieu when invading cytotoxic T cells target tumor cells that also contain healthy host cell antigens. Alternatively, the invading immune reactive cells and attendant inflammation may also damage other healthy nonmalignant host cells leading to the generation of self-reactivity. Classical immunologic mechanisms leading to loss of T cell tolerance within the tumor milieu include molecular mimicry, epitope spreading, and bystander activation [39, 40] (Fig. 3.1d). Supporting immunopathologic evidence for the centrality of compromised T cell tolerance in irAEs comes largely from a few well-studied cases of myositis/myocarditis [8] and pneumonitis [41]. In these case studies, T cells within end organs displaying immune-mediated damage and T cells within the tumors share the same T cell receptors, supporting such a mechanism. The second mechanism could come about through the activation of nascent self-reactive T cells in secondary lymphoid organs, peripheral tissues, or blood as the peripheral T cell repertoire of healthy individuals contains a high frequency of such cells [42]. Further detailed work on how ICIs affect this resident population of autoreactive cells is urgently needed.

Most preclinical models in rodents have added relatively little to our immunopathologic understanding of irAEs as previously noted, but one study supporting the role of pathogenic T cells in a primate model of myositis and myocarditis has added important insights regarding the role of T cells in irAEs. In this model, a regimen of high-dose combined anti-CTLA-4 and anti-PD-1 therapy in cynomolgus monkeys resulted in multiple organ toxicities with expansion of activated T cells, including central memory cells, in blood as well as target end organs including the muscle and heart [43], suggesting that T cell autoreactivity can be generated in the absence of tumor-linked immune targeting. Further work is needed to elucidate the cofactors driving irAEs in an effort to understand why these complications occur in some but not all or even the majority of patients. Such understanding will also help us craft more rational targeted therapies beyond high-dose glucocorticoids.

Genetic and Environmental Factors

The question of why some patients develop specific irAEs and why others do not is not answerable at the present time. Referring again to the traditional model of autoimmunity generation (Fig. 3.1), let us consider some of the major potential cofactors, recognizing that our knowledge of such is very incomplete [19]. First consider genetic background. Major histocompatibility complex genes are known to confer risk for the development of numerous autoimmune diseases (e.g., the shared epitope in rheumatoid arthritis). To date, limited studies performed in small numbers of patients have found relatively weak genetic associations in some irAEs including hypophysitis [44]. A small study of 102 patients with various irAEs also found no single HLA type associated with all irAEs and only nominally significant associations with two Class 2 alleles (pruritus and colitis) [45]. Two conditions for which there are strong associations with MHC antigens, type 1 diabetes and rheumatoid arthritis, which have surrogate irAEs bearing some degrees of similarity, have been investigated for MHC associations. In a series of 27 patients with type 1 diabetes, a high percentage displayed HLA-DR4 positivity, an allele that is seen in idiopathic type 1 diabetes, but other high-risk alleles seen in the idiopathic type 1 diabetic population were absent [30]. Of great interest to the rheumatology field is the work of Cappelli et al. who performed HLA typing in 27 patients with inflammatory arthritis and compared them to healthy and RA controls [46]. This report documented that irAE inflammatory arthritis patients, who were predominantly seronegative for ACPA and RF, were more likely to have one shared epitope allele that is found in ACPA-positive RA than healthy controls. No association with HLA-B27, another likely candidate, was found in this cohort. This raises interesting questions regarding the pathophysiologic role of the shared epitope in those where ACPA are absent. Clearly far larger studies in a broad array of irAEs are warranted, but these data suggest some role of MHC expression and at least some irAEs.

Another environmental factor is infection, which would include the influence of the microbiome and the use of antimicrobials. There is now a growing literature on the emerging importance of the microbiome as a correlate of the efficacy of checkpoint inhibitors [47, 48]. While no single organism has been correlated with efficacy, there are collaborative evidence from numerous studies asserting a strong association between microbiomic health and clinical response [49–52]. Antimicrobial exposure prior to ICI therapy is correlated with a poor outcome, further supporting the critical role of the microbiome in ICI mechanism of action [53]. This phenomenon has been reproduced in animal models as well [54, 55]. More work is clearly needed on the adverse events side to determine if there are similar correlations of microbiome health and toxicity of ICIs.

Finally, the role of a wide array of environmental factors including the effects of personal behaviors such as smoking, diet, stress, pollution, and other unknown factors, as well the role of the epigenome, has been hypothesized to function as risk modifiers in the progression to autoimmunity in individuals with some degree of genetic predisposition [19, 56]. To date, there is a paucity of work in this area pertaining to irAEs. A recent abstract highlights strong associations between a variety of commonly used drugs with known effects on the microbiome with antitumoral response to ICIs, but further work is awaited examining similar effects on the association with irAEs [57].

Clinical Implications and Summary

Immune-related adverse events secondary to the first generation of ICIs have transformed the interprofessional management of patients with cancer and have developed a new field of medicine. At present, most of our therapies have been derived by co-opting the therapies used to treat traditional forms of autoimmune and autoinflammatory disease based largely on clinical similarities and availability rather than granular knowledge of immunopathogenesis. Fortunately many of these currently endorsed therapeutic paradigms have served our patients well, but concerns over overzealous empiric immunosuppression and its effects on antitumoral immunity have emerged [3]. Even more importantly, the specter of some irAEs becoming chronic inflammatory diseases of indefinite duration, which has been long feared, has recently been documented: 40% of patients with inflammatory arthritis have persistent symptoms 6 or more months after ICI discontinuation [58]. Further understanding of what may represent totally new nosologic entities is urgent to craft safe and effective therapy. Finally the field of cancer immunotherapy is merely in its infancy, and the next generation of immune-based therapeutics will likely be more effective but also may come with potential costs of causing even more challenging immune toxicities.

References

1. June CH, Warshauer JT, Bluestone JA. Is autoimmunity the Achilles' heel of cancer immunotherapy? Nat Med. 2017;23(5):540–7.
2. Postow MA, Sidlow R, Hellmann MD. Immune-related adverse events associated with immune checkpoint blockade. N Engl J Med. 2018;378(2):158–68.
3. McGonagle D, et al. Mechanistic classification of immune checkpoint inhibitor Toxicity as a pointer to minimal treatment strategies of selected emergent autoimmune diseases to further improve survival. Autoimmun Rev. 2020;19(2):102456
4. Martinez-Quiles N, Goldbach-Mansky R. Updates on autoinflammatory diseases. Curr Opin Immunol. 2018;55:97–105.
5. Kahlenberg JM, Kang I. The Clinicopathologic significance of Inflammasome activation in autoimmune diseases. Arthritis Rheumatol. 2019;
6. McGonagle D, McDermott MF. A proposed classification of the immunological diseases. PLoS Med. 2006;3(8):e297.
7. Calabrese LH, Calabrese C, Cappelli LC. Rheumatic immune-related adverse events from cancer immunotherapy. Nat Rev Rheumatol. 2018;14(10):569–79.
8. Johnson DB, et al. Fulminant myocarditis with combination immune checkpoint blockade. N Engl J Med. 2016;375(18):1749–55.
9. Young A, Quandt Z, Bluestone JA. The balancing act between cancer immunity and autoimmunity in response to immunotherapy. Cancer Immunol Res. 2018;6(12):1445–52.
10. Tivol EA, et al. Loss of CTLA-4 leads to massive lymphoproliferation and fatal multiorgan tissue destruction, revealing a critical negative regulatory role of CTLA-4. Immunity. 1995;3(5):541–7.
11. Kuol N, et al. PD-1/PD-L1 in disease. Immunotherapy. 2018;10(2):149–60.
12. Lo B, Abdel-Motal UM. Lessons from CTLA-4 deficiency and checkpoint inhibition. Curr Opin Immunol. 2017;49:14–9.
13. Lo B, et al. CHAI and LATAIE: new genetic diseases of CTLA-4 checkpoint insufficiency. Blood. 2016;128(8):1037–42.

14. Schwab C, et al. Phenotype, penetrance, and treatment of 133 cytotoxic T-lymphocyte antigen 4-insufficient subjects. J Allergy Clin Immunol. 2018;142(6):1932–46.
15. Das R, et al. Early B cell changes predict autoimmunity following combination immune checkpoint blockade. J Clin Invest. 2018;
16. Olischewsky A, et al. Dose-dependent toxicity of ipilimumab in metastatic melanoma. Eur J Cancer. 2018;95:104–8.
17. Yoo SH, et al. Low-dose nivolumab can be effective in non-small cell lung cancer: alternative option for financial toxicity. ESMO Open. 2018;3(5):e000332.
18. Nakamura Y, et al. Correlation between vitiligo occurrence and clinical benefit in advanced melanoma patients treated with nivolumab: a multi-institutional retrospective study. J Dermatol. 2017;44(2):117–22.
19. Deane KD, El-Gabalawy H. Pathogenesis and prevention of rheumatic disease: focus on preclinical RA and SLE. Nat Rev Rheumatol. 2014;10(4):212–28.
20. Huang AC, et al. T-cell invigoration to tumour burden ratio associated with anti-PD-1 response. Nature. 2017;545(7652):60–5.
21. Calabrese C, et al. Polymyalgia rheumatica-like syndrome from checkpoint inhibitor therapy: case series and systematic review of the literature. RMD Open. 2019;5(1):e000906.
22. Callahan MK, et al. Evaluation of serum IL-17 levels during ipilimumab therapy: correlation with colitis. J Clin Oncol. 2011;29(15_suppl):2505.
23. Squibb B.-M. Yervoy (Ipilimumab), immune-mediated adverse reaction management guide. 2011. http://www.yervoy.com/hcp/rems.aspx.
24. Khan S, et al. Immune dysregulation in cancer patients developing immune-related adverse events. Br J Cancer. 2019;120(1):63–8.
25. Curry JL, et al. Gene expression profiling of lichenoid dermatitis immune-related adverse event from immune checkpoint inhibitors reveals increased CD14(+) and CD16(+) monocytes driving an innate immune response. J Cutan Pathol. 2019;46(9):627–36.
26. Iwama S, Arima H. Clinical practice and mechanism of endocrinological adverse events associated with immune checkpoint inhibitors. Nihon Rinsho Meneki Gakkai Kaishi. 2017;40(2):90–4.
27. Iwama S, et al. Pituitary expression of CTLA-4 mediates hypophysitis secondary to administration of CTLA-4 blocking antibody. Sci Transl Med. 2014;6(230):230ra45.

28. Cappelli L, et al. Inflammatory arthritis and sicca syndrome induced by nivolumab and ipilimumab. Ann Rheum Dis. 2016;
29. Naidoo J, et al. Inflammatory arthritis: a newly recognized adverse event of immune checkpoint blockade. Oncologist. 2017;22(6):627–30.
30. Stamatouli AM, et al. Collateral damage: insulin-dependent diabetes induced with checkpoint inhibitors. Diabetes. 2018;67(8):1471–80.
31. Shirai T, et al. Acetylcholine receptor binding antibody-associated myasthenia gravis and rhabdomyolysis induced by nivolumab in a patient with melanoma. Jpn J Clin Oncol. 2016;46(1):86–8.
32. Cooling LL, et al. Development of red blood cell autoantibodies following treatment with checkpoint inhibitors: a new class of anti-neoplastic, immunotherapeutic agents associated with immune dysregulation. Immunohematology. 2017;33(1):15–21.
33. Mammen AL, et al. Pre-existing antiacetylcholine receptor autoantibodies and B cell lymphopaenia are associated with the development of myositis in patients with thymoma treated with avelumab, an immune checkpoint inhibitor targeting programmed death-ligand 1. Ann Rheum Dis. 2019;78(1):150–2.
34. Da Gama Duarte J, et al. Autoantibodies may predict immune-related toxicity: results from a phase I study of Intralesional Bacillus Calmette-Guerin followed by Ipilimumab in patients with advanced metastatic melanoma. Front Immunol. 2018;9:411.
35. Nielen MM, et al. Specific autoantibodies precede the symptoms of rheumatoid arthritis: a study of serial measurements in blood donors. Arthritis Rheum. 2004;50(2):380–6.
36. Calabrese LH. Sorting out the complexities of autoimmunity and checkpoint inhibitors: not so easy. Ann Intern Med. 2018;168(2):149–50.
37. Abdel-Hamid M, et al. Use of immune checkpoint inhibitors in the treatment of patients with cancer and preexisiting autoimmune disease: a systematic review. Ann Intern Med. 2017;
38. Wei SC, et al. Distinct cellular mechanisms underlie anti-CTLA-4 and anti-PD-1 checkpoint blockade. Cell. 2017;170(6):1120–33.e17
39. Pacheco Y, et al. Bystander activation and autoimmunity. J Autoimmun. 2019;103:102301.
40. Rojas M, et al. Molecular mimicry and autoimmunity. J Autoimmun. 2018;95:100–23.
41. Berner F, et al. Association of checkpoint inhibitor-induced toxic effects with shared cancer and tissue antigens in non-small cell lung cancer. JAMA Oncol. 2019;5(7):1043–7.

42. Klein L, et al. Positive and negative selection of the T cell repertoire: what thymocytes see (and don't see). Nat Rev Immunol. 2014;14(6):377–91.
43. Ji C, et al. Myocarditis in cynomolgus monkeys following treatment with immune checkpoint inhibitors. Clin Cancer Res. 2019;
44. Heaney AP, et al. HLA markers DQ8 and DR53 are associated with lymphocytic Hypophysitis and may aid in differential diagnosis. J Clin Endocrinol Metab. 2015;100(11):4092–7.
45. Hasan Ali O, et al. Human leukocyte antigen variation is associated with adverse events of checkpoint inhibitors. Eur J Cancer. 2019;107:8–14.
46. Cappelli LC, et al. Association of HLA-DRB1 shared epitope alleles and immune checkpoint inhibitor-induced inflammatory arthritis. Rheumatology (Oxford). 2018;
47. Anderson R, Rapoport BL. Immune dysregulation in Cancer patients undergoing immune checkpoint inhibitor treatment and potential predictive strategies for future clinical practice. Front Oncol. 2018;8:80.
48. Sun JY, et al. Gut microbiome and cancer immunotherapy. J Cell Physiol. 2019;
49. Gopalakrishnan V, et al. The influence of the gut microbiome on Cancer, immunity, and Cancer immunotherapy. Cancer Cell. 2018;33(4):570–80.
50. Gopalakrishnan V, et al. Gut microbiome modulates response to anti-PD-1 immunotherapy in melanoma patients. Science. 2018;359(6371):97–103.
51. Helmink BA, et al. The microbiome, cancer, and cancer therapy. Nat Med. 2019;25(3):377–88.
52. Routy B, et al. The gut microbiota influences anticancer immunosurveillance and general health. Nat Rev Clin Oncol. 2018;15(6):382–96.
53. Elkrief A, et al. The negative impact of antibiotics on outcomes in cancer patients treated with immunotherapy: a new independent prognostic factor? Ann Oncol. 2019;30(10):1572–9.
54. Goubet AG, et al. The impact of the intestinal microbiota in therapeutic responses against cancer. C R Biol. 2018;341(5):284–9.
55. Routy B, et al. Gut microbiome influences efficacy of PD-1-based immunotherapy against epithelial tumors. Science. 2018;359(6371):91–7.
56. Richardson B. The interaction between environmental triggers and epigenetics in autoimmunity. Clin Immunol. 2018;192:1–5.

57. Kostine M, et al. Commonly used drugs in rheumatology may alter anti-tumoral reponse to immune checkpoint inhibitors {abstract}. Arthritis Rheumatol. 2019;71(suppl 10). https://acrabstracts.org/abstract/commonly-used-drugs-in-rheumatology-may-alter-anti-tumoral-response-to-immune-checkpoint-inhibitors/. Accessed September 9, 2020.
58. Braaten TJ, et al. Immune checkpoint inhibitor-induced inflammatory arthritis persists after immunotherapy cessation. Ann Rheum Dis. 2019;

Part II
Immune-Related Adverse Events with Immune-Checkpoint Inhibitors

Chapter 4
Immune-Related Adverse Events with Immune Checkpoint Inhibitors: Arthritis

Laura C. Cappelli and Clifton O. Bingham III

Introduction

Immune-related adverse events (irAEs), due to immune checkpoint inhibitors (ICIs), can present similarly to several different rheumatic diseases [1, 2]. Inflammatory arthritis (IA), due to ICIs, is the irAE most likely to be encountered by rheumatologists and has been described in case series and retrospective and prospective observational studies [3–16]. Managing patients with ICI-induced IA can be more complicated than managing patients with rheumatoid arthritis or spondyloarthritis. The context in which the arthritis develops, namely, immunotherapy treatment for cancer, affects treatment decisions. Because ICI-induced IA is a relatively new entity, there is a lack of prospective data to guide management. In this chapter, we review current

L. C. Cappelli (✉) · C. O. Bingham III
Division of Rheumatology, Johns Hopkins School of Medicine, Baltimore, MD, USA
e-mail: lcappel1@jhmi.edu; cbingha2@jhmi.edu

M. E. Suarez-Almazor, L. H. Calabrese (eds.), *Rheumatic Diseases and Syndromes Induced by Cancer Immunotherapy*,
https://doi.org/10.1007/978-3-030-56824-5_4

understanding of the epidemiology, clinical manifestations, diagnosis, and management of ICI-induced IA.

Epidemiology

Data on the prevalence of inflammatory arthritis in ICI-treated patients come mostly from retrospective studies. Clinical trial data are limited for several reasons. Arthritis is rarely classified as a severe adverse event by the Common Terminology Criteria for Adverse Events (CTCAE) [17] used to grade side effects in oncology clinical trials, so may have been underreported. Additionally, IA may have been described with a variety of terms (e.g., arthralgia, arthritis, periarthritis, pain in extremity, and joint swelling), which dilutes the ability to detect signal. In clinical trials, rates of arthralgia have ranged from 1 to 43% [2].

From retrospective studies, the prevalence of IA appears to be from 3 to 7% in ICI-treated patients [14, 18]. This may underestimate the occurrence of mild cases of arthritis, as they are less likely to be documented in the medical record or to be referred to a rheumatologist for confirmation and treatment. Prospective studies of patients treated with ICIs with dedicated screening for IA would provide a more accurate estimate of true disease burden.

Risk factors for IA are largely unknown. It is unclear whether IA occurs more commonly in particular tumor types. For other irAEs, there is an association with class of ICI; hypophysitis and colitis occur more commonly with cytotoxic T-lymphocyte-associated protein 4 (CTLA-4) blockade, while pneumonitis and thyroid disease occur more commonly with programmed death 1 (PD-1) blockade [19]. Generally, irAEs are more prevalent with combination anti-CTLA-4/anti-PD-1 therapy as opposed to monotherapy with anti-PD-1 [20]; however, there is no study to our knowledge that compares the prevalence of IA by ICI regimen.

In cohort studies and case series of ICI-induced IA, there has been a roughly equal representation of men and women, though some cohorts have a slight predominance of men [5, 6, 8, 11, 15, 18]. The age at presentation ranges widely from the 30s to 80s, but most patients are in their 50s to 70s as would be expected for an oncology population. There has been limited information concerning race or ethnicity of affected patients in the current literature.

Pathogenesis

As with other irAEs, there are little data relating to the pathogenesis of ICI-induced IA. Data presented in abstract form have shown expanded CD4 and CD8 populations with a PD-1 $^{+}$ CD38 ^{hi} CD127 $^{-}$ phenotype in synovial fluid [21] and increased Th17 cells in synovial fluid [22]. Increased senescent T cells and elevated IL-6 levels have been noted in the peripheral blood of patients with ICI-induced IA [23]. Genetic risk factors are not well elucidated, but a pilot study showed an association of HLA DRB1 shared epitope alleles with ICI-induced IA [24]. Finally, the efficacy of TNF-inhibitors and IL-6R inhibitors may suggest a role of these cytokines in pathogenesis. Future directions include studying ICI-induced IA alongside other forms of autoimmune IA, such as rheumatoid arthritis, to understand similarities and differences in pathogenesis [25]. Please also see Chap. 3 for a discussion of pathogenesis of rheumatic irAEs.

Clinical Manifestations

Arthralgia was documented in early trials of ICIs, but true inflammatory arthritis was not well described until more recently. One of the first case reports of ICI-induced IA, in 2015, described arthritis and tenosynovitis in patients treated with a PD-1 inhibitor [3]. Since that time, a heterogeneous group of clinical presentations has emerged for patients with ICI-induced IA.

Patients may present with monoarthritis (rare) or, more commonly, oligoarthritis or polyarthritis [6, 8, 9, 15, 16]. Predominant polymyalgia rheumatica-like symptoms with accompanying small joint arthritis has also been described [26]. In addition to synovitis, patients may have considerable tendon involvement, with both tenosynovitis and enthesitis noted [5, 9, 27, 28].

The reactive arthritis triad (i.e., sterile urethritis and conjunctivitis accompanying inflammatory arthritis) is another possible presentation for ICI-induced IA. Interestingly, in one study, all three patients with reactive arthritis were male, were treated with anti-CTLA-4/anti-PD-1 combination therapy, and had antecedent colitis [9]. This may be an important group to study in understanding pathogenesis not just of ICI-induced IA, but also reactive arthritis.

Inflammatory axial disease appears to be rare. Sacroiliitis was discovered incidentally on imaging of patients being treated with anti-CTLA-4 therapy [29]. Polyarthritis of the facet and costovertebral joints has also been reported [30].

Bone involvement, not necessarily limited to the joint, has also been described [31]. One case series demonstrated accelerated osteoporosis leading to multiple vertebral fractures and resorptive lesions of the shoulder, the clavicle, and a carpal bone [31].

Determinants of the clinical heterogeneity in ICI-induced IA are not well studied. In one study, whether a patient was on monotherapy with anti-PD-1/anti-PD-L1 agents or combination anti-CTLA-4 with anti-PD-1 therapy appeared to influence how the arthritis presented [9]. Those on combination therapy had more elevation in inflammatory markers, were more likely to have other irAEs, and were more likely to have the knee involved as the first joint, while those treated with monotherapy were more likely to have IA as their only irAE and to have small joint involvement [9].

Clinical features of ICI-induced IA are summarized in Table 4.1.

TABLE 4.1 Clinical features of ICI-induced IA

Clinical features	Description in ICI-induced IA
Demographic variables	Similar male and female prevalence All tumor types represented Not clear if more common with particular ICIs Age: 30–80s, with 50s–70s the most common
Symptoms	Joint pain, swelling, stiffness Fatigue Function decline, difficulty with ADLs
Patterns of joint involvement	Variable – polyarthritis and lower extremity oligoarthritis most common Axial disease is rare
Other exam findings	Tendon involvement including stenosing tenosynovitis (trigger fingers)
Laboratory results	Blood: Elevated inflammatory markers Most autoantibodies negative Synovial fluid: Inflammatory with neutrophil predominance
Imaging	Synovitis with power Doppler Joint effusions Erosions Enethesitis, enthesophytes Tendinitis
Long-term prognosis	Both resolution and persistence after ICI cessation reported Patients may have permanent erosive damage (rare)

Diagnosis

ICI-induced IA should be suspected in patients receiving ICIs who present with new musculoskeletal symptoms, including joint pain, swelling, stiffness, or functional decline.

Some patients with preexisting musculoskeletal issues, such as osteoarthritis or old injuries, may have a difficult time discerning whether they are experiencing new symptoms. One cohort of patients described a phenotype of "activated osteoarthritis" due to ICIs, where patients had a worsening of symptoms in joints already affected by osteoarthritis with synovitis on exam [18]. This entity is important to keep in mind, particularly in older patients.

Laboratory Testing

In active disease, inflammatory markers are elevated in a majority, but not in all patients. Autoantibodies associated with RA, that is, rheumatoid factor and anti-cyclic citrullinated peptide antibodies, have been negative in most patients with ICI-induced IA [4, 5, 11]. There is a series of patients with seropositive RA, where some patients had antibodies in pre-ICI treatment serum without having previous symptoms of arthritis [7]. Joint aspirations have yielded an inflammatory joint fluid with neutrophil predominance [10, 28]. There are no reports to date of novel autoantibodies associated with ICI-induced IA.

Imaging

Patients with ICI-induced IA have been evaluated with ultrasound, radiographs, and MRIs of the affected joints. Erosive disease can develop early in the course of IA in some patients [10]. Ultrasound imaging has shown synovitis with power Doppler signal, erosions, tendinitis, enthesitis, and enthesophytes [28, 32]. Interestingly, enthesophytes can occur in atypical parts, such as the proximal interphalangeal joint [28]. Musculoskeletal ultrasound or MRI may be useful in patients in whom the examination is unclear or in those with concomitant osteoarthritis to differentiate active inflammatory joint disease. Radiographs can identify comorbid osteoarthritis or can be used to monitor disease over time, but may be normal early in disease.

Differential Diagnosis

Crystalline arthritis should be considered, particularly in patients with characteristic joint involvement or risk factors for pseudogout or gout. Recurrent pseudogout with ICI therapy has been described [33].

Paraneoplastic inflammatory arthritis is a possibility, particularly in patients with symptoms predating ICI therapy or when developing around the time of their cancer diagnosis.

Metastasis to a joint is also important to consider in this population. A case of elbow metastasis in the setting of ICI-induced IA has been reported [34].

Rarely, patients may have an underlying autoimmune disease or subclinical autoimmune disease that is manifesting only after ICI therapy. In our experience, patients with skin psoriasis, who did not previously have psoriatic arthritis, may develop IA on ICI therapy.

Management

Management of IA is dictated by the severity of presentation and current clinical context. A multidisciplinary discussion with the patient, their oncologist, and any other relevant specialists for other irAEs is critical when forming a treatment plan. An overview of treatment by severity is illustrated in Fig. 4.1. Generally, mild cases are managed with non steroidal anti-inflammatory drugs (NSAIDs) or intra-articular steroids, while moderate to severe symptoms require systemic corticosteroids. Patients who do not respond to corticosteroids or who are unable to taper can be escalated to conventional synthetic disease modifying antirheumatic drugs (DMARDs) or biologic DMARDs [4–6, 11, 35].

As with all patients who are being treated with corticosteroids and other forms of immunosuppression, infection moni-

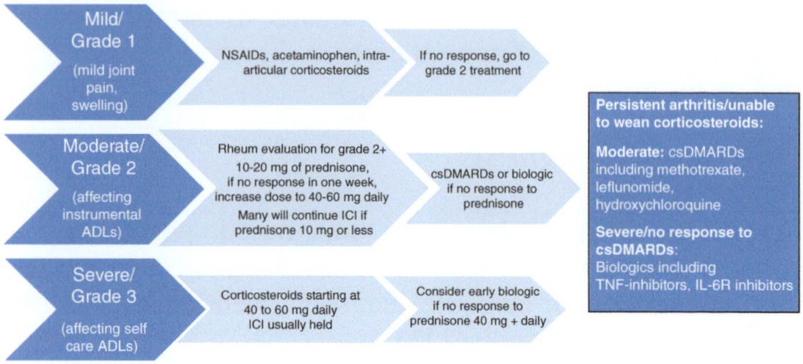

FIGURE 4.1 Treatment of ICI-induced IA based on severity and persistence

toring is important. Patients should be screened for tuberculosis and viral hepatitis if there is consideration of TNF-inhibition, methotrexate, or other DMARD use. There are emerging cases of tuberculosis infection with ICI therapy; hence, patients may be at even higher risk than those with traditional autoimmune disease treated with DMARDs [36]. Bone health is another important issue for patients who have often had more than one course of corticosteroids and may be on extended therapy. Moreover, the description of accelerated osteoporosis in some ICI-treated patients raises additional concerns for long-term steroid use [31].

Immunosuppression and Tumor Response

There is conflicting evidence as to whether immunosuppression with corticosteroids blunts tumor response to ICI therapy. Studies from melanoma and other tumors show that treatment of irAEs with immunosuppression does not seem to affect tumor response or survival [37, 38]. Baseline corticosteroids greater than the equivalent of prednisone 10 mg daily, however, have been shown to be detrimental in non-small cell lung cancer outcomes [39]. Additionally, those with hypophysitis from ipilimumab, who received high-dose steroids, had worsened survival [40]. The timing of administration and dose of corticosteroids are likely important factors. Generally, we try to use the least amount of immunosuppression for greatest functional benefit when treating patients with ICI-induced IA.

Data on non-corticosteroid immunosuppression are more limited. In a cohort of 60 patients with ICI-induced IA, there was no difference in tumor progression in those treated with conventional synthetic antirheumatic drugs (csDMARDs) or biologics as compared to those patients who did not receive these forms of immunosuppression [11]. Another study in patients with steroid-refractory irAEs and melanoma, however, showed decreased survival in those treated with TNF-inhibitors [41]. Patients with preexisting autoimmune disease on baseline immunosuppression of any type, however, had worsened tumor response to therapy in a nationwide study from France [42].

Usually, ICIs are held in patients receiving high-dose steroids or biologics. There are, however, limited reports of patients receiving biologic DMARDs for IA concurrently with ICI therapy (IA treated with IL-6R inhibition [35]). A recent case series demonstrated successful use of TNF-inhibitors concurrently with ICIs in gastrointestinal irAEs [43]. This strategy needs more investigation, but may spare prolonged steroid exposure in patients with severe ICI-induced IA.

Prognosis

Though many patients have a self-limited course, ICI-induced IA can persist after ICI cessation. In one study of 60 patients with at least one visit after ICI cessation, 53% had symptoms or arthritis at their last follow-up with rheumatology, and 20 out of 41 patients (48.8%) with follow-up 6 months after ICI cessation still had active IA [11]. Longer duration of ICI therapy and receiving combination anti-PD-1/anti-CTLA-4 therapy were independent risk factors for persistent arthritis.

Patients with ICI-induced IA need to understand not only the prognosis of their arthritis but also what the development of IA means for their cancer therapy. Indeed, in aggregate analyses of irAEs, there has been a positive association with irAE development and improved cancer prognosis [37, 44, 45]. Specifically relevant to rheumatologists, one study has shown that patients with rheumatic irAEs may have better response to ICI therapy than those without rheumatic irAEs [15].

Conclusions and Future Directions

There is growing recognition of IA as a consequence of ICI therapy. ICI-induced IA is clinically heterogeneous and may involve any joint in the body. Imaging with ultrasound and MRI has shown synovitis, effusions, erosions, tenosynovitis, enthesitis, and enthesophytes. Evaluation may fail to show traditional autoantibodies, with increased acute phase reactants in most cases. Some patients respond to steroids and NSAIDs alone, but many may require DMARDs, including biologics. Patients may have a self-limited or chronic course of ICI-induced IA. Risk factors for developing IA due to ICIs, operative mechanisms, predictors of persistence, and optimal treatment regimens require further study.

Case Study

Clinical Description A 59-year-old woman, with a history of melanoma, presented to rheumatology clinic for evaluation of new joint swelling and pain. Her melanoma was diagnosed a year and a half earlier when she had a scalp lesion biopsied. A wide local excision was performed, with one sentinel node positive for melanoma. The multidisciplinary melanoma team at our institution recommended nivolumab therapy, which she started 13 months prior to rheumatology clinic presentation. She remained on the nivolumab for 12 months with minimal issues; she experienced a mild rash but no other irAEs. She had no evidence of melanoma at the end of her nivolumab therapy. A month after stopping nivolumab, she noticed swelling in both knees. She had difficulty squatting, particularly at work where she worked with small children. Her knees progressively got worse, with symptoms of pain and stiffness worst in the morning. She was referred to rheumatology by her oncologist after 1 month of symptoms. Examination showed warm, slightly erythematous knees and large bilateral knee effusions.

Diagnostic tests Joint aspiration was performed, showing a white blood cell count of 15,380 cells/cu mm (92% neutrophils). Labs showed a negative RF, negative anti-CCP, an elevated CRP of 11 mg/dL, and an ESR of 53 mm/h.

Management She received intra-articular steroids in both knees. Four weeks later, she was back in clinic with continued knee pain and new joint involvement of her right ankle and left elbow. She was started on a prednisone at 40 mg daily, with plans to taper over the next 6–8 weeks. One month later, she returned to clinic on 20 mg of prednisone. She had persistent synovitis in the elbow, ankle, knees, and now had new involvement of two metacarpophalangeal joints. Given her lack of response to 40 mg of prednisone and active symptoms on 20 mg daily, methotrexate was initiated as a steroid-sparing agent at 15 mg weekly and titrated to 20 mg weekly. After over 3 months of methotrexate therapy, she was still unable to taper off steroids. At that time, adalimumab, a TNF-inhibitor, was started. She finally had significant improvement in joint swelling, pain, and stiffness and was able to taper and discontinue her prednisone.

Outcome She has remained on adalimumab for 6 months with good control of her arthritis and no recurrence of melanoma.

This case highlights several important points in terms of the clinical presentation and management of ICI-induced IA. First, the patient presented 13 months after the start of

ICI therapy, which is not uncommon in ICI-induced IA, but is unusual for some other irAEs, such as skin rash and colitis, which tend to occur during the first 3 months of treatment [46]. Second, she had large joints affected initially, but then had an additive course. This is a pattern we see commonly in practice as we evaluate patients longitudinally. Third, the patient received a full year of nivolumab therapy; longer duration of ICI use has been shown to be a risk factor for persistence of inflammatory arthritis [11]. Finally, the patient was unable to taper off steroids, and thus she needed treatment with other DMARDs. She had an inadequate response to methotrexate and was only able to discontinue prednisone with the initiation of a TNF-inhibitor. For patients with severe arthritis, TNF-inhibitors or IL-6R inhibitors are often required for improvement in symptoms [11, 35].

References

1. Calabrese LH, Calabrese C, Cappelli LC. Rheumatic immune-related adverse events from cancer immunotherapy. Nat Rev Rheumatol. 2018;14(10):569–79.
2. Cappelli LC, Gutierrez AK, Bingham CO, Shah AA. Rheumatic and musculoskeletal immune-related adverse events due to immune checkpoint inhibitors: a systematic review of the literature. Arthritis Care Res. 2017;69(11):1751–63.
3. Chan MM, Kefford RF, Carlino M, Clements A, Manolios N. Arthritis and tenosynovitis associated with the anti-PD1 antibody pembrolizumab in metastatic melanoma. J Immunother(Hagerstown, Md: 1997). 2015;38(1):37–9.
4. Calabrese C, Kirchner E, Kontzias K, Velcheti V, Calabrese LH. Rheumatic immune-related adverse events of checkpoint therapy for cancer: case series of a new nosological entity. RMD Open. 2017;3(1):e000412.
5. Smith MH, Bass AR. Arthritis after cancer immunotherapy: symptom duration and treatment response. Arthritis Care Res. 2019;71(3):362–6.
6. Leipe J, Christ LA, Arnoldi AP, Mille E, Berger F, Heppt M, et al. Characteristics and treatment of new-onset arthritis after checkpoint inhibitor therapy. RMD Open. 2018;4(2):e000714.

7. Belkhir R, Burel SL, Dunogeant L, Marabelle A, Hollebecque A, Besse B, et al. Rheumatoid arthritis and polymyalgia rheumatica occurring after immune checkpoint inhibitor treatment. Ann Rheum Dis. 2017;76(10):1747–50.
8. Mooradian MJ, Nasrallah M, Gainor JF, Reynolds KL, Cohen JV, Lawrence DP, et al. Musculoskeletal rheumatic complications of immune checkpoint inhibitor therapy: a single center experience. Semin Arthritis Rheum. 2019;48(6):1127–32.
9. Cappelli LC, Brahmer JR, Forde PM, Le DT, Lipson EJ, Naidoo J, et al. Clinical presentation of immune checkpoint inhibitor-induced inflammatory arthritis differs by immunotherapy regimen. Semin Arthritis Rheum. 2018;48(3):553–7.
10. Cappelli LC, Gutierrez AK, Baer AN, Albayda J, Manno RL, Haque U, et al. Inflammatory arthritis and sicca syndrome induced by nivolumab and ipilimumab. Ann Rheum Dis. 2017;76(1):43–50.
11. Braaten TJ, Brahmer JR, Forde PM, Le D, Lipson EJ, Naidoo J, et al. Immune checkpoint inhibitor-induced inflammatory arthritis persists after immunotherapy cessation. Ann Rheum Dis. 2020;79(3):332–8.
12. Lidar M, Giat E, Garelick D, Horowitz Y, Amital H, Steinberg-Silman Y, et al. Rheumatic manifestations among cancer patients treated with immune checkpoint inhibitors. Autoimmun Rev. 2018;17(3):284–9.
13. Ramos-Casals M, Maria A, Suarez-Almazor ME, Lambotte O, Fisher BA, Hernandez-Molina G, et al. Sicca/Sjogren's syndrome triggered by PD-1/PD-L1 checkpoint inhibitors. Data from the International ImmunoCancer Registry (ICIR). Clin Exp Rheumatol. 2019;37(Suppl 118(3)):114–22.
14. Kostine M, Rouxel L, Barnetche T, Veillon R, Martin F, Dutriaux C, et al. Rheumatic disorders associated with immune checkpoint inhibitors in patients with cancer-clinical aspects and relationship with tumour response: a single-centre prospective cohort study. Ann Rheum Dis. 2018;77(3):393–8.
15. Mitchell EL, Lau PKH, Khoo C, Liew D, Leung J, Liu B, et al. Rheumatic immune-related adverse events secondary to anti-programmed death-1 antibodies and preliminary analysis on the impact of corticosteroids on anti-tumour response: a case series. Eur J Cancer. (Oxford, England: 1990). 2018;105:88–102.
16. Richter MD, Crowson C, Kottschade LA, Finnes HD, Markovic SN, Thanarajasingam U. Rheumatic syndromes associated with

immune checkpoint inhibitors: a single-center cohort of sixty-one patients. Arthritis Rheumatol(Hoboken, NJ). 2019;71(3):468–75.
17. U.S. Department of Health and Human Services N, NCI. Common Terminology Criteria for Adverse Events (CTCAE) Version 5.0 2017. Available from: https://ctep.cancer.gov/protocolDevelopment/electronic_applications/docs/CTCAE_v5_Quick_Reference_8.5x11.pdf.
18. Buder-Bakhaya K, Benesova K, Schulz C, Anwar H, Dimitrakopoulou-Strauss A, Weber TF, et al. Characterization of arthralgia induced by PD-1 antibody treatment in patients with metastasized cutaneous malignancies. Cancer Immunol Immunother. 2018;67(2):175–82.
19. Khoja L, Day D, Wei-Wu Chen T, Siu LL, Hansen AR. Tumour- and class-specific patterns of immune-related adverse events of immune checkpoint inhibitors: a systematic review. Ann Oncol. 2017;28(10):2377–85.
20. Xing P, Zhang F, Wang G, Xu Y, Li C, Wang S, et al. Incidence rates of immune-related adverse events and their correlation with response in advanced solid tumours treated with NIVO or NIVO+IPI: a systematic review and meta-analysis. J Immunother Cancer. 2019;7(1):341.
21. Wang R, Chan K, Cunningham-Bussel A, Donlin L, Vitone G, Tirpack A, Benson C, Keras G, Jonsson A, Brenner M, Bass A, Rao D. Mass cytometry Immunophenotyping of synovial fluid from checkpoint inhibitor related arthritis [abstract]. Arthritis Rheumatol. 2019;71(suppl 10). https://acrabstracts.org/abstract/mass-cytometry-immunophenotyping-of-synovial-fluid-from-checkpoint-inhibitor-related-arthritis/. Accessed June 2, 2020
22. Kim S, Tayar J, Suárez-Almazor M, Lu H, Zhao Y, Liu Z, Rodriguez E, Neelapu S, Wang J, Shah A, Tannir N, Gibbons D, Garcia-Manero G, Tawbi H, Hwu P, Futreal A, Diab A, Nurieva R. Enrichment of IL-17-producing CD4+ T cells in synovial fluid from patients with arthritis after anti-CTLA-4 and anti-PD-1 combination therapy [abstract]. Arthritis Rheumatol. 2019;71(suppl 10)). https://acrabstracts.org/abstract/enrichment-of-il-17-producing-cd4-t-cells-in-synovial-fluid-from-patients-with-arthritis-after-anti-ctla-4-and-anti-pd-1-combination-therapy/. Accessed June 2, 2020
23. Thanarajasingam U, Zhu X, Zhou X, Jaquith J, Li Y, Zeng H. Inflammatory arthritis induced by immune checkpoint inhibitor therapy: a distinct clinical entity and immunologic phenotype [abstract]. Arthritis Rheumatol. 2019;71(suppl 10). https://acrabstracts.org/abstract/inflammatory-arthritis-induced-by-

immune-checkpoint-inhibitor-therapy-a-distinct-clinical-entity-and-immunologic-phenotype/. Accessed June 2, 2020
24. Cappelli LC, Dorak MT, Bettinotti MP, Bingham CO, Shah AA. Association of HLA-DRB1 shared epitope alleles and immune checkpoint inhibitor-induced inflammatory arthritis. Rheumatology (Oxford). 2019;58(3):476–80.
25. Cappelli LC, Thomas MA, Bingham CO 3rd, Shah AA, Darrah E. Immune checkpoint inhibitor-induced inflammatory arthritis as a model of autoimmune arthritis. Immunol Rev. 2020;294(1):106–23.
26. Kuswanto WF, MacFarlane LA, Gedmintas L, Mulloy A, Choueiri TK, Bermas BL. Rheumatologic symptoms in oncologic patients on PD-1 inhibitors. Semin Arthritis Rheum. 2018;47(6):907–10.
27. Murakami S, Nagano T, Nakata K, Onishi A, Umezawa K, Katsurada N, et al. Tenosynovitis induced by an immune checkpoint inhibitor: a case report and literature review. Intern Med. (Tokyo, Japan). 2019;58(19):2839–43.
28. Albayda J, Dein E, Shah AA, Bingham CO 3rd, Cappelli L. Sonographic findings in inflammatory arthritis secondary to immune checkpoint inhibition: a case series. ACR Open Rheumatol. 2019;1(5):303–7.
29. Bronstein Y, Ng CS, Hwu P, Hwu WJ. Radiologic manifestations of immune-related adverse events in patients with metastatic melanoma undergoing anti-CTLA-4 antibody therapy. AJR Am J Roentgenol. 2011;197(6):W992–w1000.
30. Feist J, Murray A, Skapenko A, Schulze-Koops H. A rare side effect of checkpoint inhibitor therapy: Nivolumab induced axial polyarthritis of the facet and costovertebral joints. Arthritis Rheumatol. (Hoboken, NJ). 2019;71(11):1823.
31. Moseley KF, Naidoo J, Bingham CO, Carducci MA, Forde PM, Gibney GT, et al. Immune-related adverse events with immune checkpoint inhibitors affecting the skeleton: a seminal case series. J Immunother Cancer. 2018;6(1):104.
32. Inamo J, Kaneko Y, Takeuchi T. Inflammatory tenosynovitis and enthesitis induced by immune checkpoint inhibitor treatment. Clin Rheumatol. 2018;37(4):1107–10.
33. Kim ST, Bittar M, Kim HJ, Neelapu SS, Zurita AJ, Nurieva R, et al. Recurrent pseudogout after therapy with immune checkpoint inhibitors: a case report with immunoprofiling of synovial fluid at each flare. J Immunother Cancer. 2019;7(1):126.
34. Albayda J, Bingham CO 3rd, Shah AA, Kelly RJ, Cappelli L. Metastatic joint involvement or inflammatory arthritis? A

conundrum with immune checkpoint inhibitor-related adverse events. Rheumatology (Oxford). 2018;57(4):760–2.
35. Kim ST, Tayar J, Trinh VA, Suarez-Almazor M, Garcia S, Hwu P, et al. Successful treatment of arthritis induced by checkpoint inhibitors with tocilizumab: a case series. Ann Rheum Dis. 2017;76(12):2061–4.
36. Picchi H, Mateus C, Chouaid C, Besse B, Marabelle A, Michot JM, et al. Infectious complications associated with the use of immune checkpoint inhibitors in oncology: reactivation of tuberculosis after anti PD-1 treatment. Clin Microbiol Infect. 2018;24(3):216–8.
37. Judd J, Zibelman M, Handorf E, O'Neill J, Ramamurthy C, Bentota S, et al. Immune-related adverse events as a biomarker in non-melanoma patients treated with programmed cell death 1 inhibitors. Oncologist. 2017;22(10):1232–7.
38. Horvat TZ, Adel NG, Dang TO, Momtaz P, Postow MA, Callahan MK, et al. Immune-related adverse events, need for systemic immunosuppression, and effects on survival and time to treatment failure in patients with melanoma treated with Ipilimumab at Memorial Sloan Kettering Cancer Center. J Clin Oncol Off J Am Soc Clin Oncol. 2015;33(28):3193–8.
39. Arbour KC, Mezquita L, Long N, Rizvi H, Auclin E, Ni A, et al. Impact of baseline steroids on efficacy of programmed cell Death-1 and programmed death-ligand 1 blockade in patients with non-small-cell lung cancer. J Clin Oncol Off J Am Soc Clin Oncol. 2018;36(28):2872–8.
40. Faje AT, Lawrence D, Flaherty K, Freedman C, Fadden R, Rubin K, et al. High-dose glucocorticoids for the treatment of ipilimumab-induced hypophysitis is associated with reduced survival in patients with melanoma. Cancer. 2018;124(18):3706–14.
41. Verheijden RJ, May AM, Blank CU, Aarts MJB, van den Berkmortel FWPJ, van den Eertwegh AJM, de Groot JWB, Boers-Sonderen MJ, van der Hoeven JJM, Hospers GA, Piersma D, van Rijn RS, Ten Tije AJ, van der Veldt AAM, Vreugdenhil G, van Zeijl MCT, Wouters MWJM, Haanen JBAG, Kapiteijn E, Suijkerbuijk KPM. Association of anti-TNF with decreased survival in steroid refractory ipilimumab and anti-PD1-treated patients in the Dutch Melanoma Treatment Registry. Clin Cancer Res. 2020;26(9):2268–74.
42. Tison A, Quere G, Misery L, Funck-Brentano E, Danlos FX, Routier E, et al. Safety and efficacy of immune checkpoint inhibitors in patients with cancer and preexisting autoim-

mune disease: a Nationwide, multicenter cohort study. Arthritis Rheumatol(Hoboken, NJ). 2019;71(12):2100–11.
43. Badran YR, Cohen JV, Brastianos PK, Parikh AR, Hong TS, Dougan M. Concurrent therapy with immune checkpoint inhibitors and TNFalpha blockade in patients with gastrointestinal immune-related adverse events. J Immunother Cancer. 2019;7(1):226.
44. Haratani K, Hayashi H, Chiba Y, Kudo K, Yonesaka K, Kato R, et al. Association of immune-related adverse events with nivolumab efficacy in non-small-cell lung cancer. JAMA Oncol. 2018;4(3):374–8.
45. Freeman-Keller M, Kim Y, Cronin H, Richards A, Gibney G, Weber JS. Nivolumab in resected and Unresectable metastatic melanoma: characteristics of immune-related adverse events and association with outcomes. Clin Cancer Res. 2016;22(4):886–94.
46. Weber JS, Kahler KC, Hauschild A. Management of immune-related adverse events and kinetics of response with ipilimumab. J Clin Oncol Off J Am Soc Clin Oncol. 2012;30(21):2691–7.

Chapter 5
Immune-Related Adverse Events with Immune Checkpoint Inhibitors: Polymyalgia Rheumatica

Cassandra Calabrese

Introduction

Immune checkpoint inhibitor (ICI) therapy has led to a paradigm shift in the field of oncology, producing significant survival benefits in patients with an ever-growing list of malignancies. Their use, however, is attended by a spectrum of immune-related adverse events (irAEs), both general and rheumatic, which threaten their overall effectiveness. A critical and presently unanswered question is what proportion of rheumatic irAEs represents the occurrence of classic rheumatic diseases or, alternatively, represents new clinical variants with potentially different pathogenesis, clinical course, and treatment responsiveness. A syndrome resembling polymyalgia rheumatica (PMR) has been described in the setting of ICI; however, little is known about this entity.

C. Calabrese (✉)
Department of Rheumatologic and Immunologic Diseases, Cleveland Clinic Foundation, Cleveland, OH, USA
e-mail: calabrc@ccf.org

M. E. Suarez-Almazor, L. H. Calabrese (eds.), *Rheumatic Diseases and Syndromes Induced by Cancer Immunotherapy*, https://doi.org/10.1007/978-3-030-56824-5_5

Epidemiology

While PMR has become one of the most commonly reported inflammatory rheumatic irAEs, despite clinical descriptions, its incidence remains unknown [1–3]. A pharmacovigilance study using VigiBase, the World Health Organization's global database of individual case safety reports, demonstrated a fivefold increased risk for developing PMR with ICI therapy versus cancer patients not receiving immunotherapy [4]. Similar to traditional PMR, ICI-related PMR occurs in older adults [5]. It is likely that most rheumatic irAEs are underreported, and there are many reasons for this. First, the majority of clinical trials report irAEs that are Common Terminology Criteria for Adverse Events grade 3 (e.g., severe) or higher, and PMR does not have to require hospitalization to be severely debilitating to the patient. Also, there is no standard coding for rheumatic symptoms. Furthermore, there is no diagnostic laboratory test for PMR, leaving clinicians to rely on the presence of a suggestive clinical picture with elevated inflammatory markers and a glucocorticoid response to establish the diagnosis.

Pathogenesis

The pathogenesis of rheumatic irAEs, including PMR, remains largely speculative as most irAE studies have been clinical in nature. Several candidate mechanisms have been proposed for the immunopathogenesis of irAEs (discussed in Chap. 3), and it is felt that generalized immune activation from immune checkpoint neutralization may play a role in ICI-related PMR; however, further investigations in this area are needed [6].

Clinical Manifestations

The clinical presentation of ICI-related PMR is very similar to that of de novo PMR, including prominent morning stiffness and pain and stiffness involving the shoulder and hip girdle. The American College of Rheumatology (ACR) and European League Against Rheumatism (EULAR) created a provisional set of classification criteria for PMR [7] (Table 5.1), which Calabrese C et al. used to determine how many cases of ICI-related PMR provided adequate information to apply these criteria, through a systemic literature review [5]. Out of 49 cases, 37 (75%) had sufficient data to reliably apply the EULAR/ACR criteria, and of these, 28 (75%) fulfilled complete criteria for PMR. A number of cases demonstrated clinical features unusual for PMR, including the presence of other joint involvement (most

Table 5.1 Provisional classification criteria for PMR scoring algorithm

Feature	Points without ultrasound (0–6)	Points with ultrasound (0–8)
Morning stiffness lasting >45 min	2	2
Hip pain or limited range of motion	1	1
Absence of RF or ACPA	2	2
Absence of other joint involvement	1	1
≥ 1 shoulder with subdeltoid bursitis and/or biceps tenosynovitis and/or glenohumeral synovitis and ≥ 1 hip with synovitis and/or trochanteric bursitis	n/a	1
Both shoulders with subdeltoid bursitis, biceps tenosynovitis, or glenohumeral synovitis	n/a	1

Required to apply algorithm: age ≥ 50 years, bilateral shoulder aching, and abnormal CRP and/or ESR

A score ≥ 4 is categorized as PMR without ultrasound, and a score of ≥5 is categorized as PMR if ultrasound findings are included commonly knees, followed by hands and elbows), normal inflammatory markers in six cases, and a requirement for initial glucocorticoid dose of more than 20 mg in 37%.

Rarely, giant cell arteritis (GCA) has been described to occur with ICI-related PMR as an irAE [8, 9], as well as reports of isolated GCA [10]. Two cases were attributed to ipilimumab monotherapy [8] and another to nivolumab[9]. Interestingly, the PD-1/PD-L1 axis has been implicated in the development of GCA in the general population [11]. All of these cases presented with classic GCA features including jaw claudication, vision loss, temporal headaches, and scalp tenderness.

Remitting seronegative synovitis with pitting edema (RS3PE), a syndrome characterized by tenosynovitis of extensor tendons of the wrist and pitting edema of the dorsum of the hands and less commonly the feet, is considered by many to be part of the PMR spectrum as well as a possible paraneoplastic phenomenon [12]. Several cases of RS3PE have been reported in the setting of ICI, all secondary to anti-PD-1/L1 therapy [13–15]. All of these cases of RS3PE were felt to be secondary to immunotherapy, rather than a paraneoplastic process, and all cases responded to low-dose glucocorticoids.

Diagnosis

The diagnostic evaluation for ICI-related PMR mirrors that for de novo PMR. The American Society of Clinical Oncology (ASCO) clinical practice guidelines for irAEs include a section on recommended diagnostic workup for "polymyalgia-like syndrome" [16]. In all the irAE guidelines, the diagnosis and management recommendations are based on Common Terminology Criteria for Adverse Events (CTCAE) grading system [17], which ranges from grade 1 through grade 5 (grade 1, mild; grade 2, moderate; grade 3, severe; grade 4, life-threatening; grade 5, death). The majority of clinical trials report irAE events that are grade 3 or higher, meaning they require hospitalization. For presumed PMR of any grade, the diagnostic workup should include the following: a completed rheumatologic history, an examination of all joints and skin, checking for symptoms of giant cell arteritis, and laboratory evaluation including antinuclear antigen, rheumatoid factor, anti-CCP, erythrocyte sedimentation rate (ESR), and C-reactive protein (CRP) [16]. If the PMR is grade 2 or higher, early referral to a rheumatologist is recommended. Monitoring of ESR and CRP should be done for all patients.

While there are no specific guidelines for advanced imaging of patients with suspected ICI-related PMR, in case reports where imaging has been utilized, classic findings were seen on shoulder and/or hip ultrasound, including subdeltoid bursitis and biceps tenosynovitis [5]. There are case reports describing classic temporal artery histopathology for giant cell arteritis (active arteritis, intimal proliferation, disruption of the internal elastic lamina) in patients with concomitant PMR and GCA who underwent temporal artery biopsy [8, 9].

Differential Diagnosis

The differential diagnosis includes ICI-related inflammatory arthritis and myositis, as well as mechanical pain such as rotator cuff tear. It should be noted that inflammatory arthritis has been described to occur in patients with PMR as an overlap-type syndrome [5].

Management

There are no controlled trials for any agent to treat irAEs, including ICI-related PMR, and at present current guidelines are based largely on consensus opinion. Several sets of guidelines have been published which specially address the management of inflammatory arthritis [16, 18] and myositis and polymyalgia rheumatica-like syndrome [16]. The ASCO guidelines have specific recommendations for the manage-

Table 5.2 Treatment recommendations for ICI-related PMR, based on grade of toxicity

Grade 1	Grade 2	Grade 3–4
Continue ICI Initiate treatment with acetaminophen and/or NSAIDs (if not contraindication)	May hold ICI and resume upon symptom control and prednisone <10 mg/d Should initiate prednisone 20 mg/d or equivalent. If symptoms improve, start to taper dose after 3–4 weeks If no improvement, or need for higher-dose GC after 4 weeks, escalate to grade 3 Referral to rheumatology	Hold ICI and may resume, in consultation with rheumatology, if recovery to ≤ grade 1[a] Referral to rheumatology Initiate prednisone 20 mg/d or equivalent. If no improvement or need for prolonged courses of higher dose GC, consider GC-sparing agent (MTX, tocilizumab)[b]

Adapted from ASCO guidelines

GC glucocorticoid, *MTX* methotrexate, *ICI* immune checkpoint inhibitors

[a]Cases of PMR recurrence upon rechallenge with ICI have been reported

[b]IL-6 inhibition has rarely been associated with intestinal perforation and should not be used in patients with ICI-related colitis or gastrointestinal metastases

ment of PMR (Table 5.2). The majority of patients respond well to prednisone 20 mg equivalent daily or less; however, it should be noted that some patients require higher-than-expected doses of glucocorticoids, and some may require a steroid-sparing agent, such as tocilizumab [5, 19].

Conclusions and Future Directions

A burning question in the field of rheumatic irAEs is whether diseases which closely resemble de novo autoimmune disease states are actually examples of the classical forms of such disorders or new entities, and such is the case with PMR secondary to ICI therapy. Based on case reports and case series thus far, it appears that a meaningful proportion of ICI-related PMR cases fall outside of what appears to be reasonable in terms of their overall clinical picture suggesting that at least some may represent a new clinical entity. Moving forward, there is an urgency for prospective registry-based studies with uniform assessment and reporting of data.

Case Study

Clinical Description A 60-year-old female with stage IV metastatic melanoma was started on pembrolizumab. She had no other significant past medical history, including no history of preexisting musculoskeletal issues. Within 10 h of her first pembrolizumab infusion, she awoke at 1 am with acute-onset severe stiffness and pain, most prominently involving her bilateral hip girdles. She required assistance to get out of bed. Symptoms improved somewhat with acetaminophen, and she received a second dose of pembrolizumab 200 mg 3 weeks later with subsequent worsening of her symptoms, with pain and stiffness spreading to involve the shoulders, neck, thighs, buttocks, and knees. She was seen by her oncologist, who noted that her knees appeared swollen. She had great difficulty rising from a seated position and with walking due to pain. She started using a cane. She noted profound stiffness and symptoms were exacerbated after periods of inactivity. She denied headaches, vision changes, or jaw pain. Subsequent doses of pembrolizumab were held, and she was referred to rheumatology clinic for evaluation.

Diagnostic Tests Laboratory evaluation revealed an erythrocyte sedimentation rate (ESR) of 118 mm/h, C-reactive protein (CRP) of 9.2 mg/dL, rheumatoid factor of 45 IU/mL, negative anti-citrullinated peptide protein, and normal creatine kinase. MRI of the right shoulder revealed evidence of rotator cuff tendinosis, with severe supraspinatus and subacromial subdeltoid bursitis.

Management Eight weeks after symptom onset, she was started on prednisone 1 mg/kg, and within hours she felt nearly 100% better. She quickly became symptom-free, no longer needing a cane to walk. One week after starting prednisone, repeat ESR was 27 mm/h and CRP 0.7 mg/dL. Prednisone dose was tapered by 10 mg every 3 days to 20 mg daily. She continued to feel well, and prednisone dose was further tapered by 2.5 mg every 2 weeks and was able to successfully reach a dose of 2.5 mg daily.

Outcome Pembrolizumab was held indefinitely due to severe presentation of what was felt to be PMR secondary to immunotherapy, with atypical features including explosive acute onset, involvement of the knee joints, positive rheumatoid factor, and need for higher initial dose of prednisone than typical PMR cases. Unfortunately, 6 months after her last dose of pembrolizumab, she was found to have new brain metastases, for which she received gamma knife radiation; however, central nervous system involvement by tumor progressed, and the patient died.

References

1. Cappelli LC, Gutierrez AK, Bingham CO 3rd, Shah AA. Rheumatic and musculoskeletal immune-related adverse events due to immune checkpoint inhibitors: a systematic review of the literature. Arthritis Care Res. (Hoboken) 2017;69(11):1751–1763. https://doi.org/10.1002/acr.23177.
2. Suarez-Almazor ME, Kim ST, Abdel-Wahab N, Diab A. Review: immune-related adverse events with use of checkpoint inhibitors for immunotherapy of Cancer. Arthritis Rheumatol. 2017;69(4):687–99. https://doi.org/10.1002/art.40043.

3. Calabrese C, Kirchner E, Kontzias K, Velcheti V, Calabrese LH. Rheumatic immune-related adverse events of checkpoint therapy for cancer: case series of a new nosological entity. RMD Open. 2017;3(1):e000412. https://doi.org/10.1136/rmdopen-2016-000412.
4. Salem JE, Manouchehri A, Moey M, et al. Cardiovascular toxicities associated with immune checkpoint inhibitors: an observational, retrospective, pharmacovigilance study. Lancet Oncol. 2018;19(12):1579–89. https://doi.org/10.1016/S1470-2045(18)30608-9.
5. Calabrese C, Cappelli LC, Kostine M, Kirchner E, Braaten T, Calabrese L. Polymyalgia rheumatica-like syndrome from checkpoint inhibitor therapy: case series and systematic review of the literature. RMD Open. 2019;5(1) https://doi.org/10.1136/rmdopen-2019-000906.
6. Calabrese LH, Calabrese C, Cappelli LC. Rheumatic immune-related adverse events from cancer immunotherapy. Nat Rev Rheumatol. 2018;14(10):569–79. https://doi.org/10.1038/s41584-018-0074-9.
7. Dasgupta B, Cimmino MA, Maradit-Kremers H, et al. 2012 provisional classification criteria for polymyalgia rheumatica: a European League Against Rheumatism/American College of Rheumatology collaborative initiative. Ann Rheum Dis. 2012;71(4):484–92. https://doi.org/10.1136/annrheumdis-2011-200329.
8. Goldstein BL, Gedmintas L, Todd DJ. Drug-associated polymyalgia Rheumatica/Giant cell arteritis occurring in two patients after treatment with Ipilimumab, an antagonist of CTLA-4. Arthritis Rheumatol. 2014;66(3):768–9. https://doi.org/10.1002/art.38282.
9. Betrains A, Blockmans DE. Immune checkpoint inhibitor-associated polymyalgia Rheumatica/Giant cell arteritis occurring in a patient after treatment with Nivolumab. J Clin Rheumatol. 2019;1 https://doi.org/10.1097/RHU.0000000000001012.
10. Micaily I, Chernoff M. An unknown reaction to pembrolizumab: giant cell arteritis. Ann Oncol Off J Eur Soc Med Oncol. 2017;28(10):2621–2. https://doi.org/10.1093/annonc/mdx306.
11. Watanabe R, Zhang H, Berry G, Goronzy JJ, Weyand CM. Immune checkpoint dysfunction in large and medium vessel vasculitis. Am J Physiol Circ Physiol. 2017;312(5):H1052–9. https://doi.org/10.1152/ajpheart.00024.2017.
12. Cantini F, Salvarani C, Olivieri I, et al. Remitting seronegative symmetrical synovitis with pitting oedema (RS3PE) syn-

drome: a prospective follow up and magnetic resonance imaging study. Ann Rheum Dis. 1999;58(4):230–6. https://doi.org/10.1136/ard.58.4.230.
13. Wada N, Uchi H, Furue M. Case of remitting seronegative symmetrical synovitis with pitting edema (RS3PE) syndrome induced by nivolumab in a patient with advanced malignant melanoma. J Dermatol. 2017;44(8):e196–7. https://doi.org/10.1111/1346-8138.13840.
14. Ngo L, Miller E, Valen P, Gertner E. Nivolumab induced remitting seronegative symmetrical synovitis with pitting edema in a patient with melanoma: a case report. J Med Case Rep. 2018;12(1):48. https://doi.org/10.1186/s13256-018-1579-1.
15. Yamamoto S, Fujita S, Mukai T. Paraneoplastic remitting seronegative symmetrical synovitis with pitting edema syndrome should be treated with low-dose prednisolone during Pembrolizumab therapy. Intern Med. 2019:3902–19. https://doi.org/10.2169/internalmedicine.3902-19.
16. Brahmer JR, Lacchetti C, Schneider BJ, et al. Management of immune-related adverse events in patients treated with immune checkpoint inhibitor therapy: American Society of Clinical Oncology clinical practice guideline. J Clin Oncol. 2018;4. https://doi.org/10.1200/JCO.2017.77.6385.
17. Common Terminology Criteria for Adverse Events (CTCAE) v4.0. https://www.acrin.org/Portals/0/Administration/Regulatory/CTCAE_4.02_2009-09-15_QuickReference_5x7.pdf. Accessed March 6, 2018.
18. Puzanov I, Diab A, Abdallah K, et al. Managing toxicities associated with immune checkpoint inhibitors: consensus recommendations from the Society for Immunotherapy of Cancer (SITC) toxicity management working group. J Immunother Cancer. 2017;5(1):1–28. https://doi.org/10.1186/s40425-017-0300-z.
19. Leipe J, Mariette X. Management of rheumatic complications of ICI therapy: a rheumatology viewpoint. Rheumatology (Oxford). 2019;58(7):vii49–58. https://doi.org/10.1093/rheumatology/kez360. Ro te volori ut ut mossendam fugiamusciur autem.

Chapter 6
Myositis

Andrew L. Mammen

Introduction

Myositis is a rare, but potentially serious, side effect of immune checkpoint inhibitors (ICIs). Although ICI-induced myositis shares certain features of spontaneously occurring myositis (e.g., polymyositis), it also has some unusual clinical features that may cause diagnostic confusion. In addition, some patients with myositis as an immune-related adverse event (irAE) also have myasthenia gravis and/or myocarditis. Fortunately, once correctly diagnosed, many of these patients respond well to immunosuppressive therapy. In this chapter, we will review what is known about the epidemiology of ICI-induced myositis, describe the clinical features and diagnosis of these patients, and discuss therapeutic strategies for treating patients with this irAE.

A. L. Mammen (✉)
Laboratory of Muscle Stem Cells and Gene Expression, National Institute of Arthritis and Musculoskeletal and Skin Diseases, National Institutes of Health, Bethesda, MD, USA
e-mail: andrew.mammen@nih.gov

M. E. Suarez-Almazor, L. H. Calabrese (eds.), *Rheumatic Diseases and Syndromes Induced by Cancer Immunotherapy*,
https://doi.org/10.1007/978-3-030-56824-5_6

Epidemiology

Myositis is a relatively rare irAE. For example, one retrospective analysis of 33 checkpoint inhibitor clinical trials revealed that less than 1% of patients developed weakness as a result of treatment [1]. A subsequent study utilizing VigiBase, the World Health Organization database of individual safety case reports, showed that among the 15,334 ICI-associated adverse events reported in the year 2017, 87 (0.57%) were myositis [2]. A more recent study using the same database provided similar results: among 54,085 ICI-related adverse drug reactions, myositis occurred in just 345 (0.6%) [3]. Despite the low probability of myositis as an irAE, with the increased use of ICIs for various malignancies, the absolute number of myositis cases has increased in recent years; while there were only 20 cases between 2008 and 2015, 47 cases were reported in 2016, 90 cases were documented in 2017, and 184 cases were diagnosed in 2018 [3].

Certain ICI classes are more strongly associated with the development of myositis than others. For example, using case/non-case analyses, one large study found that myositis was more likely to occur in patients receiving anti-PD-1/PD-L1 monotherapy compared with anti-CTLA-4 monotherapy (OR = 2.4, 95% CI: 1.6 to 3.5) [3]. Furthermore, as with other types of irAEs, myositis was more likely to occur in patients receiving ICI combination therapy than in those receiving ICI monotherapy (OR = 1.8, 95% CI: 1.3 to 2.4). Although lung and skin cancers are most commonly associated with myositis as an ICI-related adverse event [3], the frequent use of these medications for these indications may account for this observation. Interestingly, although the PD-L1 inhibitor avelumab is associated with a 0.3% risk of myositis in patients with other solid tumors [4], 4 out of 8 thymoma patients treated with this drug developed myositis [5]. This high prevalence of myositis may be related to the well-established propensity for autoimmunity, including myositis, in patients with thymoma.

Importantly, patients with ICI-associated myositis have an increased risk of presenting with co-existing myasthenia gravis and/or myocarditis. Overall, among 345 patients reported to have myositis in VigiBase, 41 (11.9%) had myasthenia gravis, and 39 (11.3%) had myocarditis [3]. Conversely, another large study demonstrated that among 177 patients with ICI-associated myasthenia gravis, 29 (16.4%) had myositis, 12 (6.8%) had myocarditis, and 8 (4.5%) had both [6].

Pathogenesis

Analyses of muscle biopsies from patients with ICI-associated myositis provide some clues about the pathogenesis of this entity. For example, numerous reports have documented that muscle biopsies from these patients are infiltrated by CD8+ and CD4+ T cells [7–14]. Furthermore, two case reports showed that T cell populations infiltrating skeletal muscle had undergone clonal expansion [7, 8]. Importantly, some of these infiltrating T cells are PD-1-positive [11, 13], and one study showed that muscle cells overexpress PD-L1 on their sarcolemmal surface [11]. Taken together, these findings suggest that ICI-associated myositis is a T cell-driven process that occurs when autoreactive lymphocytes are released from inhibition and attack the skeletal muscle.

It remains unclear why a few patients develop myositis when treated with ICIs, while most do not. However, two small case series provide evidence that patients with pre-existing autoimmunity may be at increased risk. For example, several Japanese patients who developed myositis and myasthenia gravis following treatment with nivolumab had pre-existing anti-acetylcholine receptor autoantibodies without pre-existing CK elevations or weakness [14]. Similarly, among the thymoma patients treated with avelumab (described above), the presence of anti-acetylcholine receptor and other thymoma-associated autoantibodies (e.g., anti-striational autoantibodies) were present in all of those who developed myositis and in none of those who did not [5]. In addition, among thymoma patients treated with avelumab, only those who developed myositis had pre-existing B-cell lymphopenia. Future studies will be required to determine whether pre-existing autoantibodies and/or immune cell subset dysregulation can predict which non-thymic tumor patients are at increased risk for myositis following ICI administration.

Clinical Manifestations

Patients with pure ICI-associated myositis (i.e., without co-existing myasthenia gravis or myocarditis) typically present after one or two rounds of ICI infusions with myalgias, followed by symmetric proximal muscle weakness, ptosis, and/or oculomotor weakness with diplopia [9, 13]. Distal weakness, dysphonia, dyspnea, and fatiguability are less common, and both Raynaud phenomenon and cutaneous manifestations are absent [9, 13].

Diagnosis

Laboratory studies reveal elevated muscle enzymes (ranging from mild elevations to >10,000 IU/L) and negative testing for anti-acetylcholine receptor, anti-muscle-specific tyrosine kinase, and myositis-specific autoantibodies. Electrophysiologic studies show evidence of an irritable myopathy. However, repetitive nerve stimulation studies and single-fiber electromyography are normal, even in those with typical myasthenic features, such as ptosis and diplopia. Muscle biopsies reveal T cell infiltrates (as discussed above) as well as abundant CD68+ macrophages [8, 9, 13]. Although most patient biopsies have very few infiltrating CD20+ B cells [8, 9, 13], occasional patients may have more prominent collections of these cells [11]. In addition, muscle cells in patients with ICI-associated myositis have increased sarcolemmal expression of MHC I class antigens [9–11, 13].

Patients with myositis and co-existing myasthenia gravis may present with more significant diaphragmatic weakness. For example, in one case series describing the clinical manifestations of such patients, 5 out of 10 required ventilatory support [11]. Prominent neck extensor weakness (i.e., dropped head), ocular symptoms, and dysphagia may also be more common in patients with both myositis and myasthenia gravis.

In unfortunate patients with both myositis and myocarditis, the electrocardiogram may reveal intraventricular conduction delay followed by complete heart block [8], and echocardiograms may show a reduction of the ejection fraction. Laboratory studies may be notable for elevated troponin T levels (as seen in patients with various types of skeletal myopathy) as well as elevated troponin I levels (which are not seen in patients with myositis alone) [15]. Cardiac muscle biopsies show infiltration of the myocardium with CD8+ T cells more than CD4+ T cells [8, 14].

Differential Diagnosis

There is a broad differential diagnosis for patients who become weak after ICI therapy. For example, checkpoint inhibitor therapy has been associated with a variety of neurological and neuromuscular irAEs that includes non-infectious encephalitis and/or myelitis, cerebral artery vasculitis, Guillain-Barre syndrome, and chronic inflammatory demyelinating polyneuropathy [6]. While a muscle biopsy showing lymphocytic infiltrates is the gold standard for establishing a diagnosis of ICI-associated myositis, the presence of elevated serum muscle enzyme levels and a myopathic EMG may be sufficient to establish the presence of myositis in many patients. Electrophysiologic studies are also essential for excluding a neuropathic process or neuromuscular junction defect. Muscle imaging (e.g., magnetic resonance imaging) may also be helpful in showing the presence of an inflammatory process. In selected patients, brain and/or spinal imaging may be advisable to rule out a central process.

Management

Since authoritative guidelines have yet to be established for the treatment of ICI-associated myositis, recommendations regarding management are based on published reports [7, 9–11, 13, 14] as well as the author's experience. In all cases, ICI treatment should be discontinued and oral corticosteroid therapy should be initiated at a dose of 0.5–2 mg/kg/day, depending on the severity of weakness. In patients with more severe disease or who are not responsive to oral steroids, intravenous methylprednisolone, intravenous immunoglobulin, methotrexate, plasma exchange, cyclosporine, and tacrolimus have all been used with variable success. In patients with co-existing myasthenia gravis, pyridostigmine, intravenous immunoglobulin, and/or plasma exchange are most often utilized.

There is limited information about response to treatment in patients with ICI-associated myositis without co-existing myasthenia gravis. In one study of 10 such patients, 4 of whom also had myocarditis, all patients improved with treatment and CK levels normalized in a median of 44 days after diagnosis (range 6–96 days) [13]. Despite the good outcomes reported in this case series, the largest study utilizing VigiBase found that the overall fatality rate for patients with ICI-related myositis is 22.3% [3]. Although co-existing myasthenia gravis only modestly increases the fatality rate to 26.8%, patients with both ICI-associated myositis and myocarditis have a fatality rate of 51.3% [3].

In some cases, the development of irAEs may also be associated with a potent anti-tumor response. For example, among 8 thymoma patients treated with avelumab, 4 developed myositis that resolved with immunosuppressive therapy; each of these also had a clinical response [16]. This raises the question of whether it may be advisable to rechallenge such patients with ICIs. A recent report described two patients, one with Merkel cell carcinoma and another with melanoma, who developed myositis after treatment with avelumab and ipilimumab, respectively [17]. Following treatment with steroids, each patient recovered and was retreated with ICIs without recurrence of myositis.

Conclusions and Future Directions

Myositis has now emerged as a rare, but important, irAE. While many patients with checkpoint inhibitor-triggered myositis do not have other irAEs, a significant number develop co-existing myasthenia gravis and/or myocarditis. Whether occurring alone or along with other irAEs, myositis should be treated with corticosteroids along with other immunosuppressive treatments as needed. Future studies will be required to predict which patients are at increased risk for developing myositis when treated with ICIs, to determine optimal prevention and treatment strategies, and to establish whether ICI rechallenge is safe in patients who develop myositis as an irAE.

Case Study

A 61-year-old man with metastatic melanoma was treated with ipilimumab along with novilumab. Eighteen days later, the patient developed myalgias, proximal muscle weakness, ptosis, and dysphagia. Laboratory testing revealed a serum CK level of ~14,000 IU/L, elevated troponin T levels, normal serum troponin I levels, and absent anti-acetylcholine receptor autoantibodies. An electrocardiogram was normal. Electromyography showed spontaneous fibrillation potentials and myopathic motor units consistent with an inflammatory myopathy. Repetitive nerve stimulation testing showed no evidence of a neuromuscular junction defect. A left deltoid muscle biopsy was performed and demonstrated numerous CD8+ T cells infiltrating the endoymysium and upregulation of class I MHC on the surface of myofibers.

The patient was diagnosed with ICI-associated myositis without evidence for co-existing myocarditis or myasthenia gravis. He was treated with intravenous methylprednisolone 1 g/day for 3 days and was subsequently started on oral prednisone at a dose of 1 mg/kg/day. The patient's strength began to improve within 1 week of treatment and the CK normalized over the course of an additional 3 weeks. The oral prednisone was tapered and then withdrawn over 8 weeks, during which time there was no recurrence of weakness or elevated CK levels.

Funding This work was supported by the Intramural Research Program of the National Institute of Arthritis and Musculoskeletal and Skin Diseases of the National Institutes of Health.

References

1. Cappelli LC, Gutierrez AK, Bingham CO 3rd, Shah AA. Rheumatic and musculoskeletal immune-related adverse events due to immune checkpoint inhibitors: a systematic review of the literature. Arthritis Care Res. (Hoboken). 2017;69:1751–63.
2. Anquetil C, Salem JE, Lebrun-Vignes B, et al. Immune checkpoint inhibitor-associated myositis. Circulation. 2018;138:743–5.
3. Nguyen T, Maria ATJ, Ladhari C, et al. Rheumatic disorders associated with immune checkpoint inhibitors: what about myositis? An analysis of the WHO's adverse drug reactions database. Ann Rheum Dis. 2020; (published online ahead of print), [2020 Feb 17]; https://doi.org/10.1136/annrheumdis-2020-217018.
4. Gulley JL, Rajan A, Spigel DR, et al. Avelumab for patients with previously treated metastatic or recurrent non-small-cell lung cancer (JAVELIN Solid Tumor): dose-expansion cohort of a multicentre, open-label, phase 1b trial. Lancet Oncol. 2017;18:599–610.
5. Mammen AL, Rajan A, Pak K, et al. Pre-existing antiacetylcholine receptor autoantibodies and B cell lymphopaenia are associated with the development of myositis in patients with thymoma treated with avelumab, an immune checkpoint inhibitor targeting programmed death-ligand 1. Ann Rheum Dis. 2019;78:150–2.
6. Johnson DB, Manouchehri A, Haugh AM, et al. Neurologic toxicity associated with immune checkpoint inhibitors: a pharmacovigilance study. J Immunother Cancer. 2019;7:134.

7. Kimura T, Fukushima S, Miyashita A, et al. Myasthenic crisis and polymyositis induced by one dose of nivolumab. Cancer Sci. 2016;107:1055–8.
8. Johnson DB, Balko JM, Compton ML, et al. Fulminant myocarditis with combination immune checkpoint blockade. N Engl J Med. 2016;375:1749–55.
9. Matas-Garcia A, Milisenda JC, Selva-O'Callaghan A, et al. Emerging PD-1 and PD-1L inhibitors-associated myopathy with a characteristic histopathological pattern. Autoimmun Rev. 2020;19:102455.
10. Valenti-Azcarate R, Esparragosa Vazquez I, Toledano Illan C, Idoate Gastearena MA, Gallego Perez-Larraya J. Nivolumab and Ipilimumab-induced myositis and myocarditis mimicking a myasthenia gravis presentation. Neuromuscul Disord. 2020;30:67–9.
11. Uchio N, Taira K, Ikenaga C, et al. Inflammatory myopathy with myasthenia gravis: Thymoma association and polymyositis pathology. Neurol Neuroimmunol Neuroinflamm. 2019;6:e535.
12. Moreira A, Loquai C, Pfohler C, et al. Myositis and neuromuscular side-effects induced by immune checkpoint inhibitors. Eur J Cancer. 2019;106:12–23.
13. Touat M, Maisonobe T, Knauss S, et al. Immune checkpoint inhibitor-related myositis and myocarditis in patients with cancer. Neurology. 2018;91:e985–e94.
14. Suzuki S, Ishikawa N, Konoeda F, et al. Nivolumab-related myasthenia gravis with myositis and myocarditis in Japan. Neurology. 2017;89:1127–34.
15. Schmid J, Liesinger L, Birner-Gruenberger R, et al. Elevated cardiac troponin T in patients with skeletal myopathies. J Am Coll Cardiol. 2018;71:1540–9.
16. Rajan A, Heery CR, Thomas A, et al. Efficacy and tolerability of anti-programmed death-ligand 1 (PD-L1) antibody (Avelumab) treatment in advanced thymoma. J Immunother Cancer. 2019;7:269.
17. Delyon J, Brunet-Possenti F, Leonard-Louis S, et al. Immune checkpoint inhibitor rechallenge in patients with immune-related myositis. Ann Rheum Dis. 2019;78:e129.

Chapter 7
Sicca Syndromes

Blake M. Warner and Alan N. Baer

Introduction

Biologic agents that block immune checkpoints have shown success in treating certain cancer subtypes [1]. These immune checkpoint inhibitors (ICIs) demonstrate remarkable efficacy by augmenting the anti-tumor immune response via interruption of negative costimulation of T cells [1, 2]. Currently approved targets include the cytotoxic T-lymphocyte antigen 4 (CTLA4), programmed cell death 1 (PD-1), and programmed cell death ligand 1 (PD-L1).

B. M. Warner (✉)
Salivary Disorders Unit, National Institute of Dental and Craniofacial Research, Bethesda, MD, USA

Sjögren's Syndrome Clinic, National Institute of Dental and Craniofacial Research, Bethesda, MD, USA
e-mail: blake.warner@nih.gov

A. N. Baer
Sjögren's Syndrome Clinic, National Institute of Dental and Craniofacial Research, Bethesda, MD, USA

Division of Rheumatology, Johns Hopkins University School of Medicine, Baltimore, MD, USA
e-mail: alanbaer@jhmi.edu

M. E. Suarez-Almazor, L. H. Calabrese (eds.), *Rheumatic Diseases and Syndromes Induced by Cancer Immunotherapy*,
https://doi.org/10.1007/978-3-030-56824-5_7

ICI therapies can induce the development of clinically significant inflammatory lesions of specific organ systems in up to 60% of patients [3, 4], often mandating cessation of the ICI therapy and/or treatment with immunosuppressive agents. The distribution and frequency of these immune-related adverse events (irAEs) are dependent in part on the specificity and mode of action of the agent [3–6]. These lesions most commonly affect endocrine glands, skin, gastrointestinal tract, and liver, but other organs may also be affected including the salivary and lacrimal glands [7]. irAEs may occur *de novo* or as exacerbations of previously diagnosed organ-specific or systemic autoimmune diseases. Although the pathogenesis is still under intense investigation, these lesions are thought to arise from activation of autoreactive T-cells or other autoimmune pathways [2, 7].

"Sicca syndrome" is clinically used to describe dryness of more than one mucosal surface, generally that of the eyes and mouth. It was once synonymous with Sjögren's syndrome, a systemic autoimmune disease defined clinically by dryness of the mouth (salivary hypofunction) and eyes (keratoconjunctivitis sicca), and pathologically by periductal lymphocytic infiltrates in the salivary and lacrimal glands [8]. However, sicca syndrome can have a variety of other etiologies, including the effects of anti-cholinergic drugs, head and neck radiation, glandular amyloid infiltration, viral sialadenitis (e.g., human immunodeficiency virus, hepatitis C virus), sarcoidosis, and IgG4-related sialadenitis or dacryoadenitis [9]. Sicca syndrome was first reported as a complication of ICI therapy (i.e., ICI-induced sicca) in four patients treated with ipilimumab and/or nivolumab [10]. Since this initial publication, additional case studies and case series of ICI-induced sicca have been reported (detailed below). In this chapter, we outline the epidemiology, the clinical presentation, and diagnosis, including distinct subsets of patients, possible pathogenesis, and our approach to management of ICI-induced sicca. We summarize our report with a case study of a representative patient who developed this irAE.

Epidemiology

Seven ICI drugs were approved between March 2011 and December 2019 for a variety of malignancies (reviewed in Chap. 2). Likewise, from 2011 to 2018, the estimated number of cancer patients in the United States eligible for ICI drugs increased from 1.5% to approximately 44% [11]. Expanded clinical use of ICIs is expected to precipitate an increase in the prevalence of irAEs. This use will also expand given the approximately 1.7 million new cancer cases in the United States annually [12]. Due to the nascency of this emerging field, it is difficult to predict fully the cumulative impact on public health as the number of patients who develop irAEs with chronic sequelae increases.

Systematic reviews on the epidemiology of irAEs are in the early phases of reporting. The true rates of irAEs and drug-specific differences in likelihood or distribution of irAEs, especially those considered mild, have not yet been clearly defined. This reflects underreporting or lack of recognition of some irAEs as clinically important (e.g., dry mouth). Most clinical trials report only common terminology and criteria for adverse events (CTCAE) grade 3 or higher adverse events and those events are found in >10–15% of patients rather than all adverse events [13, 14]. The CTCAE system for cataloging adverse events fails to capture the full range of irAEs, having been designed for cancer chemotherapeutic trials. Rationale for under reporting may be the perceived benignity of the adverse event, lack of apparent relatedness to the ICI therapy, or a delayed onset of the irAE (>1 year after initiation) after the study window. However, organ damage or sustained autoimmunity may persist long after the cessation of immunotherapy, especially in poorly-regenerative organs, such as the salivary and lacrimal glands. In our experience, ICI-induced sicca patients are similar to those with Sjögren's syndrome in their experience of long-lasting glandular dysfunction, leading to chronic clinical problems and impaired quality of life. In order to understand the full spectrum and accurate rates of irAEs in the context of ICI, it is our opinion that all irAEs should be reported in clinical trials, using reporting systems upgraded to include the full spectrum of rheumatic irAEs.

Reports of "dry mouth" and or "dry eyes" were rare in clinical trials of ipilimumab for metastatic melanoma (~1%) [5, 15]. "Dry mouth" has been reported as a side effect in clinical trials examining nivolumab and pembrolizumab with or without ipilimumab as treatments for melanoma (4–16%) [5, 15, 16], renal cell carcinoma (3–11%) [17], and thymic epithelial tumors (5%) [18]. The incidence of irAEs, including ICI-induced sicca, has been estimated in several systematic reviews [19, 20]. In general, ipilimumab monotherapy exhibited very low risk of "dry mouth" (~1%) whereas anti-PD-1 monotherapies exhibited intermediate rates (5–6%), with combination therapy exhibiting the highest rates (12%); the overall rate of "dry mouth" was estimated to be 5.4% [19]. Risk of developing dry mouth may be dose-dependent. A study examining pembrolizumab monotherapy (10 mg/kg) showed a nearly doubling of the rate of sicca using an every-two-week regimen versus an every-three-week regimen [15]. Similarly, a dose-finding study of nivolumab in renal cell carcinoma showed a dose-dependent increase in sicca at the 0.3, 2, and 10 mg/kg doses at 3%, 6%, and 11%, respectively [17]. It is possible that there are differences with respect to the risk of developing ICI sicca based upon malignancy type; however, there are too few studies and too much variation across the reported clinical trials to provide accurate estimates in this regard.

Pathogenesis

Deciphering the mechanisms of specific irAEs is an important line of research investigation. Landmark studies of rare life-threatening irAEs, such as hypophysitis [21], cardiac myositis [22], and encephalitis [23], have revealed specific mechanisms associated with these organs. It is generally accepted that activation of T cells and release of cytokines are central to organ-specific inflammation. However, the mechanism(s) underlying the establishment of organ-specific autoimmune-like disease (e.g., *de novo* development of Sjögren's syndrome) is not clear. Several possible mechanisms for irAEs have been proposed and the pattern and severity of irAEs may be specific both to the organ and the ICI agent.

Variability in the pattern and severity between CTLA4 and PD-1/PD-L1 targeting therapies may reflect the normal tissue distribution of the targets. CTLA4 inhibition primarily activates T cells centrally, whereas PD-1/PD-L1 results in peripheral T cell activation. In our experience, ICI-induced sicca is more common with PD-1/PD-L1 targeted therapies. This suggests several possible mechanisms: (i) activation of tumor-specific T cells that recognize a shared antigen between salivary and/or lacrimal glands and tumor; (ii) breach of immune tolerance to endogenous tissue antigens distinct from the tumor, leading to T cell or antibody-mediated tissue damage, and lastly, (iii) breach of immune tolerance to low-level expression of anergic exogenous antigens (e.g., viral peptides).

First, enhanced T cell activity against organs expressing a shared antigen between normal and tumor tissue may lead to T cell-mediated damage, as is seen in melanoma and the development of vitiligo [24, 25]. The salivary glands express 77% of the human transcriptome, and ~2300 proteins are secreted in saliva [26]. With this expansive protein synthesis repertoire, it is likely that some salivary-specific proteins are recognized as tumor antigens after ICI-induced tumor immunity is established. Second, tolerance to antigenic self-peptides may be lost within the periphery, leading to salivary- or lacrimal-specific immunity. For example, expression of PD-L1 and other targets within the peripheral tissues may lead to their complement-mediated destruction and the development of autoimmune disease. This mechanism has been demonstrated for hypophysitis [21]. Lastly, tissue-resident T cells that are tolerant to low-level, chronic viral infections (e.g., Epstein-Barr virus [EBV]) in the salivary glands may lose tolerance with ICI therapy and then elicit a vigorous anti-viral response with glandular damage. This could be postulated from a single patient who developed ICI-induced encephalitis with enrichment of EBV-specific T cell receptors and EBV+ lymphocytes in the affected tissues [23]. The authors suggest that tissue damage may have been due to proliferation and infiltration of highly oligoclonal T cells with a receptor repertoire indicative of an activated memory cytotoxic $CD4^+$ phenotype [23].

In our cohort, significantly more patients with sicca were treated with anti-PD-1 or anti-PD-L1 therapies than anti-CTLA4 alone [33]. This may be due to referral bias; however, dry mouth and salivary hypofunction have been reportedly more common, with the former in other studies as well [5, 15]. This phenomenon may reflect the specificity of PD-1 for its ligand (PD-L1 or PD-L2) within the peripheral tissue and tumor microenvironment. Blockade of PD-1/PD-L1 ligation results in tissue-specific interruption of immune tolerance and the expansion of self-reactive T cells and ultimately the secretion of effector cytokines. These data are supported by immunophenotyping data from our laboratory and others showing increased T cell (CD4 > CD8) infiltration, including variable numbers of T cells expressing PD-1 and in three cases, salivary epithelial cells expressing PD-L1 (manuscript in preparation). Moreover, it is well documented that PD-1/PD-L1 expression can restrain a previously overactive immune system [27]. IFN-gamma is a potent inducer of PD-L1 and acts to restrict inflammatory responses in normal tissues [28]. In the context of PD-L1 blockade, this checkpoint is overcome and activated T cells may attack normal tissues. Studies of T cell exhaustion in chronic infection show that PD-1 functions to limit effector T cell–mediated inflammatory injury. PD-1 blockade has been shown to reactivate exhausted effector T cells through engagement of activating transcription factors [29]. This can occur in the setting of chronic viral infections. Salivary glands are known reservoirs for chronic viral infections, such as HCV, EBV, and others. However, it remains to be demonstrated if exhausted virus-specific T cells are contributing to the pathogenesis of ICI sicca.

Histopathology

Several reports have now described the histopathologic changes in the salivary glands induced by anti-PD-1 and anti-PD-L1 therapy in subjects with ICI sicca [10, 19, 30–33]. Despite expected variance in histological presentation, the most common features of inflammation and injury found in the salivary glands of ICI sicca are remarkably consistent. The authors examined the histopathology of the minor salivary glands in 19 patients with ICI sicca [30]. In general, three histopathologic patterns were present: mild non-specific chronic sialadenitis with acinar atrophy and fibrosis (focus score [FS] = 0); mild-to-moderate sialadenitis with focal lymphocytic sialadenitis (FLS) with atrophy and fibrosis (FS =1–4); and severe sialadenitis (FS >4 or diffuse lymphocytic sialadenitis) with injury to the ducts and acini. Features of epithelial injury include: nuclear enlargement, anisonucleosis, and irregular distribution, apoptosis, fibrosis, acinar atrophy, luminal mucin inspissation, and rupture mucin extravasation. Immunohistochemistry demonstrated increased numbers of CD3+ T cells, a slight predominance of CD4+ compared with CD8+ T cells, with very few of CD20+ B cells in contrast with the immune cell infiltrates of SS [19, 30, 32]. PD-1 was variably positive in the lymphocytes in ICI patients' salivary glands, whereas PD-L1 was positive in the epithelium in areas of dense inflammation and, in some inflammatory cells, in only the most severe sialadenitis cases.

Pringle et al. (2020) published an in-depth case report investigation of a single patient with severe ICI sicca induced by anti-PD-L1 therapy and reported both the histopathological and immunohistochemical studies to expertly describe the changes to the functional epithelial structures in the parotid gland underpinning the glandular dysfunction characteristic of ICI sicca [32]. What was striking was the total absence of conventional acinar structures and replacement with more primitive intercalated duct-like structures; changes that are very rare in both healthy individuals and even SS patients. Immunohistochemical studies included the use of salivary differentiation markers, cytokeratin 7 (CK7), and aquaporin-5 (AQP5), the canonical water channel located on the apical lumen of acinar cells. The authors noted mislocalization of AQP5 in the acini-like clusters and varied expression of both AQP5 and CK7. We can confirm that some patients with prolonged anti-PD-L1 therapy may, in fact, exhibit marked atrophy and profound architectural distortion of the parotid gland parenchyma, which was discovered on postmortem in a single subject from our original 19-subject report (Patient 14, *unpublished data*). It may be this loss of functional parenchyma that underlies the severe dysfunction observed in ICI sicca.

Literature Review of Reported Cases

The 89 patients reported to date with ICI-induced sicca syndrome are heterogeneous in their case definition (Table 7.1). They can be grouped into the following three categories: (1) those with *de novo* development of oral and/or ocular dryness without systemic manifestations typically ascribed to Sjögren's syndrome (n = 54); (2) those with *de novo* development of ocular and oral dryness, in association with systemic manifestations typical of Sjögren's syndrome (n = 28); and (3) those who have a flare of a recognized preexisting rheumatic disease, with ocular and oral dryness being a major component of the ensuing clinical picture (n = 6). In addition to these patients with sicca syndrome, one patient developed central nervous system manifestations associated with the characteristic autoantibodies and had a labial gland histopathology of Sjögren's syndrome, but lacked sicca symptoms [34]. This heterogeneity in case definition mandates caution in combining case series to determine cardinal features of ICI-induced sicca.

Among the 89 reported patients with oral and/or ocular sicca developing in the context of ICI therapy, the median age was 61.5 years, with 51 (58%) men. The underlying malignancies included melanoma (n = 35) and carcinomas of the lung

Table 7.1 Three predominant subsets of ICI-induced sicca within 88 cases

Subset	Reference	Case number or identifier (age/gender)
ICI-induced sicca without systemic symptoms	Ortiz Brugués et al. [31]	1,2,3,4,5, 6, 7, 8,9, 10, 11, 12, 13, 14, 15
	Ramos-Casals et al. [19]	3, 6, 8, 15, 16,22
	Richter et al. [46]	12, 13, 14
	Narvaez et al. [35]	46F, 63 M
	Calabrese et al. [48]	8, 9
	Teyssonneau et al. [49]	Single case
	Cappelli et al. [10]	13
	Warner et al. [30]	1, 2, 3, 5, 6, 7, 8, 9, 10, 11, 12, 13, 14, 15, 17, 18, 19, 20
	Takahashi et al. [33]	Single case
	Noble et al. [50]	1
	Nguyen et al. [39]	1, 2
	Zimmer et al. [51]	49F
	Pringle et al. [32]	Single case

(continued)

Table 7.1 (continued)

ICI-induced sicca with systemic symptoms	Ramos-Casals et al. [19]	1, 2, 4, 5, 9, 10, 11, 12, 13, 14, 17, 18, 20, 21, 24, 25, 26
	Leipe et al. [52]	13
	Calabrese et al. [48]	7, 10, 11
	LeBurel et al. [53]	2, 3
	LeBurel et al. [38]	6
	Cappelli et al. [10]	10, 12 (case 11 duplicate reported in Warner et al. – patient #1)
	Smith et al. [37]	3, 10
ICI-induced sicca in the setting of preexisting rheumatic disease	Ramos-Casals et al. [19]	7, 23
	LeBurel et al. [53]	1
	Warner et al. [30]	4, 16
	Richter et al. [46]	17

(n = 18), kidney (n = 12), colon (n = 2), endometrium (n = 2), gastroesophageal junction (n = 1), cervix (n = 2), pancreas (n = 2), prostate (n = 1), thymus (n = 3), parotid gland (n = 1), oral cavity (n = 3), and bladder (n = 1). Neoplasms included chordoma (n = 1) and recurrent respiratory papillomatosis (n = 4). The ICI treatment patients were receiving at the onset of the sicca symptoms included anti-PD-1 alone (n = 47) or in combination with an anti-CTLA4 agent

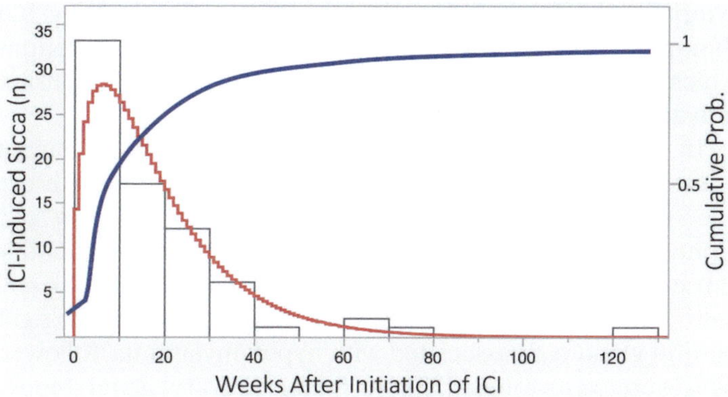

FIGURE 7.1 Histogram and cumulative probability plots of the distribution of cases by time to onset of sicca after initiation of immune checkpoint inhibitors. Histogram (columns and redline; left axis) depicting the time to the development of sicca and a cumulative probability plot (blue line, right axis). The median time to the development of sicca after the initiation of immune checkpoint inhibitors is ~10 weeks. Data abstracted from published cases (Table 7.1), where data on time to the development of sicca was available

(n = 18), pegylated IL-10 (n = 1), or an investigational ICI (n = 4); anti-PD-L1 alone (n = 15) or in combination with BRAF and MEK inhibitors (n = 1) or TGF-beta (n = 1); and anti-CTLA4 alone (n = 1). The median interval between the onset of ICI treatment and the onset of sicca symptoms was 10 weeks (range 2–68 weeks) (Fig. 7.1). Forty-one patients had dry mouth and dry eye symptoms, thirty-nine had dry mouth alone, and eight had dry eye symptoms alone.

Subsets of ICI-Induced Sicca

De novo Development of Oral and/or Ocular Dryness Without Systemic Manifestations

The most common form of ICI-induced sicca syndrome is represented by the 54 patients who developed prominent symptoms of dry mouth and/or dry eye while receiving ICI therapy. They did not have extraglandular manifestations which typify Sjögren's syndrome, such as interstitial nephritis, polyarthritis, or annular erythema.

In the majority of the 54 reported cases, the predominant feature is oral sicca, either alone or in combination with dry eye symptoms. A small number of patients reported dry eye alone. This may represent a reporting bias. Two patients in this subset had acute swelling of their salivary glands, including one with SSB antibodies [10]. A third patient developed right parotid gland pain associated with hyperamylasemia, followed by severe xerostomia [33]. A minor salivary gland biopsy showed diffuse lymphocytic infiltration and acinar loss.

Salivary hypofunction was documented in 22/23 subjects in whom it was formally measured. In three patients, this hypofunction was documented by the finding of abnormal salivary gland scintigraphy [33, 35]. In the authors' series, there were 18 patients in this subset, with 17 having whole unstimulated saliva flow (WUSF) of less than 1.5 mL/15 min; seven of these patients exhibited no WUSF [30]. The median WUSF was 0.47 mL/15 min (range 0–2.48). Thus, CTCAE severity for "dry mouth" was grade 3 in 17 patients and grade 2 in 1 patient, as judged by WUSF (Table 7.2).

Dry eye disease was documented by abnormal tear flow (Schirmer I test of ≤5 mm in one eye) in 6 of 21 patients in whom it was tested. The median Schirmer test result in the worst of the two eyes was 9.5 mm/5 min (range 3–22).

Autoantibodies against SSA/Ro, a common marker of Sjögren's syndrome, were detected in 3 of 47 patients in whom they were tested. Other autoantibodies were detected in a few selected patients including anti-SSB/La antibodies (3/47 patients), rheumatoid factor (2/30 patients), and anti-Scl-70 antibodies (1 patient). In our cohort, a highly sensitive and specific technology, luciferase immunoprecipitation system (LIPS), was used to test for the presence of other serum autoantibodies. We confirmed the results of the serologic tests done in our hospital laboratory and identified additional patients (n = 2) with positivity to Ro60 [36]. However, there

Table 7.2 CTCAE version 5.0 for grading immune checkpoint inhibitor-induced sicca

Gastrointestinal disorders				
CTCAE term	Grade 1	Grade 2	Grade 3	Grade 4/5
"Dry mouth"				
Subjective:	Symptomatic (e.g., dry or thick saliva) without significant dietary alteration	Moderate symptoms; oral intake alterations (e.g., copious water, other lubricants, diet limited to purees and/or soft, moist foods)	Inability to adequately aliment orally; tube feeding or TPN indicated	-
Objective:	Unstimulated saliva flow >0.2 ml/min	Unstimulated saliva 0.1 to 0.2 ml/min	Unstimulated saliva <0.1 ml/min	
Definition: A disorder characterized by reduced salivary flow in the oral cavity				
Eye disorders				
CTCAE term	Grade 1	Grade 2	Grade 3	Grade 4/5

(continued)

Table 7.2 (continued)

"Dry eye"				
	Asymptomatic; clinical or diagnostic observations only; symptoms relieved by lubricants	Symptomatic; moderate decrease in visual acuity (best corrected visual acuity 20/40 and better or 3 lines or less decreased vision from known baseline)	Symptomatic with marked – decrease in visual acuity (best corrected visual acuity worse than 20/40 or more than 3 lines of decreased vision from known baseline, up to 20/200); limiting self-care ADL	–
Definition: A disorder characterized by dryness of the cornea and conjunctiva				

were no consistent patterns of antibody positivity found across the ICI-induced sicca patients [36].

Salivary gland ultrasonography was performed on 20 patients, and showed generally mild changes in the major glands, including parenchymal heterogeneity with hyperechogenic bands and scattered ovoid hypoechoic lesions [10, 30]. Hypoechoic lesions occupied more than 50% of the parotid and submandibular gland parenchyma in one patient with SSB/La antibodies and parotid gland swelling that developed in the context of ICI therapy [10]. In a patient with nivolumab-induced sialadenitis of the right parotid, increased 18F-FDG avidity was noted in the affected gland on PET imaging as well as decreased technetium-99 m pertechnetate accumulation on scintigraphy [33]. However, ultrasonography of the gland was normal.

Minor salivary gland biopsies were reported in 36 patients; focal lymphocytic sialadenitis with a focus score ≥ 1 was present in 8 patients, non-specific mild chronic sialadenitis (Chisholm-Mason or Greenspan grade 2 or less) in 25 patients, and severe diffuse lymphocytic infiltration in 3 patients.

Various approaches to clinical management were used. Among 35 reported patients, the ICI was discontinued in 26 patients at the time of sicca symptoms manifestation. The ICI was stopped in 14 patients in response to the advent of the sicca symptoms, in 6 because of tumor progression, in 4 because of other irAEs, and in 2 due to completion of the study protocol. Among 11 patients, in whom the ICI was discontinued and only symptomatic and/or topical measures used for the sicca manifestations, there was improvement in all, rated as significant in 2, mild in 6, and partial in 1. Among 15 patients, in whom the ICI was discontinued and corticosteroids were administered, improvement was again noted in all, rated as significant in 5, moderate in 5, and partial/minimal in 2. In nine patients, the ICI was not held; eight received only symptomatic and/or topical measures for the sicca, while one received concomitant corticosteroids. In the eight who did not receive corticosteroids, chronic symptoms or lack of improvement were reported in five, improvement in three, and rated as mild in two.

De Novo Development of Oral and/or Ocular Dryness with Systemic Manifestations

There were 28 reported cases in which the development of sicca occurred in conjunction with systemic manifestations, leading to the diagnostic impression of ICI-induced Sjögren's syndrome. Four had concurrent salivary gland enlargement. None had a preexisting rheumatic disease. The systemic manifestations included arthritis or arthralgia (n = 12), skin rash (n = 9), interstitial pneumonitis or persistent cough (n = 4), peripheral neuropathy (n = 3), myositis (n = 3), nephritis (n = 2), cryoglobulinemia (n = 2), polymyalgia rheumatica (n = 2), central nervous system disease (n = 1), constitutional symptoms (n = 1), and low serum complement levels (n = 1). The majority of these cases were identified in the International ImmunoCancer Registry, and it is not possible to adjudicate from the reported case series whether these systemic manifestations might have had other etiologies, such as an independent irAE from the ICI, infection, or paraneoplastic phenomena [19]. One of the authors was involved in the care of a 71-year-old man with metastatic melanoma who developed acute interstitial nephritis and marked ocular and oral sicca concurrently, 34 weeks after the initiation of nivolumab. He had hyperglobulinemia, but lacked anti-SSA/Ro and SSB/La antibodies. Even though a lip biopsy did not show focal lymphocytic sialadenitis, there was clinical impression of ICI-induced Sjögren's syndrome [10]. In some patients, the primary adverse event was polyarthritis, and the concomitant presence of dry eye disease prompted a diagnosis of "secondary Sjögren's syndrome" [37].

Dry mouth symptoms were reported by 25/28 patients and objective evidence of salivary hypofunction was present in 12/15 patients. Dry eye symptoms were present in 20/28 patients and an abnormal dry eye test in 12/18 patients.

SSA/Ro antibodies were present in 8 of 22 patients in whom they were tested, a significantly greater proportion than in the subset of patients with *de novo* sicca without systemic manifestations (36% vs. 6%, $p = 0.0015$ by χ^2). In one patient, anti-SSA/Ro antibodies were also detected retrospectively prior to the onset of ICI therapy [38]. Other autoantibodies detected in this subset included SSB/La antibodies (1/18 patients), rheumatoid factor (3/17 patients), CCP antibodies (one patient), anti-EJ antibodies (one patient with pneumonitis), and cryoglobulins (n = 2).

Labial gland biopsies were reported in 12 patients; of these, focal lymphocytic sialadenitis was present in 6 (with focus score ≥ 1 reported in 5) and non-specific chronic sialadenitis in the other 6.

The 2016 ACR/EULAR classification criteria were fulfilled by 10 of 14 patients, on whom data were available with respect to objective measures of dry eye and salivary hypofunction, anti-SSA/Ro antibodies, and labial gland biopsy. In contrast to idiopathic Sjögren's syndrome, this subset of 28 ICI-induced sicca patients had male predominance (61%), older age (mean 65 years), and much lower frequency of autoantibodies. These differences were highlighted by Ramos-Casals et al. in their case series [19].

Management of these patients was primarily focused on the systemic manifestations. Among five reported patients, in whom management approaches and outcomes were detailed specifically for the sicca manifestations, the ICI was discontinued in each; of these, four received corticosteroids for the sicca manifestations and one for other irAEs. Improvement was reported in all, rated as significant in three and moderate in one.

Flare of a Recognized Preexisting Rheumatic Disease, Associated with Ocular and Oral Dryness

Six reported patients had a clinically overt preexisting rheumatic disease, including rheumatoid arthritis (n = 1), polymyositis (n = 1), spondyloarthritis (n = 2), Sjögren's syndrome (n = 1), and undifferentiated connective tissue disease (n = 1; polyarthritis, mild sicca, rheumatoid factor, and anti-SSA antibodies). Underlying malignancies included melanoma (n = 2), thymic carcinoma (n = 1), renal carcinoma (n = 2), and lung carcinoma (n = 1). All patients developed oral (n = 5) and/or ocular sicca (n = 6). Three patients also developed arthritis or arthralgia and one developed myositis in relation to the ICI therapy. SSA/Ro antibodies were positive in 4/6 patients and rheumatoid factor in 4/6 patients. Labial gland biopsies showed focal lymphocytic sialadenitis in three and severe diffuse lymphocytic infiltration in one of the five performed.

The ICI was continued in four and discontinued in two patients; two patients received corticosteroids in the context of ongoing ICI therapy and experienced minimal or no improvement.

Clinical Manifestations

Dry mouth. The patients typically note the abrupt onset of dry mouth (i.e., "…awoke one morning with a dry mouth") and most require water to chew and swallow dry foods. In the authors' series of 20 patients, physician-reported CTCAE severity for "dry mouth" was grade 2 in 15 patients and grade 1 in 5 patients, as rated by symptom criteria alone (Table 7.2). The symptoms are often worse with physical exertion or at night, with patients awakening at night with their tongue stuck to their teeth or hard palate and the requirement to drink water. Other symptoms included thick or sticky saliva, dryness of the throat with hoarseness, altered taste, and sensitivity to spicy and acidic foods. Changes in oral mucosa, indicative of salivary gland hypofunction, are evident in the majority and may include findings consistent with chronic erythematous candidiasis (Fig. 7.2). Patients may also report oral mucosal ulcerative lesions and/or mucosal burning.

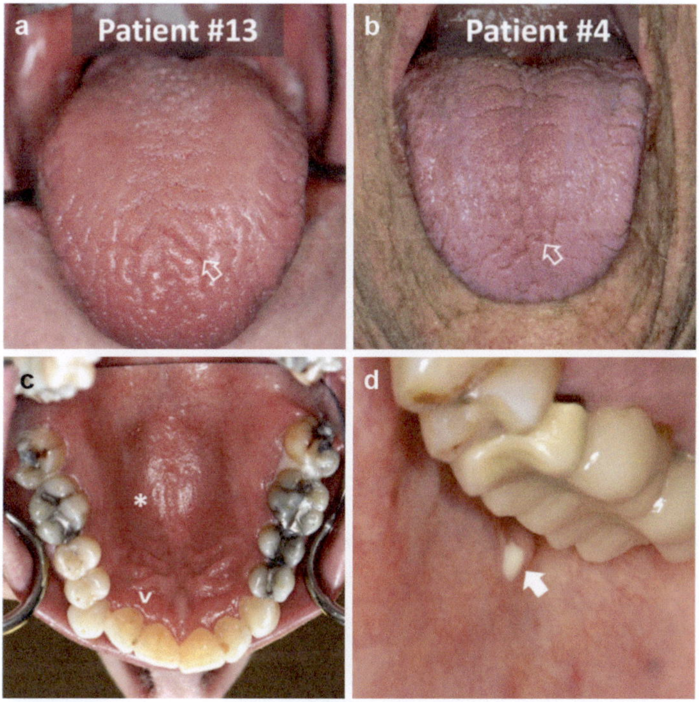

FIGURE 7.2 Examples of patient's oral cavities with ICI-induced sicca. A, C exhibits significant papillary atrophy with erythema and fissuring (open arrow). Evidence of dryness (reflectance) and inflammation (erythema) of the mucosa of the palate (*) and gingiva adjacent to the teeth (^) can be appreciated. The general erythematous appearance of the palatal and lingual mucosa is strongly indicative of erythematous candidiasis; he was treated with antifungal therapy. B, D, patient had history of preexisting rheumatoid arthritis, also exhibits papillary atrophy and fissuring (open arrow) of the dorsum of the tongue. During therapy, the patient developed strictures of the Stensen's duct and subsequent recurrent infectious parotitis (closed arrow) with *Staphylococcus aureus* and *Candidiasis* spp.; he was treated with antibiotics, irrigation of the parotid ducts, and eventual sialoendoscopic dilation of his ductal strictures. Rituximab was also used for management of his rheumatoid arthritis and possibly the sialadenitis. Figure previously published in Warner et al., 2019 [30]

Dry eye. Dry eye symptoms also arose abruptly, manifested by foreign body sensation, blurred vision, and redness of the eyes (Table 7.2). In one patient, the ocular sicca progressed within 2 weeks of presentation to corneal perforation [39].

Sialadenitis. Eight reported patients had enlargement of their parotid glands, including two with acute sialadenitis.

Diagnosis

ICI-induced sicca should be suspected when a patient reports new or worsening oral or ocular symptoms. Certain questions have high specificity for salivary hypofunction and dry eye. These include [30]:

- Do you have adequate saliva to chew and swallow a dry cracker or pretzel?
- Do you awaken at night to drink water?
- Do you have a daily, persistent feeling of sand or grit in your eyes?
- Do you need to use tear supplements four or more times a day?
- Are you able to produce tears?

Alternative etiologies for sicca (e.g., a recent prescription of a drug with anticholinergic side effects) should be excluded.

A comprehensive oral examination should be done to exclude mucositis, which can be a distinct form of irAE [40].

For patients with CTCAE grade 2 xerostomia symptoms, we recommend referral to an oral care specialist trained in the management of dry mouth (e.g., oral medicine specialist, oral oncologist, clinical oral pathologist) for comprehensive oral exam, salivary flow assessment, and labial salivary gland biopsy (Fig. 7.3). This should include an evaluation for an infectious etiology in patients with mucositis, burning mouth, or oral ulcers.

Patients with symptoms of ocular dryness (including irritation, foreign body sensation, photophobia, ocular redness) should be evaluated by an eye-care professional. The ocular sicca has the potential to progress rapidly to corneal ulceration

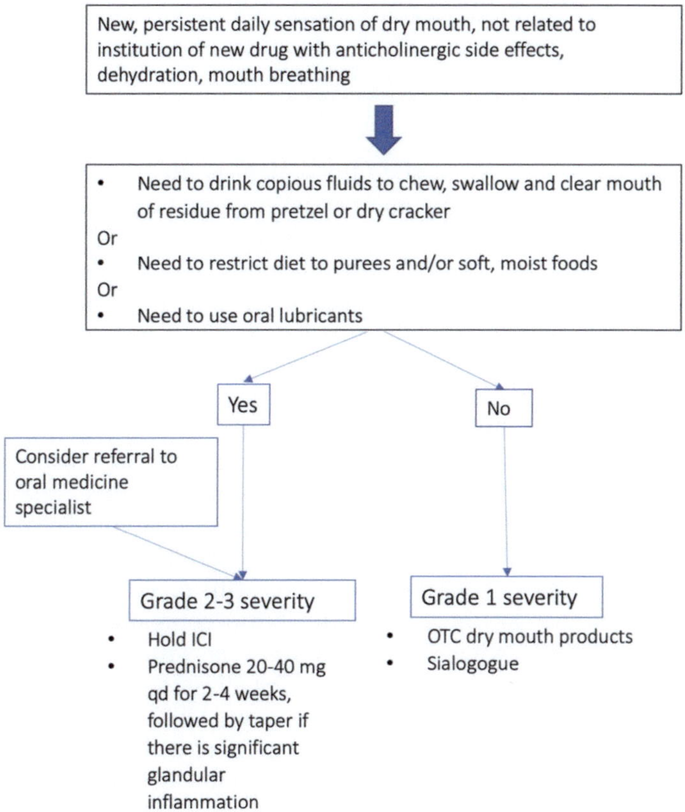

FIGURE 7.3 Assessment and management of sicca developing during the course of ICI therapy. Abbreviations: ICI, immune checkpoint inhibitor; OTC, over-the-counter; qd, quaque die (one a day). Modification of our figure previously published in Warner et al., 2019 [30]

and perforation, and thus this evaluation should be arranged as early as possible for patients with significant ocular symptoms.

Laboratory testing is indicated to assess for an underlying systemic autoimmune disease, either present before the onset of ICI therapy or induced by it. This should include testing for antinuclear antibodies (ANA), anti-SSA/Ro and anti-SSB/La antibodies (present in 70–80% of patients with Sjögren's syndrome), and rheumatoid factor. Other forms of salivary gland disease can be assessed by testing for hepatitis C, HIV, and serum IgG4 levels.

Imaging is recommended for patients with salivary gland enlargement or pain. A minor salivary gland biopsy from the labial mucosa is the preferred technique for assessing glandular inflammation and has low morbidity [41]. As described above, patients with ICI-induced sicca exhibit salivary glandular histopathology with varied degrees of inflammation. The majority have minimal inflammation (mild chronic sialadenitis). This finding does not preclude the presence of more extensive glandular damage, present without extensive inflammation, and manifested by acinar atrophy, patchy fibrosis, and architectural distortion. Some patients exhibit periductal lymphoid aggregates, with a histopathologic pattern indistinguishable from Sjögren's syndrome. This pattern was found more commonly in those with preexisting rheumatic disease and in those with sicca accompanied by systemic features, when compared to sicca without systemic features (9/18 vs. 8/36; $p = 0.038$). Finally, a severe form of sialadenitis was observed in four patients [30, 33], three with sicca but no systemic features and one with preexisting UCTD. Three of the patients had thymic carcinoma. These individuals may be a unique subset susceptible to irAEs or the exacerbation of autoimmune disease [18, 30, 42]. The mechanisms driving salivary inflammation and resultant dysfunction are currently under active investigation.

Differential Diagnosis

In the context of cancer treatment, potential etiologies for the *de novo* development of dry mouth symptoms include dehydration, anxiety, side effects of non-chemotherapeutic medications (most often those with anti-cholinergic properties), chemotherapy-induced salivary gland injury, head and neck irradiation, mouth breathing from nasal airway congestion or obstruction, and graft-versus-host disease. ICI-induced salivary hypofunction is distinguished by the often rapid development of a symptomatic dry mouth and severe loss of salivary gland function. Dry eye is also a potential problem during cancer treatment and may arise from some of the same causes as for dry mouth. Chemotherapeutic agents, such as 5-fluorouracil and docetaxel, may directly impair the maintenance of a healthy tear film.

Management

ICI-Induced Sicca Without Systemic Symptoms

Optimal management of ICI-induced sicca can be assessed primarily with data from two series, one by the authors (20 patients) [30, 43] and the other by Brugués et al. (15 patients) [31].

The authors assessed the outcome of grade 2 sicca symptoms in 11 patients in whom ICI were held/stopped and/or corticosteroids administered and follow-up data were available. Among these 11 patients, there was significant, moderate, and minimal improvement in the dry mouth symptoms in five, five, and one patient, respectively. In each category, patients improved with or without corticosteroids with cessation of ICI; however, symptoms did not resolve in any patient. Response to treatment was assessed with serial salivary flow measurements in five patients, in which all exhibited objective improvements in WUSF (median increment: 1.00 mL/15 min, range 0.19–4.39) with a median follow-up of 52 days (range 28–236 days). Only one patient reached a WUSF value above 1.5 mL/15 min. ICI therapy was resumed in seven patients. In five patients, this was done within 3 months of their last dose, allowing them to remain in their given clinical trial. This re-challenge was done while four patients were either maintained or started on prednisone to prevent worsening of their sicca. The two other patients were started on a different ICI regimen after the original ICI had been held because of sicca, after an interval of 120–872 days. Sicca symptoms remained stable with re-challenge in all but one patient, who was started on a different ICI 2.4 years after the original ICI course and had renewed dry mouth symptoms.

In the series of Brugués et al., holding the ICI due to oral symptoms was not required in any of their 15 patients [31]. However, eight patients had the ICI stopped because of tumor progression or other severe irAEs and noted slight to moderate improvement in their oral symptoms. Two of their patients noted significant relief of sicca when given a short course of high dose prednisolone for grade 3 transaminitis.

In current guidelines for management of irAEs, it is recommended that ICIs be held for most grade 2 toxicities and then resumed when symptoms and/or laboratory measures revert to grade 1 [44, 45]. Corticosteroids may be administered in addition to holding the ICI. Whether or not this management protocol should apply to ICI-induced sicca is not known, but clearly depends on whether there is significant glandular damage and/or inflammation, assessed by measures of saliva/tear flow, mucosal damage, and glandular histopathology. This is an argument for a comprehensive evaluation of all patients presenting with grade 2 toxicities.

In a multivariate analysis of a large French cohort of patients with preexisting autoimmune disease and cancer who were treated with ICI, there was a trend toward better survival in the subgroup who were managed without ICI discontinuation and without immunosuppressive therapy [46].

A stepwise approach to management is recommended, depending on the sicca severity. The sicca syndrome should be managed in accordance with practices employed for other irAEs [44, 45]. Our experience supports the following protocol for management of sicca that arises during the course of ICI therapy (Fig. 7.3) [30]. Mild (grade 1) symptoms can be managed with topical therapies (e.g., sips of water, artificial tear and saliva supplements) and sialogogues (e.g., pilocarpine and cevimeline). For patients with grade 2 or 3 symptoms, ICI therapy should be withheld and prednisone therapy initiated if there is significant glandular inflammation. Initial prednisone doses of 20–40 mg per day for 2–3 weeks, followed by a taper, was most beneficial in the authors' experience. Upon improvement of the sicca, the ICI can be resumed ideally after an interval of 3 months. In patients with persistent and severe sicca, the ICI therapy must be permanently discontinued.

ICI-Induced Sicca with Systemic Symptoms

In the reported patients, immunosuppressive treatment was utilized for management of the systemic manifestations, including glucocorticoids alone or with conventional synthetic DMARDs, biologic DMARDS, or intravenous immunoglobulin. There has been no report of the response of the sicca manifestations to these systemic therapies.

ICI-Induced Sicca in the Setting of Preexisting Rheumatic Disease

Any patient being considered for ICI treatment should be assessed for a history of a systemic autoimmune disease, including Sjögren's syndrome, rheumatoid arthritis, systemic lupus, and myositis. The presence of a preexisting autoimmune disease does not preclude ICI treatment, but the patient should be made fully aware of the risk of a flare and should be observed closely for such an occurrence, best in concert with the patient's rheumatologist [47]. We do not recommend screening patients for the presence of rheumatic disease autoantibodies in the absence of a history of a prior autoimmune systemic rheumatic disease or symptoms suggestive of this, including persistent sicca, inflammatory arthritis, past salivary gland enlargement, unexplained serositis, etc.

Conclusions and Future Directions

We have summarized and reviewed clinical data of 89 cases of dry mouth and/or dry eye attributed to ICI therapies. This review has highlighted several important findings:

- ICI-induced sicca lacks an established case definition. The resultant clinical heterogeneity may hinder its recognition and analysis. These findings may also imply different underlying pathophysiologic mechanisms. Patients with ICI-induced sicca can be broadly classified as: (1) ICI-induced sicca without systemic symptoms, (2) ICI-induced sicca with systemic symptoms, or (3) ICI-induced sicca in the setting of preexisting rheumatic disease.
- Management recommendations are based on expert opinion. Well-designed prospective studies are needed to assess the impact of various irAE therapies on the long-term outcome of sicca and other irAEs.
- Current grading criteria (i.e., CTCAE v5.0, Table 7.2) do not capture the full clinical spectrum of certain irAEs, including ICI-induced sicca. The severity of irAE can be influenced by subjective or objective criteria [30, 43]. Since sicca is a common symptom in the older population with a variety of causes, more specific definitions of sicca symptoms and signs are needed to enhance the capture of this symptom complex when it relates to ICI therapy.
- The dry mouth experienced in our cohort was appreciably abrupt and severe in most patients. The pattern of dysfunction was less suggestive of a medication-induced dry mouth (reversible); instead the function of the major salivary glands was severely (CTCAE Grade 3) reduced, often irreversibly.

Important questions persist for ICI-induced sicca. First, we remain uncertain as to its risk factors, such as the influence of genetics, comorbidities, or type of ICI. We know that patients with established autoimmune diseases (i.e., Sjögren's syndrome) are likely to experience worsening of their symptoms with ICI therapy. For the majority of patients, however, we are unable to predict who will develop this complication. The NCI is currently sponsoring a multi-center prospective clinical trial to assess the safety (including irAEs) of the anti-PD-1 antibody, nivolumab, in patients with specific autoimmune diseases (AIM-NIVO; NCT03816345, recruiting). This study promises to define the safety and efficacy of checkpoint inhibitors in patients who have both an established autoimmune disease and an indicated malignancy. However, prospective studies are needed to examine salivary and lacrimal function and glandular inflammation in all patients initiating ICI therapy, not just those with background autoimmunity. Goals for such a study would be discovery of a genetic signature of risk, early biomarkers of gland inflammation (similar to the rapid rise in TSH for thyroiditis), or imaging modalities (gallium-67 scan) that can identify early glandular inflammation. Second, the mechanisms driving ICI-induced sicca are largely unknown, but are being enthusiastically investigated. It is entirely possible that, due to the described clinical heterogeneity, several mechanisms may be driving both salivary and lacrimal hypofunction, leading to objective dysfunction. Third, longitudinal studies of ICI-induced sicca are needed to establish the (*i*) the chronicity of this irAE, (*ii*) the impact on quality of life, or (*iii*) the increased cost to the US health-care system.

Case Study

A 72-year-old man was diagnosed with metastatic melanoma during an evaluation for a left lower lobe lung mass, discovered incidentally on CT imaging of the abdomen. On PET/CT imaging, there was FDG-avidity of the left lower lobe lung lesion as well as asymmetric uptake in the brain. A wedge resection of the left lower lobe lung mass showed malignant melanoma, with negative resection margins and absence of visceral pleural involvement. On brain MRI, there was an anterior right frontal lobe lesion with no edema. The patient underwent stereotactic radiosurgery. Eleven weeks later, he began treatment with nivolumab. He began to note prominent dryness of his mouth 11 weeks after initiating nivolumab therapy, making it hard for him to chew and swallow dry foods without liquids or sustain long conversations. There was no salivary gland enlargement or pain. He did not have symptoms of dry eye. With persistence of the oral sicca for 2 weeks, his oncologist took him off the nivolumab and started prednisone 10 mg qd and pilocarpine. Higher steroid doses were avoided due to the patient's diabetes. The patient was evaluated formally for the sicca manifestations 5 weeks after the onset of his sicca symptoms.

Stage III colon cancer had been diagnosed 11 years earlier and treated with colectomy and 6 months of FOLFOX adjuvant chemotherapy. He had been free of detectable recurrence since that time.

His past medical history was notable for collagenous colitis, coronary artery disease, type 2 diabetes mellitus, hypertension, and lower extremity peripheral vascular disease. He quit smoking 40 years earlier.

On examination, the lips were dry and stuck to the teeth. There was absent sublingual pooling. Saliva was frothy and pasty. The dental mirror stuck to the buccal mucosa. There was no glossitis or salivary gland enlargement.

Laboratory studies documented normal blood counts, ESR 8 mm/hr., creatinine 1.23 mg/dl, normal hepatic function tests, glucose 327 mg/dl, hemoglobin A1c 7.2%, and TSH 2.75. IgG was 1229, IgA 313, and IgM 35 mg/dl. C3 was 117 and C4 16 mg/dl. ANA was 1.0 units (negative 0.9 units and less), rheumatoid factor was negative. Antibodies to extractable nuclear antigens (including SSA/Ro and SSB/La) and DNA were negative.

Salivary gland ultrasonography revealed bilateral parotid and submandibular glands showed heterogeneity of the parenchyma without discrete ovoid hypoechoic foci, which were interpreted as indeterminate.

Schirmer's test without anesthesia showed 8 mm wetting/5 min in the right eye and 5 mm in the left eye. Whole unstimulated saliva flow was 0 mL/15 min. Minor salivary

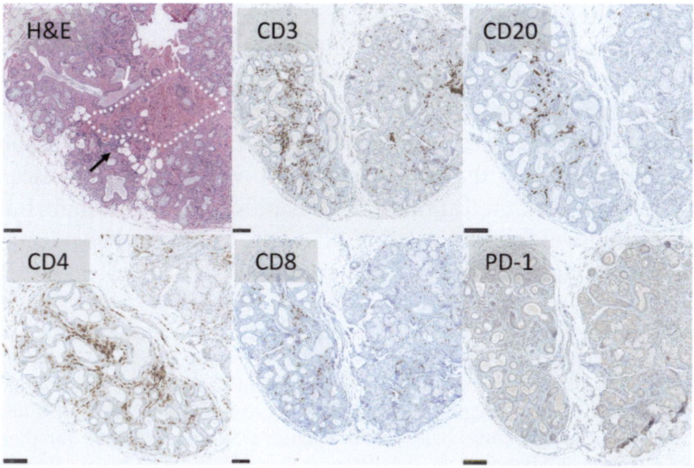

FIGURE 7.4 Representative photomicrographs of labial minor salivary glands from a patient with immune checkpoint inhibitor-induced sicca. Glass slides were scanned at 40X using the Hamamatsu S60 Digital Slide Scanner and visualized using the NDP Viewer. Representative scanned slide images at 10X digital resolution were obtained to denote characteristic features of immune checkpoint inhibitor-induced sialadenitis in the labial minor salivary glands. On H&E, note the overall distortion of the salivary gland architecture with increased eosinophilic fibrosis (dashed outline) and amphiphilic inspissated mucous lakes congesting dilated ducts (white arrow). Scattered foci of inflammation are present (>1.0 foci/4 mm^2; ex: black arrow) with a background of non-specific chronic sialadenitis. Overall, most of the acinar bundles are atrophied and numerically sparse. There is a predominance of CD3 positive T cells (CD4 > CD8) with some scattered B cells (atypically numerous). Few weakly-positive PD-1 lymphocytes are present in areas of inflammation

gland biopsy showed focal lymphocytic sialadenitis with mild fibrosis and atrophy (Fig. 7.4). Tarpley class 1, Greenspan grade 3, and focus score 1. Glandular distortion, including dilatation of the ducts, acinar atrophy, and inspissation of the mucin was noted. The inflammatory infiltrate was predominantly composed of T cells with CD4:CD8 of 2–3:1.

Few scattered B cells were present. Sparse PD-1 positive cells were detected in areas of inflammation.

The patient noted improvement to the point that symptoms were tolerable but still present (moderate). The prednisone was tapered off over the course of 6 weeks. Nivolumab was reinitiated in the patient after a10-week break. His sicca symptoms remained stable after resuming the nivolumab, but he then developed intractable diarrhea, prompting its permanent discontinuation 18 weeks after it was resumed.

Acknowledgments This work was supported by the National Institute of Dental and Craniofacial Research Division of Intramural Research. We would like to thank Dr. Peter Burbelo for this thoughtful editing of the manuscript. We acknowledge and thank the clinical support team of the National Institute of Dental and Craniofacial Research Sjögren's Syndrome Clinic for their organization of the patient visits and data collection. We thank the oncologists at Johns Hopkins Medical Institute and the NIH National Cancer Institute Center for Cancer Research for the referral of patients and active collaborations. Lastly, we thank the participation of our subjects in the research protocols. It is only through partnerships with patients that clinical research progress can be made.

References

1. Topalian SL, Drake CG, Pardoll DM. Immune checkpoint blockade: a common denominator approach to cancer therapy. Cancer Cell. 2015;27:450–61.
2. June CH, Warshauer JT, Bluestone JA. Is autoimmunity the Achilles' heel of cancer immunotherapy? Nat Med. 2017;23:540–7.
3. Tison A, et al. Safety and efficacy of immune checkpoint inhibitors in patients with cancer and preexisting autoimmune disease: a nationwide, multicenter cohort study. Arthritis Rheumatol. 2019;71:2100–11.
4. Boutros C, et al. Safety profiles of anti-CTLA-4 and anti-PD-1 antibodies alone and in combination. Nat Rev Clin Oncol. 2016;13:473–86.
5. Hodi FS, et al. Nivolumab plus ipilimumab or nivolumab alone versus ipilimumab alone in advanced melanoma (CheckMate 067): 4-year outcomes of a multicentre, randomised, phase 3 trial. Lancet Oncol. 2018;19:1480–92.

6. Brahmer JR, et al. Safety and activity of anti-PD-L1 antibody in patients with advanced cancer. N Engl J Med. 2012;366: 2455–65.
7. Tocut M, Brenner R, Zandman-Goddard G. Autoimmune phenomena and disease in cancer patients treated with immune checkpoint inhibitors. Autoimmun Rev. 2018;17:610–6.
8. Moutsopoulos HM, et al. Sjögren's syndrome (Sicca syndrome): current issues. Ann Intern Med. 1980;92:212–26.
9. Baer AN, et al. Rare diagnosis of IgG4-related systemic disease by lip biopsy in an international Sjögren syndrome registry. Oral Surg Oral Med Oral Pathol Oral Radiol. 2013;115:e34–9.
10. Cappelli LC, et al. Inflammatory arthritis and sicca syndrome induced by nivolumab and ipilimumab. Ann Rheum Dis. 2017;76:43–50.
11. Haslam A, Prasad V. Estimation of the percentage of US patients with Cancer who are eligible for and respond to checkpoint inhibitor immunotherapy drugs. JAMA Netw Open. 2019;2:e192535.
12. Siegel RL, Miller KD, Jemal A. Cancer statistics, 2019. CA Cancer J Clin. 2019;69:7–34.
13. Hammers HJ, et al. Safety and efficacy of Nivolumab in combination with Ipilimumab in metastatic renal cell carcinoma: the CheckMate 016 study. J Clin Oncol. 2017;35:3851–8.
14. Hellmann MD, et al. Nivolumab plus ipilimumab in advanced non-small-cell lung cancer. N Engl J Med. 2019;381:2020–31.
15. Robert C, et al. Pembrolizumab versus Ipilimumab in advanced melanoma. N Engl J Med. 2015;372:2521–32.
16. Long GV, et al. Standard-dose pembrolizumab in combination with reduced-dose ipilimumab for patients with advanced melanoma (KEYNOTE-029): an open-label, phase 1b trial. Lancet Oncol. 2017;18:1202–10.
17. Motzer RJ, et al. Nivolumab for metastatic renal cell carcinoma: results of a randomized phase II trial. J Clin Oncol. 2015;33:1430–7.
18. Giaccone G, et al. Pembrolizumab in patients with thymic carcinoma: a single-arm, single-centre, phase 2 study. Lancet Oncol. 2018;19:347–55.
19. Ramos-Casals M, et al. Sicca/Sjögren's syndrome triggered by PD-1/PD-L1 checkpoint inhibitors. Data from the international Immuno Cancer registry (ICIR). Clin Exp Rheumatol. 2019;37(Suppl 118):114–22.

20. Abdel-Rahman O, et al. Immune-related ocular toxicities in solid tumor patients treated with immune checkpoint inhibitors: a systematic review. Expert Rev Anticancer Ther. 2017;17:387–94.
21. Iwama S, et al. Pituitary expression of CTLA-4 mediates hypophysitis secondary to administration of CTLA-4 blocking antibody. Sci Transl Med. 2014;6:230ra45.
22. Mammen AL, et al. Pre-existing antiacetylcholine receptor autoantibodies and B cell lymphopaenia are associated with the development of myositis in patients with thymoma treated with avelumab, an immune checkpoint inhibitor targeting programmed death-ligand 1. Ann Rheum Dis. 2019;78:150–2.
23. Johnson DB, et al. A case report of clonal EBV-like memory CD4+ T cell activation in fatal checkpoint inhibitor-induced encephalitis. Nat Med. 2019;25:1243–50.
24. Hua C, et al. Association of vitiligo with tumor response in patients with metastatic melanoma treated with Pembrolizumab. JAMA Dermatol. 2016;152:45–7.
25. Attia P, et al. Autoimmunity correlates with tumor regression in patients with metastatic melanoma treated with anti–cytotoxic T-lymphocyte Antigen-4. JCO. 2005;23:6043–53.
26. Loo JA, Yan W, Ramachandran P, Wong DT. Comparative human salivary and plasma proteomes. J Dent Res. 2010;89:1016–23.
27. Francisco LM, Sage PT, Sharpe AH. The PD-1 pathway in tolerance and autoimmunity. Immunol Rev. 2010;236:219–42.
28. Schönrich G, Raftery MJ. The PD-1/PD-L1 Axis and virus infections: a delicate balance. Front Cell Infect Microbiol. 2019;9:1593–14.
29. Chen J, et al. NR4A transcription factors limit CAR T cell function in solid tumours. Nature. 2019;567:530–4.
30. Warner BM, et al. Sicca syndrome associated with immune checkpoint inhibitor therapy. Oncologist. 2019;24:1259–69.
31. Ortiz Brugués A, et al. Sicca syndrome induced by immune checkpoint inhibitor therapy: optimal management still pending. Oncologist. 2019-0467-5. 2019; https://doi.org/10.1634/theoncologist.2019-0467.
32. Pringle S, et al. Lack of conventional acinar cells in parotid salivary gland of patient taking an anti-PD-L1 immune checkpoint inhibitor. Front Oncol. 2020;10:420.
33. Takahashi S, Chieko X, Sakai T, Hirose S, Nakamura M. Nivolumab-induced sialadenitis. Respirol Case Rep. 2018;6:e00322.

34. Ghosn J, et al. A severe case of neuro-Sjögren's syndrome induced by pembrolizumab. J Immunother Cancer. 2018;6:110.
35. Narváez J, et al. Rheumatic immune-related adverse events in patients on anti-PD-1 inhibitors: fasciitis with myositis syndrome as a new complication of immunotherapy. Autoimmun Rev. 2018;17:1040–5.
36. Burbelo PD, et al. Profiling autoantibodies against salivary proteins in sicca conditions. J Dent Res. 2019;98:772–8.
37. Smith MH, Bass AR. Arthritis after Cancer immunotherapy: symptom duration and treatment response. Arthritis Care Res(Hoboken). 2018;71:362–6.
38. Le Burel S, et al. Prevalence of immune-related systemic adverse events in patients treated with anti-programmed cell death 1/anti-programmed cell death-ligand 1 agents: a single-Centre pharmacovigilance database analysis. Eur J Cancer. 2017;82:34–44.
39. Nguyen AT, Elia M, Materin MA, Sznol M, Chow J. Cyclosporine for dry eye associated with Nivolumab: a case progressing to corneal perforation. Cornea. 2016;35:399–401.
40. Acero Brand FZ, et al. Severe immune mucositis and esophagitis in metastatic squamous carcinoma of the larynx associated with pembrolizumab. J Immunother Cancer. 2018;6:22.
41. Kim J, et al. A validated method of labial minor salivary gland biopsy for the diagnosis of Sjögren's syndrome. Laryngoscope. 2016;126:2041–6.
42. Rajan A, et al. Efficacy and tolerability of anti-programmed death-ligand 1 (PD-L1) antibody (Avelumab) treatment in advanced thymoma. J Immunother Cancer. 2019;7:269.
43. Warner B, Baer A. In Reply. The Oncologist. 2019-0515-2. 2019; https://doi.org/10.1634/theoncologist.2019-0515.
44. Eigentler TK, et al. Diagnosis, monitoring and management of immune-related adverse drug reactions of anti-PD-1 antibody therapy. Cancer Treat Rev. 2016;45:7–18.
45. Brahmer JR, Lacchetti C, Thompson JA. Management of immune-related adverse events in patients treated with immune checkpoint inhibitor therapy: American Society of Clinical Oncology clinical practice guideline summary. J Oncol Pract. 2018;14:247–9.
46. Richter MD, et al. Rheumatic syndromes associated with immune checkpoint inhibitors: a single-center cohort of sixty-one patients. Arthritis Rheumatol. 2019;71:468–75.

47. Johnson DB, Sullivan RJ, Menzies AM. Immune checkpoint inhibitors in challenging populations. Cancer. 2017;123:1904–11.
48. Calabrese C, Kirchner E, Kontzias A, Velcheti V, Calabrese LH. Rheumatic immune-related adverse events of checkpoint therapy for cancer: case series of a new nosological entity. RMD Open. 2017;3:e000412.
49. Teyssonneau D, Cousin S, Italiano A. Gougerot-Sjogren-like syndrome under PD-1 inhibitor treatment. Ann Oncol. 2017;28:3108.
50. Noble CW, et al. Ocular adverse events following use of immune checkpoint inhibitors for metastatic malignancies. Ocul Immunol Inflamm. 2019;21:1–6.
51. Zimmer L, et al. Neurological, respiratory, musculoskeletal, cardiac and ocular side-effects of anti-PD-1 therapy. Eur J Cancer. 2016;60:210–25.
52. Leipe J, et al. Characteristics and treatment of new-onset arthritis after checkpoint inhibitor therapy. RMD Open. 2018;4:e000714.
53. Le Burel S, et al. Onset of connective tissue disease following anti-PD1/PD-L1 cancer immunotherapy. Ann Rheum Dis. 2018;77:468–70.

Chapter 8
Sarcoidosis

Xerxes Pundole, Manuel Ramos-Casals, and Olivier Lambotte

X. Pundole (✉)
Department of Health Services Research, The University of Texas MD Anderson Cancer Center, Houston, TX, USA
e-mail: xnpundole@mdanderson.org

M. Ramos-Casals
Department of Autoimmune Diseases, ICMiD, Barcelona, Spain

Sjögren Syndrome Research Group (AGAUR), Laboratory of Autoimmune Diseases Josep Font, IDIBAPS-CELLEX, Barcelona, Spain

Department of Medicine, University of Barcelona, Hospital Clínic, Barcelona, Spain
e-mail: mramos@clinic.cat

O. Lambotte
AP-HP-Paris Saclay, Médecine Interne/Immunologie Clinique, Hôpital Bicêtre, Paris, France

Université-Paris-Saclay; INSERM; CEA, Immunology of Viral Infections and Autoimmune Diseases Centre, IDMIT Department, Le Kremlin-Bicêtre, France
e-mail: olivier.lambotte@aphp.fr

M. E. Suarez-Almazor, L. H. Calabrese (eds.), *Rheumatic Diseases and Syndromes Induced by Cancer Immunotherapy*,
https://doi.org/10.1007/978-3-030-56824-5_8

Introduction

Despite the success of immune checkpoint inhibitors (ICIs) in cancer treatment, their use has been rapidly associated with the development of immune-related adverse events (irAEs) [1]. Reports of rheumatic irAEs are becoming increasingly common [2, 3]. A wide spectrum of rheumatic irAEs have been recognized and include arthralgia, arthritis, polymyalgia rheumatic, myositis, sicca/Sjogrens syndrome, vasculitis, lupus erythematosus, and others. The first case of sarcoidosis was reported in 2009 [4]. Today, over a hundred cases have been reported, mainly as case reports and case series (Table 8.1) [2, 5–9].

Epidemiology

A few reviews of sarcoidosis or sarcoid-like reactions following ICI therapy have been conducted thus far. A review by Gkiozos et al. reported on 23 cases [5], Tetzlaff et al. reported on 26 cases [6], Mobini et al. reported on 36 cases [8], Abdel-Wahab et al. reported on 53 cases [2], Rambhia et al. reported on 55 cases [9], and Corenjo et al. reported on 59 cases of sarcoidosis or sarcoid-like reactions [7]. While overlapping cases were included in these reviews, cross-checking the reference lists identified at least 65 unique cases. In addition, since the most recent review, at least 19 other cases of sarcoidosis or sarcoid-like reactions have been reported [10–20].

In addition to case reports and reviews of case reports, a few single-center studies and reports of pharmacovigilance databases have reported on sarcoidosis following ICI therapy. A study designed to collect data on autoimmune diseases in patients following exposure to biologics (BIOGEAS registry) showed that of 913 patients that developed an irAE, 20 developed sarcoidosis [21]. Thirteen received

Table 8.1 Published reviews of case reports on sarcoidosis or sarcoid-like reactions in patients following treatment with ICIs

Review[a]	n	Age in years	ICI	F (%)	Primary cancer	Time to irAE
Gkiozos et al. [5]	23	NR	Anti-PD-1 (18%), anti-CTLA-4 (61%), anti-PD-L1 (4%), sequential or combination anti-PD-1 & anti-CTLA-4 (17%)	NR	Melanoma (78%), lymphoma, uterine, lung, urethral, prostate cancer (4% each)	14 weeks (median)
Tetzlaff et al. [6]	26	57 (median)	Anti-PD-1 (31%), anti-CTLA-4 (54%), anti-PD-L1 (4%), sequential or combination anti-PD-1 & anti-CTLA-4 (11%)	54	Melanoma (77%), lung (8%), melanoma & colorectal, prostate, Hodgkin lymphoma, ovarian (~4% each)	6 months (median)
Mobini et al. [8]	36	57 (median)	Anti-PD-1 (44%), anti-CTLA-4 (31%), sequential or combination anti-PD-1 & anti-CTLA-4 (25%)	67	Melanoma (83%), lung (8%), ovarian, renal, urothelial, Hodgkin lymphoma (~2% each)	NR
Abdel-Wahab et al. [2]	53	57 (median)	Anti-PD-1/PD-L1 (67%) (including 9 patients receiving combination ICI)	53	Melanoma (74%)	4.3 months (median)

(continued)

Table 8.1 (continued)

Review[a]	n	Age in years	ICI	F (%)	Primary cancer	Time to irAE
Rambhia et al. [9]	55	58 (mean)	Anti-PD-1 (45%), anti-CTLA-4 (27%), sequential or combination anti-PD-1 & anti-CTLA-4 (27%)	47	Melanoma (78%), lung (11%), Hodgkin lymphoma (4%), uterine, gallbladder, renal, prostate cancer (2% each)	8.7 months (mean)
Cornejo et al. [7]	59	59 (median)	Anti-PD-1 (59%), anti-CTLA-4 (34%), anti-PD-L1 (2%), sequential or combination anti-PD-1 & anti-CTLA-4 (5%)	55	Melanoma (81%), lung (8%), urothelial, Hodgkin lymphoma, gallbladder, prostate, uterine, renal (~1%)	5.6 months (mean)

ICI immune checkpoint inhibitor; *F* female, *n* number of patients, *NR* not reported, *irAE* immune-related adverse event

[a]In the reviews, there was significant overlap in the cases included

ipilimumab, a cytotoxic T-lymphocyte-associated antigen 4 (CTLA-4) inhibitor; four received nivolumab and three pembrolizumab, which are programmed cell death receptor (PD-1) inhibitors. A single-center retrospective study of 147 patients who received ipilimumab for the treatment of melanoma and underwent body imaging found that 8 (5%) developed sarcoid-like reactions, some mimicking pulmonary sarcoidosis [22]. In another recent single-center retrospective study of 3200 patients, who were treated with ICIs, 18 (0.6%) cases of histologically proven sarcoidosis irAEs were identified [23]. In a French registry Registre des Effets Indésirables Sévères des Anticorps Monoclonaux Immunomodulateurs en Cancérologie (REISAMIC) of grade ≥ 2 irAEs occurring in patients treated with ICIs, the prevalence of sarcoidosis was 0.2% in 868 patients receiving anti-PD-1/anti-PD-L1 monotherapy [24].

Evaluation of the US Food and Drug Administration pharmacovigilance database showed safety signals for sarcoidosis, cutaneous sarcoidosis, and pulmonary sarcoidosis in relation with pembrolizumab monotherapy and in combination with ipilimumab [3]. Safety concerns were also identified for sarcoidosis in relation with ipilimumab and avelumab monotherapy. Similar safety concerns of sarcoidosis adverse event were also identified in the World Health Organization pharmacovigilance database (VigiBase) in relation with anti-PD-1 and anti-CTLA-4 inhibitors [25].

Based on the findings from case reports, sarcoidosis and sarcoid-like reactions seem to occur more frequently in patients treated with ICIs for melanoma (~80%), and in those receiving anti-PD-1 inhibitor therapy versus those receiving anti-CTLA-4 inhibitor therapy. A handful of cases following combination ICI therapy have also been reported. The median age of patients is estimated to be approximately 57 years, and a slight female predominance is noted (Table 8.1).

Pathogenesis

Primary sarcoidosis is a multisystem disorder of unknown etiology. It is characterized by a hyper reactive T helper-1 (Th-1) immune response that results in the development of non-caseating granulomas [26]. The lungs are affected in 90% of cases, and other tissues commonly involved include the skin, eyes, and lymph nodes. Herein we discuss the immunopathogenesis of sarcoidosis and sarcoid-like reactions associated with the use of ICIs.

Ipilimumab was the first approved ICI that blocks CTLA-4. By overcoming CTLA-4–mediated T lymphocyte suppression, T cells remain activated for a prolonged period, which restores T cell proliferation, consequently amplifying T cell–mediated immunity [27]. A multicenter phase 2 study demonstrated an increased expression of Th1-associated markers following treatment with ipilimumab. [28] Lymphocytes and Th1 cells are abundant in sarcoidosis and considered vital in the development of sarcoid granulomas [29]. The increase in lymphocytes with an increased expression of Th1-associated markers following ipilimumab therapy could be one mechanism by which a sarcoidosis-like reaction is induced.

T helper 17 (Th17) cells play a role in granuloma development phase and in the progression to fibrosis [30]. In a single-center analysis of 10 primary sarcoidosis patients' peripheral blood and bronchoalveolar lavage fluid, a decrease in regulatory T (Treg) cells and an increase in Th17 cells were observed, resulting in an imbalance in the Th17/Treg cell ratio [31]. In melanoma patients treated with tremelimumab (an anti-CTLA-4 inhibitor), Th17 cells in peripheral blood were increased [32]. Increase in Th17 cells is another proposed mechanism by which a sarcoidosis-like reaction can be induced.

A study designed to determine the effects of PD-1 pathway blockade on sarcoidosis $CD4^+$ T-cell proliferative capacity revealed increased $PD\text{-}1^+$ $CD4^+$ T cell counts systemically and in local environments of pulmonary sarcoidosis patients

[33]. Blockade of the PD-1 pathway restores CD4+ T-cell proliferative capacity to that of healthy subjects. These findings suggest that PD-1 plays a role in the immunopathogenesis of sarcoidosis. Thus, it seems paradoxical that the use of ICIs that inhibit PD-1 and PD-L1 enhance the Th1 T cell–mediated response and stimulate the development of sarcoidosis. This paradoxical response may involve interleukin-17-producing CD4+Th17 cells that are known to be expanded in sarcoidosis [34, 35]. Furthermore, a study by Lomax et al. found abnormally high counts of circulating Th17.1 cells in patients with melanoma prior to receiving anti-PD-1 checkpoint inhibitor therapy and prior to the onset of clinically symptomatic sarcoidosis [36]. It can be theorized that the effects of Th17.1 cells may be amplified following anti-PD-1 therapy and result in the development of sarcoidosis.

Interestingly, melanoma patients were those most frequently identified as having sarcoidosis or sarcoid-like reactions following ICI therapy (Table 8.1). This may be attributable to the fact that ICIs were first approved for use in melanoma patients, and their use is more widespread than in any other cancer types. It is, however, possible that the immunogenic nature of melanoma predisposes patients to develop irAEs following ICI therapy [37–39]. In particular, an anti-tumor response is enhanced with the use of ICIs, which results in melanoma cell death. As a consequence, tumor neoantigens are further revealed, which, when presented on host antigen-presenting cells, may fuel a Th-1 innate immune response, thus providing an environment conducive for the development of sarcoidosis [6]. Furthermore, independent of the use of ICIs, a higher incidence of sarcoidosis has been reported in patients with melanoma compared to the general population [40].

In summary, ICIs can dysregulate the immune system; however, the precise mechanistic link remains unknown. Thus, it remains unclear if ICIs truly cause sarcoidosis, render patients receiving ICIs to be more susceptible to development of sarcoidosis, or if these are distinct entities from sarcoidosis.

Clinical Manifestations

The mean age at diagnosis of sarcoidosis was 58 years in the most recent review of case reports [9]. Patients were, therefore, slightly older than in primary sarcoidosis, in whom the mean age of onset is between 47 and 51 years [41]. The male/female ratio is about 1 [9], which is different compared with primary sarcoidosis with a lower ratio [41]. The mean interval between ICI initiation and sarcoid-like reactions was between 5.6 and 8.7 months in a series by Cornejo et al. and Rambhia et al., respectively [7, 9].

As in primary sarcoidosis, sites most frequently involved include the hilar and mediastinal lymph nodes, the lungs, and/or the skin. Hilar and mediastinal lymph nodes were involved in 65% to 80% of the cases reported [5, 6, 9]. Lung involvement was present in 33% to 60%. Symptoms were nonspecific with mild dyspnea and cough. All radiographic stages consisted of stage I or stage II; some rare patients had stage III [23]. No patient showed stage IV. An important point is only part of the patients are symptomatic [6, 42]. This means that sarcoidosis was suspected in front of lymph nodes enlargement and abnormal glucose uptake on computed tomography (CT) scan and positron emission tomography (PET) scans. An abnormal PET scan was indeed always identified in mediastinal sarcoidosis and could guide biopsies. The early diagnosis could explain why lung involvement was not severe with normal lung functions in spirometry in nearly all patients (some had mild reduced CO diffusion) [5, 6].

In addition to thoracic involvement, the skin is also frequently involved (54.5%) [9] and is an easily accessible area to obtain a biopsy and identify non-caseating granulomas. Skin involvement most commonly included subcutaneous lesions, such as erythema nodosum or subcutaneous nodules, on the face, neck, and arms. Cutaneous sarcoid-like reactions within tattoos have also been reported in a handful of patients [43].

Other organs are more rarely involved. One review pointed to the involvement of extrathoracic lymph nodes and spleen in approximately 17% of the cases [5]. Eye involvement was mainly uveitis. The occurrence of severe extrathoracic sarcoidosis seems to be exceedingly rare. Four cases with neurologic involvement (one polyneuropathy and one pituitary granuloma, both after ipilimumab; two cases of neurosarcoidosis, both after ipilimumab and nivolumab combination) have been reported [45, 46, 47, 48].

Rheumatologists, oncologists, and pulmonologists should keep two important points while evaluating patients with suspected sarcoid irAE following ICI therapy. First, sarcoidosis can affect several organs simultaneously, and in Chanson's the review by Rhambia et al., >50% of the patients had both hilar and mediastinal lymph node involvement and extrathoracic manifestations [9]. Second, sarcoidosis can be diagnosed simultaneously with other irAEs such as thyroiditis, hepatitis, pneumonitis, and others [7]. Fatigue is also a symptom frequently reported.

Diagnosis

Following treatment with ICIs, patients may seek medical attention with constitutional symptoms, skin lesions, or cough, or may have signs of sarcoid-like reactions seen on radiological imaging ordered for an unrelated reason or for cancer staging. The diagnosis of sarcoidosis can be challenging, especially since approximately a quarter (22%) of patients present with signs of concern for tumor progression, such as lymphadenopathy and pulmonary infiltrates [9]. The diagnosis of sarcoidosis is one of exclusion, which requires consistent clinical and imaging characteristics coupled with histopathological findings (obtained from endobronchial ultrasound (EBUS), fine needle aspiration (FNA), transbronchial lung biopsy, or extrathoracic biopsy (salivary gland, skin, lymph node biopsy) of non-caseating granulomas, in the absence of an alternative explanation (infections or other competing diagnosis) [49]. PET imaging can be useful to identify targets to biopsy. As mentioned before, when non-caseating granulomas, in the absence of other criteria, for the diagnosis of systemic sarcoidosis are identified, the term sarcoid-like reaction is commonly used [50].

Since sarcoidosis may be mimicked by a wide variety of processes, the diagnosis is established when clinical and radiologic findings are supported by histologic evidence of granulomas. Non-caseating granulomas with epithelioid cells are the histological hallmark of sarcoidosis and generally enable to distinguish it from other granulomatous diseases, but it is a non-pathognomonic feature. Mycobacterial infections and, in particular, atypical mycobacterial infection may induce non-caseating granulomas, as well as fungal diseases (coccidiodomycosis, histoplasmosis); cat scratch disease and toxoplasmosis should also be considered in the differential diagnosis of adenopathic sarcoidosis. Other diseases that can mimic sarcoidosis included chronic berylliosis (usually an occupational disease) and Blau syndrome (a very rare hereditary disease) [51]. Finally, a large list of drugs has also been involved in the so-called drug-induced sarcoidosis-like reactions, which is defined as a systemic granulomatous tissue reaction that is clinically and histopathologically indistinguishable from sarcoidosis occurring in temporal relationship with the initiation of an offending drug [52]. Among the drugs closely associated with drug-induced sarcoidosis-like reaction, immunotherapies have emerged this century as key culprits, with the main example of tumor necrosis factor (TNF)-targeted therapies, [53] that have become key immunotherapies for treating autoimmune diseases including sarcoidosis, in which TNF-targeted antibodies are used in patients with severe, refractory disease [54]. Paradoxically, more than 100 cases of sarcoidosis, triggered by anti-TNF agents, were reported until 2017 [21]. In recent years, immune-mediated granulomatous diseases such as sarcoidosis, granuloma annulare, and granulomatous panniculitis or dermatitis have been increasingly reported as emerging toxicities in patients treated with cancer immunotherapies [7], mainly related to the use of ICIs and less frequently with kinase inhibitors [55]. Until now, the majority of cases of sarcoidosis triggered by ICIs are isolated reports which can result in publication bias, given the tendency to report more serious cases, or those with a greater diagnostic complexity.

Differential Diagnosis

Similar to the diagnosis of sarcoidosis, a diagnosis of ICI-related sarcoidosis or sarcoid-like reactions cannot be established unless alternative causes for granulomatous inflammation have been reasonably excluded, with certain specific etiologies requiring particular attention [52]. A close collaboration between clinical physicians and radiologists is essential to reach an accurate diagnosis, but always evaluating the major differential diagnoses [56], which are drug-induced pneumonitis, tumor progression, and pulmonary infections.

Drug-Induced Pneumonitis

The use of ICIs has been frequently related to the development of non-granulomatous interstitial lung diseases, such as organizing pneumonia, hypersensitivity pneumonitis, nonspecific interstitial pneumonia, and inflammatory bronchiolitis [57], and, therefore, it might be difficult to differentiate between pulmonary sarcoidosis and pneumonitis [58]. ICI-related pneumonitis commonly presents with new or worsening respiratory symptoms, showing in imaging studies a diffuse or multifocal lung disease, while sarcoidosis is mainly diagnosed in asymptomatic patients or with mild respiratory symptoms, often showing focal consolidations with surrounding ground-glass opacities [59]. This radiological pattern is distinct from that of pneumonitis, which most commonly presents bilateral multifocal areas of consolidations (cryptogenic organizing pneumonia pattern) or interstitial lung disease with interlobular septal thickening and ground-glass opacities in a subpleural and basilar distribution (non specific interstitial pneumonia pattern) [56]. The presence of bilateral hilar adenopathies is probably the key sign strongly suggesting an interstitial lung disease-related sarcoidosis, together with the presence of other extrathoracic key features (erythema nodosum (Fig. 8.1) and subcutaneous nodules (Fig. 8.2)).

Cancer Progression

As ICIs are used for the treatment of malignancies, it is important to recognize that drug-induced sarcoidosis-like reactions can mimic a malignancy in terms of roentgenographic and PET scan findings [52]. A neoplastic involvement of lymph nodes disclosed by CT/PET studies can mimic sarcoidosis; therefore, in patients under ICI treatment, new or growing

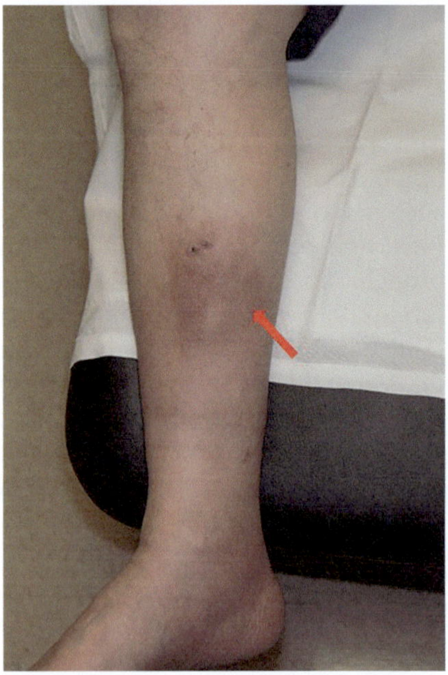

Figure 8.1 Erythema nodosum of the leg indicated by an arrow

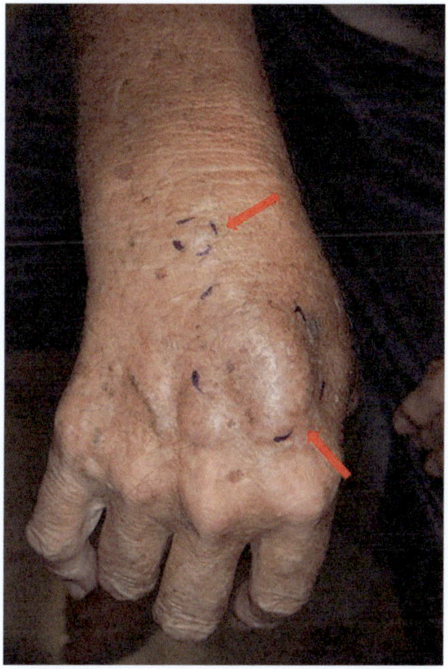

FIGURE 8.2 Subcutaneous nodules on the hand indicated by arrows

lymph node enlargements or the appearance of organ-specific nodules or masses should always require histopathological characterization. Granulomatous inflammation occurring in patients with cancer is often called "sarcoid reaction" or "sarcoid-like lymphadenopathy" [60]. Sarcoid-like reaction is thought to be caused by immunological hypersensitivity to antigens derived from tumor cell leading to granuloma formation. Sarcoid-like reactions can be reported concomitantly in biopsies obtained from the cancerous organ, the draining lymph nodes of the cancerous organ, or in cancerous metastasis, especially in patients with seminomas (50%), Hodgkin's disease (14%), B-cell lymphoma (7%), and carcinomas (4%), and it has also been observed in breast, gastric, colonic, and head and neck cancers [60]. In patients with testicular germ cell tumors, the coexistence of a non-caseating granulomatous disease is common. Schmidt et al. [61] have recently reported that, in 15 patients with a suspected tumor thoracic relapse on CT imaging, cancer relapse was confirmed in only one third of cases, while 53% showed non-caseating granulomas and 14% reactive lymphadenitis, with the coexistence of small lymphocytic lymphoma that did not have any prognostic impact on overall survival. Minimal invasive techniques such as endobronchial ultrasound-guided transbronchial fine needle aspiration can assist in the cytopathologic exclusion of malignant thoracic manifestations. Sarcoid-like reactions have been also reported in patients with lung cancer both in the lung parenchyma and in the regional lymph nodes (1–15%) [60].

Infection

Since many offending drugs that cause drug-induced sarcoid-like reaction are immunosuppressive, a thorough search for granulomatous infections, such as mycobacterial and fungal infections, must be conducted [52, 56]. The exclusion of pulmonary infections can also be challenging based on imaging alone, and clinical correlation is crucial [59].

Management

Once a patient is diagnosed with sarcoidosis or sarcoid-like reaction following ICIs, the most challenging decision that needs to be made is if a patient can continue anti-cancer treatment with ICIs. The Society for Immunotherapy and Cancer (SITC) established a multidisciplinary Toxicity Management Working Group, which developed recommendations to standardize the management of irAEs. [62]

In patients with pulmonary sarcoidosis, the working group recommends withholding ICIs, especially in patients with grade ≥ 2, extrapulmonary disease involving ocular, myocardial, neurological, or renal systems, or in patients with sarcoid-related hypercalcemia. Treatment for pulmonary sarcoid irAE should be considered if evidence of (1) progressive radiographic change; (2) pulmonary symptoms which are persistent and/or troublesome; (3) deterioration in lung function (decline of total lung capacity of ≥10%, forced vital capacity of ≥15%; diffusing capacity of the lungs for carbon monoxide of ≥20%); (4) concomitant extrapulmonary organ system involvement; or (5) sarcoid-related hypercalcemia. These recommendations were based on expert opinion, as no studies focusing on the management of sarcoidosis or sarcoid-like reactions following ICIs have been conducted. The working group recommends treatment with prednisone 1 mg/kg (or intravenous equivalent of methylprednisolone) for grade 2 sarcoidosis or cases severe enough to require hospitalization. Steroids should be tapered over 2–4 months, depending on the patient's response. Methotrexate is the molecule to be used in the setting of steroid-dependent or refractory sarcoidosis [63]. Hydroxychloroquine can be used also as cyclophosphamide, the latter in the setting of life-threatening symptoms (exceptional in the setting of sarcoidosis following ICI).

Overall, based on the recommendations of the SITC working group and our own clinical experience, the presence of sarcoidosis or sarcoid-like reactions following ICIs does not necessarily mandate therapy unless patients present with significant symptoms and organ dysfunction. In a review of case reports by Cornejo et al., in most patients (94%) with a reported outcome, an improvement or complete resolution of sarcoid-like reactions was noted [7]. ICI therapy was interrupted or discontinued in 49%, systemic steroids were used in 57%, and no therapy or minimal therapy with topical steroids was required in 24% of the cases. In patients with reported tumor response, 43% achieved a complete response, 37% experienced progression of metastatic disease, and 20% had stable disease. In patients with progression of metastatic disease, 38% of the patients' ICI therapy was interrupted or discontinued compared to 36% in patients with partial or complete tumor response. Given the lack of data, the natural history of patients with sarcoidosis or sarcoid-like reactions is not well established.

Prognosis

The mild clinical and radiological expression of sarcoidosis triggered by ICIs is parallel to their benign prognosis. The absolute predominance of the most benign radiological stages (I and II, both associated with spontaneous healing in most cases) [64] and the high frequency of asymptomatic cases contributed undoubtedly to the benign prognosis of sarcoidosis following ICIs, with a lower frequency in using systemic corticosteroids (<40%) and a total lack of requirement for immunosuppressants/biologics with respect to primary sarcoidosis [65]. The reason for this benign presentation is unclear but could be related to the close imaging monitorization of these patients that might facilitate a very early diagnosis in many cases in asymptomatic stages of disease development. This good prognosis has been described in drug-induced sarcoidosis-like reactions related to other drugs, in which sarcoidosis commonly resolved spontaneously after the withdrawal of the offending agent [52], as is reported in some cases related to ICIs [6, 7, 9]. Therefore, clinicians should weigh the benefit of continuing ICIs, considering the good prognosis of triggered sarcoidosis with most patients developing radiological stages I-II, cutaneous involvement, and taking into account a rate of relapse of 20% [58], and especially when the main reasons for discontinuing the ICIs are unrelated to sarcoidosis severity (the development of other concomitant irAEs and the lack of neoplastic response). With respect to the use of ICIs in patients previously diagnosed with sarcoidosis, data available among 17 patients with pre-existing sarcoidosis that started ICIs show that 3 (18%) had a relapse of the disease following ICI therapy [66–72].

Conclusions and Future Directions

In conclusion, sarcoidosis and sarcoid-like reactions following ICIs, albeit rare, can have adverse consequences on the morbidity and mortality of cancer patients receiving

ICIs. Rheumatologists should be vigilant about sarcoidosis and sarcoid-like reactions, and multidisciplinary collaboration between rheumatologists, oncologists, and pulmonologists is needed, as these adverse events may be misinterpreted as treatment failure or tumor progression based on imaging findings alone. A biopsy should be strongly considered when possible to differentiate irAE from tumor progression. Risk factors for predicting sarcoidosis and sarcoid-like reactions following ICIs, refining diagnostic criteria and optimal management strategies, need further investigation.

Case Study

Clinical description A 21-year-old male patient presented with loss of central vision in his left eye. He was diagnosed with uveal melanoma in 2010. He underwent enucleation and prosthetic eye placement. Within the following year his disease progressed, and metastases were noted in the lung. He underwent partial right lower lobe resection. In 2018, he developed brain metastasis, at which time he underwent right fronto-parietal craniotomy. In early 2019, he underwent gamma knife stereotactic radiosurgery. He was initiated on ipilimumab and nivolumab combination therapy. He developed fever 100.5 °F after each dose. After the fourth dose, he developed cough and a nodular skin rash in addition to the fever. His ICI therapy was held and underwent further investigation.

Diagnostic tests A CT scan of the chest showed innumerable micronodules throughout both lungs. He underwent a bronchoscopy, which revealed diffuse cobblestoning of the airways, and pathology of endobronchial and transbronchial biopsies revealed caseating granulomas. All fungal and bacterial studies were negative. Skin biopsy of a nodular rash revealed granulomatous dermatitis. A diagnosis of sarcoidosis induced by ipilimumab and nivolumab combination was the most likely explanation for his presentation and findings.

Management He was initiated on 60 mg of prednisone daily. He responded well, his respiratory symptoms improved, prednisone dose was reduced to 20 mg over a 4-week period. His clinical course was complicated by headache, tinnitus, and blurry vision. He underwent magnetic resonance imaging (MRI) of the brain, and neurologic vasculitis was suspected. He responded well to high dose steroids. His symptoms did not completely improve, and he was started on 10 mg methotrexate per week in addition to the 20 mg of prednisone.

Outcome His respiratory symptoms and skin rash improved; however, repeat MRI showed increasing lesions and biopsy revealed metastasis of melanoma. After 5 months of combination ICI therapy cessation, he was restarted on single-agent nivolumab. He also received spinal and whole brain radiation. At this time, he was also receiving 7.5 mg prednisone per day and 12 mg per week of methotrexate. He had a fluctuating clinical course and, unfortunately, his disease progressed. He was recently initiated on a trial of intravenous and intrathecal nivolumab. As of the writing of this case, he has not had a relapse of sarcoidosis following switching to single-agent nivolumab.

This case highlights a few critical points in terms of clinical presentation and management. Our patient was in his twenties, which is much younger than the cases reported in reviews. He developed fever after the first dose of combination ICI therapy and developed cough after 4 doses. While these symptoms are typically encountered, the presentation was soon after ICI initiation compared to approximately 5 to 8 months in other reported cases. As mentioned before, the presentation of sarcoidosis, on imaging, can mimic tumor progression, and clinical presentation along with histopathological diagnosis is needed to diagnose sarcoidosis, as was in this case. In previous reports, sarcoidosis irAE has been managed with steroids alone; however, this case also needed addition of methotrexate for disease control. Interestingly, after resolution of sarcoidosis symptoms, the patient was switched to single-agent nivolumab and no symptoms of a sarcoidosis irAE were noted.

References

1. Michot JM, Bigenwald C, Champiat S, Collins M, Carbonnel F, Postel-Vinay S, et al. Immune-related adverse events with immune checkpoint blockade: a comprehensive review. Eur J Cancer. 2016;54:139–48.
2. Abdel-Wahab N, Suarez-Almazor ME. Frequency and distribution of various rheumatic disorders associated with checkpoint inhibitor therapy. Rheumatology (Oxford). 2019;58(Supplement_7):vii40–vii8.
3. Pundole XN, Sarangdhar M, Suarez-Almazor ME. Rheumatic and musculoskeletal adverse events with immune checkpoint inhibitors: data from the United States Food and Drug Administration adverse event reporting system. J Immunotherapy Precis Oncol. 2019;2(3):65.
4. Eckert A, Schoeffler A, Dalle S, Phan A, Kiakouama L, Thomas L. Anti-CTLA4 monoclonal antibody induced sarcoidosis in a metastatic melanoma patient. Dermatology. 2009;218(1): 69–70.
5. Gkiozos I, Kopitopoulou A, Kalkanis A, Vamvakaris IN, Judson MA, Syrigos KN. Sarcoidosis-like reactions induced by checkpoint inhibitors. J Thorac Oncol. 2018;13(8):1076–82.
6. Tetzlaff MT, Nelson KC, Diab A, Staerkel GA, Nagarajan P, Torres-Cabala CA, et al. Granulomatous/sarcoid-like lesions associated with checkpoint inhibitors: a marker of therapy response in a subset of melanoma patients. J Immunother Cancer. 2018;6(1):14.
7. Cornejo CM, Haun P, English J 3rd, Rosenbach M. Immune checkpoint inhibitors and the development of granulomatous reactions. J Am Acad Dermatol. 2019;81(5):1165–75.
8. Mobini N, Dhillon R, Dickey J, Spoon J, Sadrolashrafi K. Exclusive cutaneous and subcutaneous Sarcoidal granulomatous inflammation due to immune checkpoint inhibitors: report of two cases with unusual manifestations and review of the literature. Case Rep Dermatol Med. 2019;2019:6702870.

9. Rambhia PH, Reichert B, Scott JF, Feneran AN, Kazakov JA, Honda K, et al. Immune checkpoint inhibitor-induced sarcoidosis-like granulomas. Int J Clin Oncol. 2019;24(10):1171–81.
10. Lafon M, Blaye C, Kind M, Bechade D, Chassaigne F, Italiano A, et al. Sarcoidosis-like reaction in metastatic triple negative breast cancer treated by anti-PD-L1. Breast J. 2019;25(5):971–3.
11. Tsuchiya K, Karayama M, Sato T, Yasui H, Hozumi H, Suzuki Y, et al. Simultaneous occurrence of sarcoidosis and anti-neutrophil cytoplasmic antibody-associated Vasculitis in a patient with lung Cancer. Intern Med. 2019;58(22):3299–304.
12. Min ST, Nordman IIC, Tran HA. Hypercalcaemia due to sarcoidosis during treatment with Avelumab for metastatic Merkel cell carcinoma. Case Rep Oncol. 2019;12(2):639–43.
13. Hiraki T, Hatanaka M, Arimura A, Kawahira H, Kirishima M, Kitazono I, et al. Granulomatous/sarcoid-like reactions in the setting of programmed cell death-1 inhibition: a potential mimic of disease recurrence. J Cutan Pathol. 2019;47(2):154–60.
14. Frohlich M, Wang H, Sakr L. Sarcoid-like reaction discovered on EBUS-TBNA of intrathoracic lymph nodes during immunotherapy for metastatic melanoma. J Immunother. 2019;43(2):75–8.
15. Mohammed H, Mahmood S. A Cutaneous case of checkpoint inhibitor-induced sarcoidosis. 2019.
16. Grosse A, Grosse C. Diagnostic yield of broncho-alveolar lavage for pembrolizumab induced sarcoid-like reaction of the lung. Cytopathology. 2019;30(6):686–7.
17. Rousseau PM, Raimbourg J, Robert M, Dansette D, Dreno B, Peuvrel L. First case of cutaneous sarcoidosis within tattoos under durvalumab. Int J Dermatol. 2019;58(9):E168–E70.
18. Honigman AD, Lai F, Elakis J, Prall O, Goh M, McCormack C. Pembrolizumab-induced sarcoid granulomatous panniculitis and bullous pemphigoid in a single patient. Clin Case Rep. 2019;7(4):773–5.
19. Rodriguez EF, Lipson E, Suresh K, Cappelli LC, Monaco SE, Maleki Z. Immune checkpoint blocker-related sarcoid-like granulomatous inflammation: a rare adverse event detected in lymph node aspiration cytology of patients treated for advanced malignant melanoma. Hum Pathol. 2019;91:69–76.
20. Faviez G, Bousquet E, Rabeau A, Rouquette I, Collot S, Goumarre C, et al. Sarcoid-like granulomatosis in cancer patients treated with immune checkpoints inhibitors. Rev Mal Respir. 2018;35(9):963–7.

21. Perez-De-Lis M, Retamozo S, Flores-Chavez A, Kostov B, Perez-Alvarez R, Brito-Zeron P, et al. Autoimmune diseases induced by biological agents. A review of 12,731 cases (BIOGEAS registry). Expert Opin Drug Saf. 2017;16(11):1255–71.
22. Tirumani SH, Ramaiya NH, Keraliya A, Bailey ND, Ott PA, Hodi FS, et al. Radiographic profiling of immune-related Adverse events in advanced melanoma patients treated with Ipilimumab. Cancer Immunol Res. 2015;3(10):1185–92.
23. Hans S, Dercle L, Champiat S, Voisin AL, Noemie C, Marabelle A, et al. Sarcoidosis-like reaction mimics progression in patients treated with immune checkpoint inhibitors. Ann Oncol. 2019;30
24. Le Burel S, Champiat S, Mateus C, Marabelle A, Michot JM, Robert C, et al. Prevalence of immune-related systemic adverse events in patients treated with anti-programmed cell death 1/anti-programmed cell death-ligand 1 agents: a single-Centre pharmacovigilance database analysis. Eur J Cancer. 2017;82:34–44.
25. Aubart FC, Lhote R, Amoura A, Valeyre D, Haroche J, Amoura Z, et al. Drug-induced sarcoidosis: an overview of the WHO pharmacovigilance database. J Intern Med. 2019;288(3):356–62.
26. Baughman RP, Lower EE, du Bois RM. Sarcoidosis. Lancet. 2003;361(9363):1111–8.
27. Robert C, Ghiringhelli F. What is the role of cytotoxic T lymphocyte–associated antigen 4 blockade in patients with metastatic melanoma? Oncologist. 2009;14(8):848–61.
28. Ji R-R, Chasalow SD, Wang L, Hamid O, Schmidt H, Cogswell J, et al. An immune-active tumor microenvironment favors clinical response to ipilimumab. Cancer Immunol Immunother. 2012;61(7):1019–31.
29. Moller D. Cells and cytokines involved in the pathogenesis of sarcoidosis. Sarcoidosis Vasc Diffuse Lung Dis. 1999;16(1):24–31.
30. Facco M, Cabrelle A, Teramo A, Olivieri V, Gnoato M, Teolato S, et al. Sarcoidosis is a Th1/Th17 multisystem disorder. Thorax. 2011;66(2):144–50.
31. Huang H, Lu Z, Jiang C, Liu J, Wang Y, Xu Z. Imbalance between Th17 and regulatory T-cells in sarcoidosis. Int J Mol Sci. 2013;14(11):21463–73.
32. von Euw E, Chodon T, Attar N, Jalil J, Koya RC, Comin-Anduix B, et al. CTLA4 blockade increases Th17 cells in patients with metastatic melanoma. J Transl Med. 2009;7(1):35.

33. Braun NA, Celada LJ, Herazo-Maya JD, Abraham S, Shaginurova G, Sevin CM, et al. Blockade of the programmed death-1 pathway restores sarcoidosis CD4+ T-cell proliferative capacity. Am J Respir Crit Care Med. 2014;190(5):560–71.
34. Ramstein J, Broos CE, Simpson LJ, Ansel KM, Sun SA, Ho ME, et al. IFN-γ–producing T-helper 17.1 cells are increased in sarcoidosis and are more prevalent than T-helper type 1 cells. Am J Respir Crit Care Med. 2016;193(11):1281–91.
35. Mortaz E, Rezayat F, Amani D, Kiani A, Garssen J, Adcock IM, et al. The roles of T helper 1, T helper 17 and regulatory T cells in the pathogenesis of sarcoidosis. Iran J Allergy Asthma Immunol. 2016;15(4):334–9.
36. Lomax AJ, McGuire HM, McNeil C, Choi CJ, Hersey P, Karikios D, et al. Immunotherapy-induced sarcoidosis in patients with melanoma treated with PD-1 checkpoint inhibitors: case series and immunophenotypic analysis. Int J Rheum Dis. 2017;20(9):1277–85.
37. Verdegaal EM, de Miranda NF, Visser M, Harryvan T, van Buuren MM, Andersen RS, et al. Neoantigen landscape dynamics during human melanoma-T cell interactions. Nature. 2016;536(7614):91–5.
38. Kristensen VN. The antigenicity of the tumor cell – context matters. N Engl J Med. 2017;376(5):491–3.
39. Kitano S, Nakayama T, Yamashita M. Biomarkers for immune checkpoint inhibitors in melanoma. Front Oncol. 2018;8:270.
40. Seve P, Schott AM, Pavic M, Broussolle C, Gilis L, Thomas L. Sarcoidosis and melanoma: a referral center study of 1,199 cases. Dermatology. 2009;219(1):25–31.
41. Arkema EV, Cozier YC. Epidemiology of sarcoidosis: current findings and future directions. Ther Adv Chronic Dis. 2018;9(11):227–40.
42. Bronstein Y, Ng CS, Hwu P, et al. Radiologic manifestations of immune-related adverse events in patients with metastatic melanoma undergoing anti-CTLA-4 antibody therapy. AJR Am J Roentgenol. 2011;197(6):992–1000.
43. Kluger N. Tattoo reactions associated with targeted therapies and immune checkpoint inhibitors for advanced cancers: a brief review. Dermatology. 2019;235(6):522–4.
44. Judson MA, Costabel U, Drent M, Wells A, Maier L, Koth L, et al. The WASOG sarcoidosis organ assessment instrument: an update of a previous clinical tool. Sarcoidosis Vasc Diffuse Lung Dis. 2014;31(1):19–27.

45. Dunn-Pirio AM, Shah S, Eckstein C. Neurosarcoidosis following Immune Checkpoint Inhibition. Case Rep Oncol. 2018;11(2):521–6.
46. Tan I, Malinzak M, Salama AKS. Delayed onset of neurosarcoidosis after concurrent ipilimumab/nivolumab therapy. J Immunother Cancer. 2018;6(1):77.
47. Luke JJ, Lezcano C, Hodi FS, Murphy GF. Antitumor granuloma formation by CD4 T cells in a patient with rapidly progressive melanoma experiencing spiking fevers, neuropathy, and other immune-related toxicity after treatment with ipilimumab. J Clin Oncology. 2015;33(6):e32–e35.
48. Murphy KP, Kennedy MP, Barry JE, et al. New-onset mediastinal and central nervous system sarcoidosis in a patient with metastatic melanoma undergoing CTLA4 monoclonal antibody treatment. Oncol Res Treat. 2014;37(6):351–3.
49. Society AT. Statement on sarcoidosis. Joint statement of the American Thoracic Society (ATS), the European Respiratory Society (ERS) and the world Association of Sarcoidosis and Other Granulomatous Disorders (WASOG) adopted by the ATS Board of directors and by the ERS executive committee. Am J Respir Crit Care Med. 1999;160(2):736–55.
50. Cohen PR, Kurzrock R. Sarcoidosis and malignancy. Clin Dermatol. 2007;25(3):326–33.
51. Prasse A. The diagnosis, differential diagnosis, and treatment of sarcoidosis. Dtsch Arztebl Int. 2016;113(33–34):565.
52. Chopra A, Nautiyal A, Kalkanis A, Judson MA. Drug-induced sarcoidosis-like reactions. Chest. 2018;154(3):664–77.
53. Ramos-Casals M, Perez-Alvarez R, Xaubet A, Bosch X, Group BS. Pulmonary disorders induced by monoclonal antibodies in patients with rheumatologic autoimmune diseases. Am J Med. 2011;124(5):386–94.
54. Brito-Zerón P, Pérez-Alvarez R, Pallarés L, Retamozo S, Baughman RP, Ramos-Casals M. Sarcoidosis: an update on current pharmacotherapy options and future directions. Expert Opin Pharmacother. 2016;17(18):2431–48.
55. Ramos-Casals M, Lambotte O, Kostine M, Calabrese L, Suarez-Almazor M, Bingham C, et al. THU0628 immune-related adverse events induced by cancer immunotherapies. Big data analysis of 13,051 cases (immunocancer international registry): BMJ Publishing Group Ltd; 2019.
56. Nishino M, Sholl LM, Awad MM, Hatabu H, Armand P, Hodi FS. Sarcoid-like granulomatosis of the lung related to immune-

checkpoint inhibitors: distinct clinical and imaging features of a unique immune-related adverse event. Cancer Immunol Res. 2018:canimm. 0715.2017.

57. Chopra A, Judson MA. How are cancer and connective tissue diseases related to sarcoidosis? Curr Opin Pulm Med. 2015;21(5):517–24.
58. Ramos-Casals MBJ, Callahan MK, Flores-Chávez A, Keegan N, Khamashta MA. Immune-related adverse events of checkpoint inhibitors. Nat Rev Dis Prim. 2020; In Press
59. Nishino M, Hatabu H, Sholl LM, Ramaiya NH. Thoracic complications of precision cancer therapies: a practical guide for radiologists in the new era of cancer care. Radiographics. 2017;37(5):1371–87.
60. Dagaonkar RS, Choong CV, Asmat AB, Ahmed DBA, Chopra A, Lim AY, et al. Significance of coexistent granulomatous inflammation and lung cancer. J Clin Pathol. 2017;70(4):337–41.
61. Schmidt LH, Huss S, Schuelke C, Schulze A, Evers G, Schliemann C, et al., editors. Noncaseating granulomatous diseases in germ cell cancer patients–a single-center experience. Urologic oncology: Seminars and Original Investigations: Elsevier; 2019.
62. Puzanov I, Diab A, Abdallah K, Bingham CO 3rd, Brogdon C, Dadu R, et al. Managing toxicities associated with immune checkpoint inhibitors: consensus recommendations from the Society for Immunotherapy of Cancer (SITC) toxicity management working group. J Immunother Cancer. 2017;5(1):95.
63. Raghu G, Berman JS, Govender P. Treatment of sarcoidosis. Am J Respir Crit Care Med. 2018;197(6):P9–P10.
64. Costabel U, Hunninghake G. ATS/ERS/WASOG statement on sarcoidosis. Sarcoidosis statement committee. American thoracic society. European respiratory society. World association for sarcoidosis and other granulomatous disorders. Eur Respir J. 1999;14(4):735–7.
65. Llabres M, Brito-Zerón P, Ramos-Casals M, Sellares J. Synthetic pharmacotherapy for pulmonary sarcoidosis. Expert Opin Pharmacother. 2019:1–8.
66. Abdel-Wahab N, Shah M, Lopez-Olivo MA, Suarez-Almazor ME. Use of immune checkpoint inhibitors in the treatment of patients with cancer and preexisting autoimmune disease. Ann Intern Med. 2018;169(2):133–4.
67. Danlos F-X, Voisin A-L, Dyevre V, Michot J-M, Routier E, Taillade L, et al. Safety and efficacy of anti-programmed death 1

antibodies in patients with cancer and pre-existing autoimmune or inflammatory disease. Eur J Cancer. 2018;91:21–9.

68. Gutzmer R, Koop A, Meier F, Hassel JC, Terheyden P, Zimmer L, et al. Programmed cell death protein-1 (PD-1) inhibitor therapy in patients with advanced melanoma and preexisting autoimmunity or ipilimumab-triggered autoimmunity. Eur J Cancer. 2017;75:24–32.
69. Johnson DB, Sullivan RJ, Ott PA, Carlino MS, Khushalani NI, Ye F, et al. Ipilimumab therapy in patients with advanced melanoma and preexisting autoimmune disorders. JAMA Oncol. 2016;2(2):234–40.
70. Kähler KC, Eigentler TK, Gesierich A, Heinzerling L, Loquai C, Meier F, et al. Ipilimumab in metastatic melanoma patients with pre-existing autoimmune disorders. Cancer Immunol Immunother. 2018;67(5):825–34.
71. Menzies AM, Johnson D, Ramanujam S, Atkinson V, Wong A, Park J, et al. Anti-PD-1 therapy in patients with advanced melanoma and preexisting autoimmune disorders or major toxicity with ipilimumab. Ann Oncol. 2016;28(2):368–76.
72. Tison A, Quéré G, Misery L, Funck-Brentano E, Danlos FX, Routier E, et al. Safety and efficacy of immune checkpoint inhibitors in patients with cancer and preexisting autoimmune disease: a nationwide, multicenter cohort study. Arthritis Rheumatol. 2019;71(12):2100–11.

Chapter 9
Miscellaneous Rheumatic Syndromes

Tamiko R. Katsumoto and Xavier Mariette

Introduction

Immune checkpoint inhibitors (ICIs) have revolutionized the field of oncology, showing unprecedented efficacy in advanced malignancies, such as lung cancer, renal cell carcinoma, and melanoma. CTLA-4 and PD-1/PD-L1 mediate T cell negative regulatory signaling pathways, called immune "checkpoints," and cancer cells can co-opt these pathways as a means of evading the immune response. Blocking these inhibitory checkpoints with antibodies to CTLA-4 and PD-1/PD-L1 unleashes the immune system, frequently enabling a productive anti-tumor response. However, this unbridled immune system can also cause collateral damage: virtually any organ may become susceptible to autoimmune attack, resulting in an immune-related adverse event (irAE).

T. R. Katsumoto (✉)
Division of Immunology and Rheumatology, Stanford University, Palo Alto, CA, USA
e-mail: tkatsum@stanford.edu

X. Mariette
Rhumatologie, Université Paris-Saclay, Assistance Publique – Hôpitaux de Paris, Hôpital Bicêtre, Le Kremlin Bicêtre, France
e-mail: Xavier.mariette@aphp.fr

M. E. Suarez-Almazor, L. H. Calabrese (eds.), *Rheumatic Diseases and Syndromes Induced by Cancer Immunotherapy*, https://doi.org/10.1007/978-3-030-56824-5_9

With the use of ICIs, rheumatic symptoms, such as arthralgias and myalgias, are frequent. The most commonly recognized rheumatic irAEs include inflammatory arthritis, polymyalgia rheumatica-like syndromes (PMR), myositis, and sicca syndrome, which can develop in ~5–10% of patients treated with ICIs [1, 2]. True incidence rates are challenging to determine, given the lack of prospective cohort studies as well as the likely underreporting of rheumatic irAEs in clinical trials.

Besides inflammatory arthritis, PMR, myositis, sicca syndrome, and sarcoidosis, other rheumatic irAEs, even less frequent, may occur after treatment with ICIs. Current guidelines (National Comprehensive Cancer Network, NCCN; Society for Immunotherapy of Cancer, SITC; American Society of Clinical Oncology, ASCO; and European Society for Medical Oncology, ESMO) provide algorithms on managing the most common rheumatic irAEs; however, they do not provide specific guidance on these less frequent rheumatic irAEs, such as vasculitis, lupus, scleroderma, and eosinophilic fasciitis [3–6]. Therefore, maintaining a high index of clinical suspicion is critical, as early recognition of irAEs will enable expedited referrals to rheumatology and other specialists, as appropriate. The goal is to expeditiously manage the irAEs such that cancer therapy can be optimized, and immunotherapy can be resumed, if clinically appropriate. The optimal management approach of these irAEs is a field that is very much in evolution. There are different treatment considerations based on risk/benefit, including the severity of the irAE and the potential for immunosuppression to impair anti-tumor immunity. Of note, some of these rarer rheumatic irAEs that will be discussed in this chapter can sometimes be more severe and, in some cases, life threatening, in which case discontinuation of ICI and/or more aggressive treatment of the irAE may be justified. Early recognition of irAEs and subspecialist involvement is paramount. Here we summarize the available literature on the clinical manifestations and treatment approaches for some of these less common rheumatic irAEs.

Vasculitis

Vasculitis is an infrequently reported irAE that tends to occur later than the other rheumatic irAEs [7]. Clinically available information is primarily limited to case reports. The diagnosis of vasculitis requires a high index of clinical suspicion, as symptoms may be protean and non-specific, leading to diagnostic challenges. Obtaining a tissue biopsy is often the gold standard for making a definitive diagnosis of vasculitis; however, this may not be practical in all situations. Given that vasculitis can have many mimickers, including other connective tissue diseases, infections, and paraneoplastic syndromes, it is critical to exclude these other potential etiologies. A detailed evaluation is often indicated, with some suggested tests shown in Table 9.1. An expeditious workup should be undertaken to circumvent irreversible long-term damage leading to morbidity and mortality.

Table 9.1 Evaluation of suspected ICI-related vasculitis

Initial assessment (to perform as clinically indicated):
Detailed history and physical exam, including:
Skin exam: Rash, e.g., palpable purpura, livedo reticularis, subcutaneous nodules
Rheum exam: Arthritis/arthralgia, myalgia/myositis
Neuro exam: Mono- or polyneuropathy, headache, seizures, focal neurologic deficits
Complete blood count with differential
Complete metabolic panel
Erythrocyte sedimentation rate, C-reactive protein
ANA
Rheumatoid factor, anti-cyclic citrullinated peptide antibody
Cryoglobulins

(continued)

TABLE 9.1 (continued)

Complement levels
Serum and urine electrophoresis and immunofixation
Urinalysis with microscopy (urine protein: creatinine ratio if proteinuria present)
ANCA (PR3, MPO)
Antiphospholipid antibodies: Beta 2 glycoprotein, anti-cardiolipin antibody, lupus anticoagulant
Hepatitis B and C, HIV
Blood cultures (bacterial and fungal)
Tuberculosis testing
Other tests as clinically indicated:
Biopsy of affected site (e.g., skin, nerve, temporal artery, kidney, lung)
Chest X-ray
EKG
Electromyography and nerve conduction study
Arterial duplex Doppler
Transthoracic echocardiogram
Bronchoscopy with lavage
Relevant cross-sectional imaging (e.g., chest CT, sinus CT, MR angiography)
Conventional angiography
Positron emission tomography

Vasculitis has been associated with both the anti-CTLA-4 antibody ipilimumab, as well as the PD-1 and PD-L1 inhibitors. The most commonly reported types of vasculitis are large vessel vasculitis and vasculitis of the nervous system; however, cases of small and medium vessel vasculitis have also been observed, as well as cases of organ-specific vasculitis. The exact mechanisms by which ICIs induce irAEs remain unknown; however, recent data on primary giant cell arteritis (GCA, also known as temporal arteritis) suggest that pathogenesis may be mediated by disruption of normal immune checkpoint mechanisms. Dendritic cells in the vessel walls of patients with GCA fail to express PD-L1, an important immuno-inhibitory ligand, thus leaving lesional T cells unopposed and enabling their activation to produce numerous inflammatory cytokines that may drive vasculitis [8]. Studies of granulomatous polyangiitis (GPA), an ANCA-associated vasculitis, have shown aberrant expression of PD-1 on T helper cells that may play a role in pathogenesis [9]. Polymorphisms in PD-1 and CTLA-4 have been linked with GPA [10], and genome-wide association studies have shown associations of ANCA vasculitis with CTLA-4 polymorphisms [11]. Thus, there are many provocative mechanisms by which immune checkpoint inhibition may be linked to the development of vasculitis and other irAEs.

A recent systematic review evaluated all the available clinical data up to Feb 2018 and identified 53 cases of vasculitis associated with ICI therapy, of which 20 were confirmed based on 2012 revised Chapel Hill Consensus Conference nomenclature [7]. The median age of these patients was 53 (31–78) years and 60% had received anti-PD-1 therapy, including one who had received combination ICI therapy. The number of treatment cycles received prior to the development of vasculitis ranged from 1 to 15 with varying dosage regimens, and the median time from the initiation of ICI to the onset of the irAE was 3 (1.2–6) months. In most cases, the vasculitis was treated by stopping the ICI and/or administering a course of oral or intravenous glucocorticoids. No fatalities due to vasculitis were noted in these 20 patients.

Large Vessel Vasculitis

A recent study evaluated adverse drug reactions reported in the VigiBase, a WHO pharmacovigilance database of global deduplicated individual case safety reports (ICSRs) [12]. ICI therapy was found to be associated with a significantly higher reporting rate for vasculitis (including GCA) as compared with the overall database. There were 82 vasculitis adverse events that were reported in patients who had received ICIs, and vasculitis was more frequently seen with those receiving anti-PD1/PD-L1 (single agent or combination ICI) compared with those receiving anti-CTLA-4 monotherapy (64 vs. 18). Of these 82 vasculitis patients, death occurred in 5 (6%), but not in patients with GCA or polymyalgia rheumatica. GCA was reported in 18 patients, with a median age of onset of 72.9 years and a median time to symptom onset of 0.7 months after ICI initiation.

To date, GCA has been the most commonly reported vasculitis irAE [12, 13, 14–16]. The reported cases of biopsy-confirmed GCA associated with ICIs presented with classic symptoms, such as occipital headache, scalp tenderness, jaw claudication, proximal myalgias, and morning stiffness, and some have had associated visual symptoms (diplopia, amaurosis fugax) [17]. Elevated inflammatory markers, ESR and CRP, were characteristically found. Cross-sectional imaging of suspected territories of involvement should be obtained, and temporal artery biopsy is considered the gold standard for diagnosis.

Cases of periaortitis have been recently reported, following 9 months of nivolumab therapy [14], after 8 doses of pembrolizumab [18], and 2 months after the third cycle of ipilimumab [19]. Periaortitis can present with systemic manifestations, including fever, chills, gastrointestinal symptoms, and abdominal pain or back pain. Cross-sectional imaging with CT or MRI can reveal soft tissue thickening around the aorta and other involved vessels. It is important to rule out infections, IgG4-related syndromes, and other autoimmune etiologies, including testing for blood cultures (bacterial and fungal), RPR, hepatitis and HIV serologies, ANA, ANCA, and IgG4. Of note, all of these cases of large vessel vasculitis tended to be highly responsive to glucocorticoids, with symptoms improving as quickly as within 1 day.

Vasculitis of the Nervous System

Aya et al. reported a patient with melanoma, who initially received anti-BRAF therapy, then ipilimumab, and finally switched to pembrolizumab [20]. Two weeks after her first pembrolizumab infusion, she developed bilateral lower extremity paresthesia in a stocking/glove distribution that rapidly progressed to severe weakness, also with a sixth cranial nerve palsy leading to diplopia. EMG nerve conduction study showed a moderate sensory peripheral neuropathy, and the muscle and nerve biopsy revealed perivascular infiltration of the small endoneural vessels consistent with a vasculitic neuropathy. The patient was treated with pulse methylprednisolone 500 mg IV for 3 days, then prednisone 50 mg a day for 6 weeks with a slow taper over 6 months, with complete functional recovery and only minimal residual paresthesia. Another case of asymmetric vasculitic neuropathy was successfully treated with pulse dose methylprednisolone 1 g for 5 days, followed by prednisone 60 mg tapered over 3 weeks [21].

There have been a few reported cases of primary angiitis of the central nervous system (PACNS), a rare vasculitic condition that is often challenging to diagnose [22, 23]. Brain MRI typically shows multifocal ischemic lesions, and confirmation of this diagnosis should ideally include a cerebral angiogram and brain biopsy, if clinically appropriate. The case presented by Laubli et al. involved prior brain irradiation, which raised the confounding diagnostic possibility of radiation necrosis that may have mimicked PACNS [24].

Other Vasculitides

The development of granulomatous polyangiitis (GPA) following ICI use is considered a rare event; however, given the potential for significant morbidity, it is important to be aware of this as a potential irAE. Van Den Brom reported a case of the rapid development of PR3 ANCA positive GPA in a woman with metastatic melanoma, who was treated initially with four cycles of ipilimumab, and then later pembrolizumab [25]. One week after her first pembrolizumab infusion, she developed fever, purpuric lesions on her feet, arthritis involving her hands, elbows, and knees, followed by progressive dyspnea, hematuria, and proteinuria with a positive PR3-ANCA. She was commenced on oral cyclophosphamide 150 mg daily and pulse methylprednisone, which induced rapid resolution of her symptoms. Nabel et al. reported a patient with pre-existing and quiescent GPA, who developed a severe flare after the first week of pembrolizumab [26].

Following three infusions of ipilimumab and nivolumab, another patient with melanoma presented with symptoms of asthma and clinically was found to have hypereosinophilia, pulmonary infiltrates, paranasal sinus abnormalities, and arthritis with negative ANCAs [27]. No tissue biopsy was obtained, but her clinical presentation was thought to be most consistent with eosinophilic granulomatous polyangiitis (EGPA). She responded well to treatment with inhaled corticosteroids, a long-acting beta agonist, and an intra-articular steroid injection.

There have been several reported cases of digital vasculitis associated with ICIs, where the time of onset has ranged from 3 to 26 weeks [28–32]. Only one of the reported cases showed complete resolution with prednisone 1 mg/kg and ICI discontinuation [30]. One case presented with Type III cryoglobulins, a positive ANA 1:160 and + SSA antibody with arterial thrombosis and capillaritis on histopathological evaluation, with partial resolution following prednisone 1 mg/kg, ICI discontinuation, as well as calcium channel blocker, iloprost, and aspirin [32]. This patient probably presented with Sjögren's syndrome-associated cryoglobulinemia. Unfortunately, most of the other reported cases led to surgical amputation despite aggressive therapy [28]. Sympathectomy has not been reported to be successful to date.

Granulomatous vasculitis has been reported in a patient after four cycles of ipilimumab for melanoma, who presented with fatigue, night sweats, chills, and diffuse lymphadenopathy and splenomegaly [33]. Lymph node biopsy showed non-necrotizing granulomatous lymphadenitis and granulomatous vasculitis, which resolved following high dose prednisone that was tapered over 6 weeks. In addition, cases of vasculitis isolated to specific organs (testicle, uterus, and retina) have been reported that have responded to short courses of steroid therapy [34–37]. A case series of leukocytoclastic vasculitis was recently reported, with clinical response to steroid therapy (0.3–0.5 mg/kg) and hydroxychloroquine (6 mg/kg daily) and with complete clinical remission within a few days [38].

Systemic Lupus Erythematosus

Compared with other rheumatic conditions such as inflammatory arthritis and polymyalgia rheumatica, systemic lupus erythematosus (SLE) is a much less common irAE, which may be, in part, reflective of the underlying biology. In the REISAMIC Registry (Registry of Severe Adverse Reactions to Immunomodulatory Antibodies used in Oncology), the prevalence of de novo lupus was found to be 0.48% based on 5 of 1044 patients who had received anti-PD-1/PD-L1 therapy [39]. The BIOGEAS Registry (Spanish Study Group of Biological Agents in Autoimmune Diseases) reported only one case of SLE in a patient receiving ipilimumab, and no case of SLE related to anti-PD-1 therapy [40]. Among 4870 rheumatic events (arthralgia = 711) in the FDA Adverse Event Reporting System (FAERS) associated with ICIs, there were 18 cases of SLE, seven cases of cutaneous SLE, two cases of lupus-like syndrome, and one case each of lupus nephritis and central nervous system lupus (as of June 2018) [41]. Anti-PD-1/PD-L1 agents were reported to be involved in these 18 cases. Of note, the mean age was older than in classical SLE: 61 years with a female:male ratio of 1.6:1. Hospitalization occurred in four cases, with one death. The median time to onset of SLE after ICIs was 196 days. Arnaud and colleagues did not identify a pharmacovigilance signal of ICIs, inducing SLE [42].

The majority of reported cases of lupus have been subcutaneous lupus erythematosus (SCLE), sometimes associated with a negative ANA and no other systemic symptoms, and, in these cases, the diagnosis of lupus may be difficult to confirm [43–45]. Blakeway et al. report two cases of SCLE that occurred with pembrolizumab, which highlight the importance of performing not only lesional histopathology but also direct immunofluorescence staining, in order to distinguish SCLE from the more commonly reported lichenoid reactions [43]. Kosche et al. report a case of fatigue associated with a pruritic eruption on the arms, thighs, and abdomen, following two cycles of ipilimumab and nivolumab for serous ovarian carcinoma [44]. Skin biopsy revealed changes consistent with SCLE, and ANA was 1:160 (speckled) with a high titer anti-SSA/Ro antibody at >8.0 AI (normal 0–0.9 AI), but with other negative subserologies. The patient was treated with prednisone 40 mg daily with a taper over 6 weeks and hydroxychloroquine 200 mg twice daily, to which quinacrine 100 mg daily was later added. The patient restarted pembrolizumab with no significant flares of her SCLE, demonstrating that ICI-induced SCLE can generally be managed with a combination of topical steroids, antimalarials (hydroxychloroquine and/or quinacrine), and a short course of oral steroids in order to obtain rapid disease control.

Although there have been several cases of nephritis reported in association with ICIs, lupus nephritis is rare. Fadel et al. report the development of nephrotic syndrome following two infusions of ipilimumab [46]. Anti-nuclear antibodies were borderline positive, and double-stranded DNA antibodies were positive (27%, normal <20%) with normal serum complement levels. Kidney biopsy showed extramembranous and mesangial deposits of IgG, IgM, C3, and C1q, suggestive of lupus nephritis. Details of treatment are unclear, but the patient improved and showed resolution of nephrotic range proteinuria with withdrawal of ipilimumab.

Scleroderma

Barbosa et al. reported two cases of ICI-induced scleroderma with clinical presentations most consistent with diffuse and limited scleroderma, respectively [47]. The first patient developed fatigue, joint swelling, skin dryness and burning, and muscle weakness after cycle 13 of pembrolizumab for melanoma. Pembrolizumab was discontinued and he was started on prednisone 1 mg/kg daily. Weakness progressed and he rapidly developed diffuse skin tightness with a modified Rodnan skin score of 36 (out of a maximal score of 51). Symptoms were notable for the absence of Raynaud's, gastroesophageal reflux, dysphagia, diarrhea, or shortness of breath. No nailfold capillary changes, synovitis, or tendon friction rubs were noted. Skin biopsy showed mild dermal fibrosis and sclerosis with trapping of adnexal structures and minimal lymphocytic inflammation, consistent with a sclerosing process. C-reactive protein was mildly elevated, with a normal ESR and negative ANA, including anti-centromere, anti-RNP, and anti-topoisomerase (Scl-70) antibodies; however, anti-RNA polymerase 3 was not tested. Muscle enzymes were not elevated. Electromyography showed a sensorimotor polyneuropathy (primarily axonal), without evidence of myopathy, and no muscle biopsy was performed. The patient was treated with IVIG (0.4 mg/kg for 5 days monthly) mycophenolate mofetil 1000 mg twice a day, and prednisone, which was tapered within 8 weeks, with improvement in his skin and muscle strength.

The second patient was a 79-year-old male with Stage IV melanoma, who developed Raynaud's phenomenon with hand and foot stiffness and shortness of breath after cycle 5 of pembrolizumab. His modified Rodnan skin score was 12, and he was found to have mildly dilated nailfold capillaries and inspiratory crackles at the left lung base. Skin biopsies showed mild perivascular lymphocytic inflammation and deep dermal sclerosis, consistent with a sclerodermoid reaction. Autoantibodies were negative (including ANA, anti-centromere, anti-RNP, and anti-Scl-70, but RNA polymerase 3 was not tested). Echocardiogram did not show elevation in right ventricular systolic pressure. Chest CT showed patchy ground glass infiltrates in the lower lung fields. The patient was diagnosed with limited systemic sclerosis secondary to pembrolizumab and pembrolizumab-induced pneumonitis, and pembrolizumab was discontinued. The patient was treated with hydroxychloroquine 200 mg twice daily and prednisone starting at 1 mg/kg with a rapid taper, and clinical improvement in his fatigue, shortness of breath, and acral stiffness was observed within 3 weeks, along with a decrease in ground glass opacities on chest CT.

Other scleroderma-like reactions have been reported, which, in some circumstances, have required the use of steroid-sparing agents such as mycophenolate mofetil [48, 49]. Collaboration with rheumatology and dermatology is especially critical in these cases, given the rarity of scleroderma and scleroderma-like conditions. Scleroderma can be limited to the skin or, in the case of systemic sclerosis, can lead to internal organ complications such as interstitial lung disease or gastrointestinal dysmotility. There may be a heightened risk of ICI-induced pneumonitis in patients with pre-existing ILD, such that these patients should be closely monitored. Scleroderma renal crisis is a disease-specific complication to be aware of, more frequently associated with diffuse cutaneous systemic sclerosis and the anti-RNA polymerase 3 antibody that has strong associations with paraneoplastic scleroderma [50]. Scleroderma renal crisis can be precipitated by the use of high dose steroids (i.e., prednisone >15 mg/day); however, whether this risk also applies to ICI-induced scleroderma remains unknown, and the few reported cases of scleroderma to date that have been treated with high dose steroids did not develop this complication.

Eosinophilic Fasciitis

Eosinophilic fasciitis (EF), also known as Shulman syndrome, is a rare fibrosing disorder whose pathogenesis is poorly understood and is characterized by limb or trunk erythema and edema, followed by collagenous thickening of the subcutaneous fascia. Eosinophilia is variably present, typically in the early phases of disease. Although EF shares some similarities with scleroderma, there is the notable absence of sclerodactyly, Raynaud's phenomenon, telangiectasias, and dilated nailfold capillary loops. EF is characterized by inflammatory cell infiltration of the fascia, leading to thickening and fibrosis and resulting in the characteristic "groove sign" suggesting involvement deeper than that seen in scleroderma. The two major diagnostic criteria for EF, after ruling out scleroderma, are (1) swelling or induration of the skin and subcutaneous tissues and (2) fascial thickening with lymphocytes and macrophages, with or without eosinophilic infiltration on a full-thickness skin biopsy. If only one of the major criteria is present, then the presence of any two of the following minor criteria will support the diagnosis: (1) peripheral eosinophilia, (2) hypergammaglobulinemia, (3) muscle weakness, (4) groove sign, or (5) hyperintense fascia on T2-weighted images by MRI [51].

Although most cases of EF have been considered idiopathic, there have been associations with infections [52, 53], radiation therapy, burns, graft-versus-host disease, hematologic disorders, exposure to certain medications, and autoimmune diseases (such as thyroid disease, primary biliary cirrhosis, systemic lupus erythematosus, Sjogren's syndrome) [54–57]. A recent case series and review of the literature by Chan et al. describes 15 EF cases in patients undergoing treatment with ICIs, highlighting a new potential etiology of EF and the importance of being aware of this rare condition [58]. Early collaboration among oncology, rheumatology, and dermatology is critical, given the aggressive nature of EF and potential for irreversible damage without early intervention, including joint contractures that can profoundly limit mobility.

In several of these reported cases of ICI-induced EF, patients typically presented with myalgias and limb edema, often accompanied by fatigue and sometimes fever [58]. The timing of onset after treatment with ICIs ranged from 1.5 months up to 24 months, and the majority of cases involved PD-1/PD-L1 inhibition, with metastatic melanoma being the most frequent diagnosis. Peak absolute eosinophil count ranged from 600 to 5240/uL, but, in many cases, this data was not reported. An extremity MRI was performed in 11 of the 15 cases, with findings suggestive of the diagnosis of EF. Eight patients had a full-thickness skin biopsy that showed dense inflammation of the fascia by lymphocytes and plasma cells, sometimes with tissue eosinophilia. Available immunohistochemistry reports on five patients revealed a T-cell dominant (CD3+) infiltrate, in some cases with a CD4+ predominance, and others with a CD8+ predominance. The checkpoint inhibitor was discontinued in the majority of cases. Eight of the fifteen patients demonstrated complete tumor response (most of whom received high dose steroids and either methotrexate or mycophenolate mofetil for treatment of their EF), one with partial response, one with stable disease, four with disease progression, and one with no outcome reported.

There have been no randomized controlled trials in primary EF, given the rarity of this condition, and hence the optimal treatment approach in EF, including ICI-induced EF, is unknown. Glucocorticoids are the mainstay of treatment, often starting at doses of prednisone 1 mg/kg/day. Steroids are tapered as the affected skin softens, which can take weeks to months. In patients who have relapses or inadequate response to steroids alone, methotrexate is most commonly utilized (at 15–25 mg/week), and mycophenolate mofetil is also a reasonable approach. In a large cohort of 63 patients, complete response was achieved in 64% of patients treated with a combination of methotrexate and prednisone [59]; however, the responses in ICI-induced EF have been less impressive [58]. Another retrospective study of 32 patients suggested that patients who received pulse dose methylprednisolone

500–1000 mg/day had better responses [60]. Other potential agents that have been tried in EF include azathioprine, sulfasalazine, penicillamine, cyclosporine, rituximab, infliximab, tocilizumab, and tofacitinib [61–63]. Given the mechanism of ICIs, the use of T-cell-directed therapies could be more easily justified; however, there is no data available to support this recommendation. Discontinuation of ICI has occurred in most cases reported to date. Early referral to rheumatology and dermatology is critical to optimize the treatment of this challenging condition, including getting physical therapy involved early in order to prevent loss of mobility. Further experience is needed in order to identify the most effective treatment approaches in ICI-induced EF.

Conclusions and Future Directions

In conclusion, besides the most common rheumatic irAEs of inflammatory arthritis, PMR, myositis, sicca syndrome, and sarcoidosis, other rare rheumatic irAEs may occur, mainly lupus-like diseases, scleroderma-like diseases, vasculitis, and EF. It is tempting to hypothesize that the reason these rheumatic irAEs are less common after ICI treatment is because the role of T cells may be less important in these diseases, as compared to RA-like, PMR-like, myositis, or Sjögren's-like conditions. In fact, further investigation is necessary to achieve a better understanding of the pathophysiologic mechanisms underlying these irAEs and what they can teach us about these primary rheumatic autoimmune diseases independent of ICIs.

Finally, an interesting observation regarding rheumatic complications of ICIs is that the most frequent adverse events are exacerbations of back pain, tendinitis, or other mechanical pain (i.e., linked to osteoarthritis): in the study by Kostine et al., half of the rheumatic adverse events post ICIs belonged to this category [64]. Until now, we did not know if these rheumatic complications were immune-mediated or not. The rheumatologist should be aware of this when a patient is referred with musculoskeletal symptoms after ICI treatment.

References

1. Narváez J, et al. Rheumatic immune-related adverse events in patients on anti-PD-1 inhibitors: fasciitis with myositis syndrome as a new complication of immunotherapy. Autoimmun Rev. 2018;17(10):1040–5. https://doi.org/10.1016/j.autrev.2018.05.002.
2. Richter MD, Crowson C, Kottschade LA, Finnes HD, Markovic SN, Thanarajasingam U. Rheumatic syndromes associated with immune checkpoint inhibitors: a single-center cohort of sixty-one patients. Arthritis Rheumatol. 2019;71(3):468–75. https://doi.org/10.1002/art.40745.
3. Puzanov I, et al. Managing toxicities associated with immune checkpoint inhibitors: consensus recommendations from the Society for Immunotherapy of Cancer (SITC) Toxicity Management Working Group. J Immunother Cancer. 2017;5(1):1–28. https://doi.org/10.1186/s40425-017-0300-z.
4. Brahmer JR, et al. Management of immune-related adverse events in patients treated with immune checkpoint inhibitor therapy: American society of clinical oncology clinical practice guideline. J Clin Oncol. 2018;36(17):1714–68. https://doi.org/10.1200/JCO.2017.77.6385.
5. Guidelines CP. Management of toxicities from immunotherapy : ESMO Clinical Practice Guidelines for diagnosis, treatment and follow-up. Clinical Practice Guidelines. 2017;28(Supplement 4):119–42. https://doi.org/10.1093/annonc/mdx225.
6. Thompson JA, et al. Management of immunotherapy-related toxicities, version 1.2019. JNCCN J Natl Compr Cancer Netw. 2019;17(3):255–89. https://doi.org/10.6004/jnccn.2019.0013.
7. Daxini A, Cronin K, Sreih AG. Vasculitis associated with immune checkpoint inhibitors—a systematic review. Clin Rheumatol. 2018;37(9):2579–84. https://doi.org/10.1007/s10067-018-4177-0.
8. Watanabe R, Zhang H, Berry G, Goronzy JJ, Weyand CM. Immune checkpoint dysfunction in large and medium vessel vasculitis. Am J Physiol Heart Circ Physiol. 2017;312(5):H1052–9. https://doi.org/10.1152/ajpheart.00024.2017.

9. Wilde B, et al. Aberrant expression of the negative costimulator PD-1 on T cells in granulomatosis with polyangiitis. Rheumatol (United Kingdom). 2012;51(7):1188–97. https://doi.org/10.1093/rheumatology/kes034.
10. Slot MC, Sokolowska MG, Savelkouls KG, Janssen RGJH, Damoiseaux JGMC, Cohen Tervaert JW. Immunoregulatory gene polymorphisms are associated with ANCA-related vasculitis. Clin Immunol. 2008;128(1):39–45. https://doi.org/10.1016/j.clim.2008.03.506.
11. Alberici F, Martorana D, Vaglio A. Genetic aspects of anti-neutrophil cytoplasmic antibody-associated vasculitis. Nephrol Dial Transplant. 2014;30:i37–45. https://doi.org/10.1093/ndt/gfu386.
12. Salem JE, et al. Cardiovascular toxicities associated with immune checkpoint inhibitors: an observational, retrospective, pharmacovigilance study. Lancet Oncol. 2018;19(12):1579–89. https://doi.org/10.1016/S1470-2045(18)30608-9.
13. Cappelli LC, Shah AA, Bingham CO. Immune-related adverse effects of Cancer immunotherapy— implications for rheumatology. Rheum Dis Clin N Am. 2017;43(1):65–78. https://doi.org/10.1016/j.rdc.2016.09.007.
14. Roy AK, Tathireddy HR, Roy M. Aftermath of induced inflammation: acute periaortitis due to nivolumab therapy. BMJ Case Rep. 2017;2017:3–5. https://doi.org/10.1136/bcr-2017-221852.
15. Abdel-Wahab N, Shah M, Suarez-Almazor ME. Adverse events associated with immune checkpoint blockade in patients with Cancer: a systematic review of case reports. PLoS One. 2016;11(7):e0160221. https://doi.org/10.1371/journal.pone.0160221.
16. Goldstein BL, Gedmintas L, Todd DJ. Concise communication. Arthritis Rheumatol. 2014;66(3):768–9. https://doi.org/10.1002/art.38282.
17. Goldstein BL, et al. Immune checkpoint dysfunction in large and medium vessel vasculitis. J Immunother Cancer. 2019;58(1):1. https://doi.org/10.1016/j.ejim.2018.07.023.
18. Tolaymat OA, et al. Drug-associated vasculitis occurring after treatment with pembrolizumab. Rheumatology (Oxford). 2019;58(8):1501–3. https://doi.org/10.1093/rheumatology/kez051.
19. Ban B, Crowe J, Graham R. Rheumatology case report: immune-reltaed aortitis associated with ipilimumab. The Rheumatologist, 2017;11(5).

20. Aya F, Ruiz-Esquide V, Viladot M, Font C, Prieto-Gonzalez S, Prat A. Vasculitic neuropathy induced by pembrolizumab. Ann Oncol. 2017;28(2):433–4.
21. Kao JC, et al. Neurological complications associated with anti–programmed death 1 (PD-1) antibodies. JAMA Neurol. 2017;74(10):1216–22. https://doi.org/10.1001/jamaneurol.2017.1912.
22. Läubli H, et al. Cerebral vasculitis mimicking intracranial metastatic progression of lung cancer during PD-1 blockade. J Immunother Cancer. 2017;5(1):1–6. https://doi.org/10.1186/s40425-017-0249-y.
23. Bender HJ, Dimitrakopoulou-Strauss A, Enk A. Safety of the PD-1 antibody pembrolizumab in patients with high-grade adverse events under ipilimumab treatment. Ann Oncol. 2016;27(7):1353–4.
24. Sun R, et al. Anti-PD-1 Vasculitis of the central nervous system or radionecrosis? J Immunother Cancer. 2017;5(1):4–6. https://doi.org/10.1186/s40425-017-0304-8.
25. van den Brom RRH, et al. Rapid granulomatosis with polyangiitis induced by immune checkpoint inhibition. Rheumatol (United Kingdom). 2016;55(6):1143–5. https://doi.org/10.1093/rheumatology/kew063.
26. Nabel CS, et al. Anti-PD-1 immunotherapy-induced flare of a known underlying relapsing vasculitis mimicking recurrent cancer. Oncologist. 2019;24(8):1013–21. https://doi.org/10.1634/theoncologist.2018-0633.
27. Roger A, et al. Eosinophilic granulomatosis with polyangiitis (Churg-Strauss) induced by immune checkpoint inhibitors. Ann Rheum Dis. 2019;78(8):8–9. https://doi.org/10.1136/annrheumdis-2018-213857.
28. Padda A, Schiopu E, Sovich J, Ma V, Alva A, Fecher L. Ipilimumab induced digital vasculitis. J Immunother Cancer. 2018;6(1):3–7. https://doi.org/10.1186/s40425-018-0321-2.
29. Gambichler T, Strutzmann S, Tannapfel A, Susok L. Paraneoplastic acral vascular syndrome in a patient with metastatic melanoma under immune checkpoint blockade. BMC Cancer. 2017;17(1):1–5. https://doi.org/10.1186/s12885-017-3313-6.
30. Comont T, Sibaud V, Mourey L, Cougoul P, Beyne-Rauzy O. Immune checkpoint inhibitor-related acral vasculitis. J Immunother Cancer. 2018;6(1):120. https://doi.org/10.1186/s40425-018-0443-6.

31. Khaddour K, Singh V, Shayuk M. Acral vascular necrosis associated with immune-check point inhibitors: case report with literature review. BMC Cancer. 2019;19(1):1–6. https://doi.org/10.1186/s12885-019-5661-x.
32. Le Burel S, et al. Prevalence of immune-related systemic adverse events in patients treated with anti-programmed cell death 1/anti-programmed cell death-ligand 1 agents: a single-Centre pharmacovigilance database analysis. Eur J Cancer. 2017;82:34–44. https://doi.org/10.1016/j.ejca.2017.05.032.
33. Arellano K, Mosley JC, Moore DC. Case report of Ipilimumab-induced diffuse, nonnecrotizing granulomatous lymphadenitis and granulomatous Vasculitis. J Pharm Pract. 2018;31(2):227–9. https://doi.org/10.1177/0897190017699762.
34. Weiner R, Hanson B, Rehman J, Sun B. Isolated testicular vasculitis due to immune checkpoint inhibitor. no. 4. 2019. https://doi.org/10.5152/eurjrheum.2019.19061.
35. Tsui E, Gonzales JA. Retinal vasculitis associated with Ipilimumab. Ocul Immunol Inflamm. 2019;3948:1–3. https://doi.org/10.1080/09273948.2019.1610460.
36. Manusow JS, Khoja L, Pesin N, Joshua AM, Mandelcorn ED. Retinal vasculitis and ocular vitreous metastasis following complete response to PD-1 inhibition in a patient with metastatic cutaneous melanoma. J Immunother Cancer. 2015;2(1):2–5. https://doi.org/10.1186/s40425-014-0041-1.
37. Minor DR, Bunker SR, Doyle J. Lymphocytic vasculitis of the uterus in a patient with melanoma receiving ipilimumab. J Clin Oncol. 2013;31(20):2019. https://doi.org/10.1200/JCO.2012.47.5095.
38. Tomelleri A, Campochiaro C, De Luca G, Cavalli G, Dagna L. Anti-PD1 therapy-associated cutaneous leucocytoclastic vasculitis: A case series. Eur J Intern Med. 2018;57:e11–2. https://doi.org/10.1016/j.ejim.2018.07.023.
39. Michot JM, et al. Drug-induced lupus erythematosus following immunotherapy with anti-programmed death-(ligand) 1. Ann Rheum Dis. 2019;78(7):1–3. https://doi.org/10.1136/annrheumdis-2018-213677.
40. Pérez-De-Lis M, et al. Autoimmune diseases induced by biological agents. A review of 12,731 cases (BIOGEAS registry). Expert Opin Drug Saf. 2017; https://doi.org/10.1080/14740338.2017.1372421.

41. Raschi E, Antonazzo IC, Poluzzi E, De Ponti F. Drug-induced systemic lupus erythematosus: should immune checkpoint inhibitors be added to the evolving list? Ann Rheum Dis. 2019; https://doi.org/10.1136/annrheumdis-2019-215819.
42. Arnaud L, Lebrun-Vignes B, Salem JE. Checkpoint inhibitor-associated immune arthritis. Ann Rheum Dis. 2019;78(7):1–2. https://doi.org/10.1136/annrheumdis-2018-213470.
43. Blakeway EA, Elshimy N, Muinonen-Martin A, Marples M, Mathew B, Mitra A. Cutaneous lupus associated with pembrolizumab therapy for advanced melanoma: a report of three cases. Melanoma Res. 2019;29(3):338–41. https://doi.org/10.1097/CMR.0000000000000587.
44. Kosche C, Owen JL, Choi JN. Widespread subacute cutaneous lupus erythematosus in a patient receiving checkpoint inhibitor immunotherapy with ipilimumab and nivolumab. Dermatol Online J. 2019;25(10):0–3.
45. Liu RC, Sebaratnam DF, Jackett L, Kao S, Lowe PM. Subacute cutaneous lupus erythematosus induced by nivolumab. Australas J Dermatol. 2018;59(2):e152–4. https://doi.org/10.1111/ajd.12681.
46. Fadel KB, El Karoui K. Anti-CTLA4 antibody-induced lupus nephritis. N Engl J Med. 2009;361(2):211–2.
47. Barbosa NS, Wetter DA, Wieland CN, Shenoy NK, Markovic SN, Thanarajasingam U. Scleroderma induced by Pembrolizumab: a case series. Mayo Clin Proc. 2017;92(7):1158–63. https://doi.org/10.1016/j.mayocp.2017.03.016.
48. Tjarks BJ, Kerkvliet AM, Jassim AD, Bleeker JS. Scleroderma-like skin changes induced by checkpoint inhibitor therapy. J Cutan Pathol. 2018;45(8):615–8. https://doi.org/10.1111/cup.13273.
49. Shenoy N, Esplin B, Barbosa N, Wieland C, Thanarajasingam U, Markovic S. Pembrolizumab induced severe sclerodermoid reaction. Ann Oncol. 2017;28(2):432–3. https://doi.org/10.1093/annonc/mdw543.
50. Shah AA, Casciola-Rosen L. Cancer and scleroderma: a paraneoplastic disease with implications for malignancy screening. Curr Opin Rheumatol. 2015;27(6):563–70. https://doi.org/10.1097/BOR.0000000000000222.
51. Pinal-Fernandez I, Selva-O' Callaghan A, Grau JM. Diagnosis and classification of eosinophilic fasciitis. Autoimmun Rev. 2014;13(4–5):379–82. https://doi.org/10.1016/j.autrev.2014.01.019.
52. Granter SR, Barnhill RL, Hewins ME, Duray PH. Identification of Borrelia burgdorferi in diffuse fasciitis with peripheral eosinophilia: Borrelial fasciitis. Clin Pediatr. 1995; https://doi.org/10.1001/jama.272.16.1283.

53. Hashimoto Y, et al. Polymerase chain reaction of borrelia burgdorferi flagellin gene in shulman syndrome. Dermatology. 1996; https://doi.org/10.1159/000246339.
54. Bachmeyer C, Monge M, Dhôte R, Sanguina M, Aractingi S, Mougeot-Martin M. Eosinophilic fasciitis following idiopathic thrombocytopenic purpura, autoimmune hemolytic anemia and Hashimoto's disease [6]. Dermatology. 1999; https://doi.org/10.1159/000018271.
55. Imren S, Tüzüner N, Yazici H. Eosinophilic fasciitis with thyroid disease. Clin Exp Rheumatol. 1988;
56. Boiesen M, Keiding LM, Thomsen K. Eosinophilic fasciitis: report of a case with features of other autoimmune disease. Dermatology. 1983; https://doi.org/10.1159/000249768.
57. Smiley AM, Husain M, Indenbaum S. Eosinophilic fasciitis in association with thyroid disease: a report of three cases. J Rheumatol. 1980;
58. Chan KK, et al. Eosinophilic fasciitis following checkpoint inhibitor therapy: four cases and a review of literature. Oncologist. 2019; https://doi.org/10.1634/theoncologist.2019-0508.
59. Wright NA, Mazori DR, Patel M, Merola JF, Femia AN, Vleugels RA. Epidemiology and treatment of eosinophilic fasciitis: an analysis of 63 patients from 3 tertiary care centers. JAMA Dermatol. 2016; https://doi.org/10.1001/jamadermatol.2015.3648.
60. Wechsler B, et al. Concise report Eosinophilic fasciitis (Shulman disease): new insights into the therapeutic management from a series of 34 patients. 2011, p. 557–61. doi: https://doi.org/10.1093/rheumatology/ker366.
61. Lebeaux D, Sène D. Eosinophilic fasciitis (Shulman disease). Best Pract Res Clin Rheumatol. 2012;26(4):449–58. https://doi.org/10.1016/j.berh.2012.08.001.
62. Fett N, Arthur M. Eosinophilic fasciitis: current concepts. Clin Dermatol. 2018;36(4):487–97. https://doi.org/10.1016/j.clindermatol.2018.04.006.
63. Kim SR, Charos A, Damsky W, Heald P, Girardi M, King BA. Treatment of generalized deep morphea and eosinophilic fasciitis with the Janus kinase inhibitor tofacitinib. JAAD Case Rep. 2018;4(5):443–5. https://doi.org/10.1016/j.jdcr.2017.12.003.
64. Kostine M, et al. Rheumatic disorders associated with immune checkpoint inhibitors in patients with cancer-clinical aspects and relationship with tumour response: a single-Centre prospective cohort study. Ann Rheum Dis. 2018;77(3):393–8. https://doi.org/10.1136/annrheumdis-2017-212257.

Chapter 10
Non-Rheumatic Immune-Related Adverse Events

Aanika Balaji, Bairavi Shankar, and Jarushka Naidoo

Introduction

Immune-related adverse events (irAEs) from immune checkpoint inhibitors (ICIs) can result in a wide spectrum of toxicities affecting multiple organ systems (Table 10.1) [1]. Due to FDA approvals in approximately 14 different cancer indications, ICIs are being increasingly used in routine clinical practice. For oncology practitioners and the organ specialists to whom they may refer patients with irAEs, it may be a challenge to identify irAEs early and initiate appropriate management [2]. The severity of irAEs is graded utilizing the Common Terminology Criteria for Adverse Events (CTCAE version 5) [3].

A. Balaji · B. Shankar
Johns Hopkins University School of Medicine, Baltimore, MD, USA
e-mail: abalaji1@jhmi.edu; bshanka3@jhmi.edu

J. Naidoo (✉)
Department of Oncology, Sidney Kimmel Comprehensive Cancer Center Johns Hopkins University, Baltimore, MD, USA

Bloomberg-Kimmel Institute for Cancer Immunotherapy at Johns Hopkins University, Baltimore, MD, USA
e-mail: jnaidoo1@jhmi.edu

M. E. Suarez-Almazor, L. H. Calabrese (eds.), *Rheumatic Diseases and Syndromes Induced by Cancer Immunotherapy*,
https://doi.org/10.1007/978-3-030-56824-5_10

Table 10.1 A list of reported irAEs by organ system. Bolded irAEs will be further discussed in this chapter

Organ system	Spectrum of irAEs
Dermatologic	**Maculopapular rash/dermatitis**
	Pruritis
	Lichenoid dermatitis
	Oral mucositis
	Dermatitis acneiform
	Bullous pemphigoid
Ocular	**Uveitis**
	Conjunctivitis
	Episcleritis
	Orbital inflammation
	Blepharitis
Neurologic	**Autoimmune encephalitis**
	Peripheral neuropathy
	Myasthenia gravis
	Guillain-Barre syndrome
	Posterior reversible encephalopathy syndrome
	Aseptic meningitis
	Enteric neuropathy
	Transverse myelitis
	Pancerebellitis
	Cranial neuropathy
	Neurosensory hyperacusis
Cardiovascular	**Myocarditis**
	Pericarditis
Pulmonary	**Pneumonitis**
	Sarcoid-like reactions
Endocrine	**Hypothyroidism**
	Hyperthyroidism
	Hypophysitis
	Type 1 diabetes mellitus
	Thyroiditis
	Adrenal insufficiency
	Cushing's syndrome
	Hypogonadism

TABLE 10.1 (continued)

Organ system	Spectrum of irAEs
Gastrointestinal	**Colitis** **Hepatitis** **Pancreatitis** Diarrhea Small bowel enteritis
Renal	**Acute tubulointerstitial nephritis** Immune complex glomerulonephritis Thrombotic microangiopathy
Hematologic	**Thrombocytopenia** Red cell aplasia Acquired hemophilia A Cryoglobulinemia Hemophagocytic lympohistiocytosis Lymphopenia Aplastic anemia Pernicious anemia
Rheumatologic	Inflammatory arthritis Polymyalgia rheumatica Giant cell arteritis Sicca syndrome Systemic lupus erythematosus Psoriasis Vasculitis

Data from late-phase clinical trials estimate the incidence of any grade irAEs range from 15% to 90% [4, 5]. The incidence of high grade (CTCAE grade 3+) in these late-phase trials range from 10% to 42% [4, 5]. Immune-related adverse events are more common and more severe among those treated with combination ICIs [6]. Phase I trials of combination ICIs have shown 94% of patients develop any grade toxicity and 56% develop high-grade (CTCAE grade 3+) toxicities [7, 8]. The two most common classes of ICIs, cytotoxic T lymphocyte-associated antigen 4 (CTLA-4) and programmed death 1 (PD-1)/programmed cell death ligand-1

(PD-L1) therapies, are associated with different patterns of irAEs. Colitis and hypophysitis are more commonly seen with CTLA-4 therapy [9], while patients more commonly develop pneumonitis and thyroiditis with PD-1/PD-L1 therapy [10, 11]. A general outline of the approach to the diagnosis and management of patients who develop irAEs is depicted in Fig. 10.1 [12].

The management of irAEs is guided by the CTCAE grade. For patients who develop grade 1 toxicity, ICI therapy may be continued under close supervision or withheld for selected irAEs, such as pneumonitis [13]. Those who develop toxicities that are grade 2 or higher usually require ICI withholding and treatment of the irAE with corticosteroids (with the exception of selected endocrine toxicities) [14]. Higher-grade (grade 3+) require hospitalization and treatment with high-dose systemic corticosteroids [15]. Importantly, high-grade irAEs may require additional immunosuppressive therapy if there is no clinical improvement in the irAE within 48–72 hours of management [12]. A recent meta-analysis reported deaths from irAEs occurred at a rate of 0.3–1.3%, with the most fatal toxicities including pneumonitis and myocarditis [16]. If grade 2+ toxicities resolve completely or to less than grade 1, the treating provider may consider restarting ICI therapy [17].

This chapter aims to provide a practical guide to assist rheumatology practitioners in the diagnosis and management

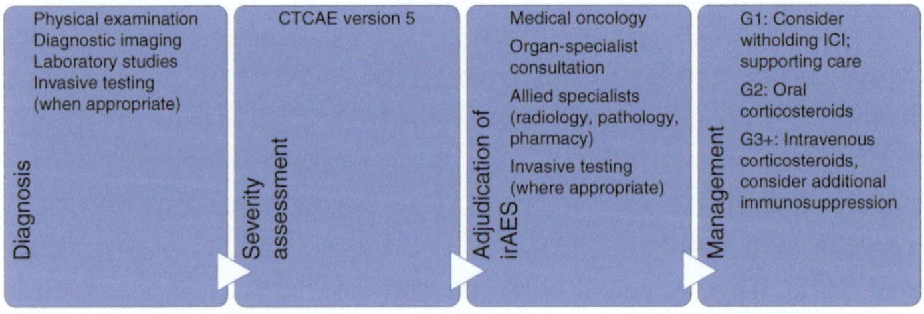

FIGURE 10.1 A workflow of the diagnosis and management of irAEs. (Figure adapted from Connolly [12])

of common non-rheumatological irAEs. Herein, we highlight current knowledge on epidemiology, risk factors, diagnostic evaluation, management, and unanswered questions for common irAEs that occur from ICIs for cancer.

Neurologic Immune-Related Adverse Events

The central nervous system (CNS) is partially safeguarded from an influx of immune cells by the blood-brain barrier [18]. Under normal circumstances, few lymphocytes are present in and cerebrospinal fluid (CSF) [18]. Brain cancers and metastases can disrupt the blood-brain barrier [19]. With the loss of the blood-brain barrier's immune protection, treatment with ICIs can lead to increased lymphocyte access to the CNS [20]. Overactivation of the immune system can lead to neurologic irAEs [21].

Neurologic irAEs are rare, occurring in less than 4% of patients with CTLA-4 therapy, 6% with PD-1/PD-L1 therapy, and 12% with combination therapy [22]. However, these figures may be an underestimation, as patients and providers may not recognize the signs and symptoms of neurologic irAEs and underreport them [19]. Grade 3+ events occur in less than 1% of patients; however, deaths from neurologic irAEs have been reported [19]. The published experience of neurologic irAEs is mainly based on large case series and isolated case reports [23–25].

Challenges in identifying and managing neurologic irAEs include nonspecific patient presentations and early identification and management of these sequelae may have a lifelong impact on patients' quality-of-life [26]. In a published case series by Fellner et al. the mean time to onset for a neurologic irAE was 8 weeks after the initiation of ICI [27]. A case series by Dubey et al. demonstrated that patients who restart ICIs after an initial neurologic irAE are at a higher risk of redeveloping their neurologic irAEs (60% relapse vs. 14% relapse rates comparing restarted ICI group to permanently discontinued ICIs) [28].

Acute Encephalitis

While prospective data on the epidemiology of encephalitis are lacking, it is estimated that approximately 0.1–0.2% of patients treated with ICIs develop autoimmune encephalitis [20]. In a review of 13 immune-related encephalitis cases by Blackmon et al., 60% of cases were associated with ipilimumab use and 20% associated with programmed cell death-1 (PD-1) monotherapy [29]. Encephalitis occurred a median 6 weeks after ICI commencement [24]. There are no known risk factors for immune-related encephalitis [30].

Clinically, patients with ICI-encephalitis may present with a range of symptoms, including headache, altered mental status, unusual behaviors, dysarthria, personality change, sensory deficits, or movement disorders [17, 31]. Differential diagnoses include infectious meningitis, viral encephalitis, brain metastases, and leptomeningeal disease [20]. Initial diagnostic tools include a thorough clinical history and physical examination with emphasis on the neurological exam [32]. Laboratory tests, such as complete blood count (CBC), comprehensive metabolic panel (CMP), pituitary hormones, ESP, C-reactive protein (CRP), antineutrophil cytoplasmic antibodies (ANCA), and thyroid studies should be sent to rule out other common causes of altered mental status. Additional studies can include anti-NMDA-receptor antibodies to rule out autoimmune encephalitis [33].

Initial, noninvasive testing includes radiologic investigations. MRI of the brain is a useful diagnostic tool, primarily to rule out the presence of focal brain metastases, hemorrhage, or stroke [34]. In case reports, MRI has identified that these patients may display abnormal T2-weighted hypo- or hyperintensity in various regions of the brain, including hypointensity of basal ganglia, enhancing bilateral temporal lobe foci, and white matter lesions in the parietal and frontal lobes in reported case series [30, 33, 35]. After treatment, MRI can also be used to track the resolution of encephalitis [29].

While a more invasive test, sampling of cerebrospinal fluid (CSF) via lumbar puncture may help to hone the differential diagnosis, in particular to rule out infectious causes of meningitis, such as enterovirus, herpesvirus, *Neisseria meningitidis*, *Streptococcus pneumoniae*, and *Listeria monocytogenes* [29, 36–38]. In 60% of encephalitis cases, the CSF displays a lymphocytic pleocytosis [29]. Electroencephalogram (EEG) assessments in patients with suspected encephalitis can identify focal or widespread slowing or subclinical epileptiform activity [34, 39].

Treatment algorithms have been created to provide differential treatments based on CTCAE grading. Table 10.2 outlines typical treatments used for encephalitis [3]. Early detection and treatment can stop and possibly reverse neurological consequences and lead to complete resolution of the irAE [21]. Many combinations of treatments have been suc-

Table 10.2 Treatment schema for immune-mediated encephalopathy based on CTCAE grade

CTCAE grade	**Symptoms**	**Management**
1	Asymptomatic	Hold ICI Close clinical monitoring of symptoms
2	Moderate: concerning symptoms for the patients	Stop ICI Start methylprednisolone 1–2 mg/kg/day Neurology consultation
3 4	Severe symptoms	Discontinue ICI permanently Hospitalization and neurology consultation Pulse IV methylprednisolone 1 g/day with IVIG 2 g/kg or plasmapheresis over 5 days Consider additional nonsteroidal immunosuppression, such as rituximab

Adapted from Brahmer et al. JCO [17]
ICI immune checkpoint inhibitor, *IV* intravenous, *IVIG* intravenous immunoglobulin

cessfully used in case reports. As current guidelines are informed largely by case series and expert consensus, prospective data are needed to optimize the diagnosis and management of ICI-encephalitis.

For grades 1–2 encephalitis, ICI therapy can be restarted once symptoms return to baseline [12, 20]. Intravenous acyclovir may be started empirically until CSF polymerase chain reaction (PCR) results return and definitely rule out herpes virus-mediated encephalitis [17]. In cases of refractory encephalitis, where methylprednisolone and IVIG have not shown benefit, case reports have detailed the successful use of both rituximab and infliximab [24, 30]. Additionally, for cases with positive autoimmune markers of encephalitis, such as positive anti-NMDA-receptor antibodies, rituximab has shown therapeutic benefit [39].

Peripheral Neuropathy and Guillain-Barre Syndrome

Nearly 1% of patients will develop peripheral neuropathy after ICI therapy [40]. The definition of peripheral neuropathy is broad and includes symmetric or asymmetric motor, sensory, or combination of both sensory and motor deficit [23]. Immune-related neuropathies can involve the cranial nerves and also encompasses Guillain-Barre syndrome, a disorder of ascending symmetric weakness with sensory deficits [41]. As of 2018, there have been 122 reported cases of Guillain-Barre syndrome (GBS) from ICIs and, of those, 13 deaths (10.7%) primarily due to ventilatory failure [34]. Therefore, even though rare, early recognition and treatment are key to preventing deaths from Guillain-Barre syndrome.

Peripheral neuropathies have a varied presentation and can include progressive symmetric or asymmetric weakness, muscular atrophy, burning pain, tingling sensations, loss of sensation, cranial nerve deficits, loss of reflexes, ataxia, and/or loss of proprioception [23, 42–44]. GBS presents as symmetrical weakness, with paresthesias and pain in the distal limbs.

Gradually, these symptoms worsen, leading to difficulties in walking, climbing stairs, and swallowing [25].

The diagnostic workup begins with a thorough neurological exam that can pinpoint focal areas of deficit. Laboratory tests can help rule out common reversible mimics of peripheral neuropathy. Commonly sent laboratory tests include CBC, CMP, thyroid function tests, vitamin B12, folate, methylmalonic acid, homocysteine, HbA1C, and HIV antibodies [45]. MRI of the brain (if suspected cranial nerve involvement) and spine can reveal nerve enhancement in addition to ruling out brain metastases, nerve compression, and infection [46]. Electrodiagnostic tools, such as compound muscle action potential and sensory nerve action potential studies, can identify locations with loss of motor and sensory function [37, 47]. For cases of suspected GBS, pulmonary function tests can identify diaphragmatic weakness [48]. Additionally, lumbar puncture in cases of GBS can show albuminocytologic dissociation in the CSF [38]. Biopsy is not commonly used in practice in the diagnosis of peripheral neuropathy; however, in multiple case reports and series, nerve biopsy samples have shown immune-cell infiltration [28, 43, 49].

Treatment algorithms are found in Tables 10.3 and 10.4, and outline common practices for treatment in peripheral neuropathy and GBS, respectively. For peripheral neuropathy, ICIs may be continued for grade 1 symptoms and temporarily held for grade 2 symptoms [17]. ICIs may be restarted if symptoms resolve or improve to grade 1 or less [38]. Severe cases of peripheral neuropathy follow the treatment algorithm outlined for GBS. A case series by Dubey et al. demonstrated treatment benefit with rituximab and plasmapheresis for corticosteroid-refractory cases of peripheral neuropathy [28].

Cases of suspected GBS are hospitalized, with access to ICU-level monitoring and treated immediately with IVIG to identify and prevent impending respiratory failure [17]. These patients require close follow-up with neurology and pulmonology services to monitor the progression of symptoms. Unlike typical GBS, where corticosteroids have not shown

Table 10.3 Treatment algorithm for immune-related peripheral neuropathy

CTCAE grade	Symptoms	Management
1	Asymptomatic	Continue ICI Screen for reversible causes of neuropathy Consider neurology consultation Consider MRI of the spine
2	Moderate: concerning symptoms for the patients, reduction in activities of daily living	Hold ICI Neurology consultation Consider electrodiagnostic studies Consider MRI of the spine or brain (if cranial nerve involvement) Begin prednisone 0.5–1.0 mg/kg/day
3, 4	Severe symptoms	See GBS management

Adapted from NCCN Guidelines version 1 [13] and Brahmer et al. JCO [17]
ICI immune checkpoint inhibitor, *MRI* magnetic resonance imaging, *GBS* Guillain-Barre syndrome

benefit, intravenous methylprednisone can be used alongside IVIG or plasmapheresis in immune-related GBS [13, 17]. ICIs are not recommended to be restarted in severe cases of peripheral neuropathy or cases of GBS [17].

Myasthenia Gravis

An estimated 0.1–0.2% of patients will develop myasthenia gravis (MG) after ICI therapy [50]. The majority of reported cases were de novo (73%), while 17% of cases were exacerbations of pre-existing autoimmune disease [51]. About 30% of those who develop MG will die from the toxicity [42], highlighting the importance of clinical recognition and the

Table 10.4 Treatment algorithm for Guillain-Barre syndrome

CTCAE grade	Symptoms	Management
2	Moderate	Discontinue ICI permanently
3, 4	Severe symptoms, respiratory failure, dysphagia, facial weakness, or rapidly progressive symptoms	Hospitalization and neurology consultations If concern for respiratory failure, consult pulmonology Frequent neurology and pulmonary assessments Pulmonary function testing at bedside IVIG 0.4 g/kg for 5 days (2 g total) or plasmapheresis for 5 days In addition to IVIG or plasmapheresis, pulse methylprednisolone 1.0 mg/kg/day for 5 days

Adapted from NCCN Guidelines version 1 [13] and Brahmer et al. JCO [17]
ICI immune checkpoint inhibitor, *IVIG* intravenous immunoglobulin

need to commence treatment early. Those who develop de novo disease are more likely to die from myasthenic crisis as compared to patients who have an exacerbation of existing disease [42]. It has been increasingly recognized that patients who develop MG from ICIs may have a high risk of developing other, concurrent irAEs [52]. Nearly 25% of those who develop MG previously treated with nivolumab will have concurrent myocarditis [53]. The onset of MG, in a large series of patients with co-occurring myocarditis and MG by Fukasawa et al. occurred at a median of 6 weeks after ICI start [54]. Other reported concurrent irAEs include thyroiditis [55], dermatitis, myositis [56], polyneuropathy, and hepatitis. A case series by Becquart et al. noted the higher incidence of MG in melanoma patients [57]. However, this association reflects the increased use of ICIs in melanoma treatment, not that there is a predisposition for MG development in melanoma patients [57].

Patients who develop MG may present with clinical symptoms that include dysphagia, diplopia, dysarthria, ptosis, limb weakness, facial edema, and dyspnea on exertion [54, 57]. Death from myasthenia gravis occurs due to ventilatory failure from rapid, worsening muscle weakening, termed myasthenic crisis [56]. Initial laboratory testing includes a CBC, CMP, thyroid studies, creatinine kinase, anti-acetylcholine receptor (AchR) antibodies, and anti-muscle-specific kinase (MuSK) antibodies [56, 58]. The specificity of anti-MuSK antibodies is low, a study of patients with nivolumab-induced myasthenia gravis revealed that no patients had elevated anti-MuSK titers [50]. Thyroid studies can help rule out cases of hypothyroidism, which may mimic some symptoms of myasthenia gravis [59]. Although anti-AchR antibodies are present in a majority of cases, their absence does not rule out a diagnosis of myasthenia gravis in a patient with corresponding clinical symptoms [54].

Diagnosing the cause of MG can help guide treatment. Up to 15% of those presenting with MG have thymomas, CT imaging can reveal if an underlying thymoma is causing a patient's current MG [60]. Additionally, CT imaging can be used to identify metastases, which may present similarly to myasthenia gravis [61]. Magnetic resonance imaging of the brain can be used to exclude the presence of brain metastases, hemorrhage, or stroke [61]. A case series by Montes et al. described other commonly used tests to successfully diagnose myasthenia gravis, such as the tensilon test, electrophysiologic testing, and repetitive nerve stimulation [61].

The Myasthenia Gravis Foundation of America (MGFA) provides clinical classification of myasthenia gravis and is used in conjunction with the CTCAE grading scale [3, 17, 61]. Table 10.5 outlines a general treatment schema for myasthenia gravis by CTCAE grade [3]. Neurology input is appreciated with suspected and confirmed cases of myasthenia gravis of all grades [17]. Pyridostigmine, an acetylcholinesterase inhibitor, is initiated to provide symptomatic relief from MG [62]. Certain medications may exacerbate MG, these medications should be avoided and include beta-blockers,

Table 10.5 Management of myasthenia gravis by CTCAE grade and MGFA classification

CTCAE grade	MGFA classification	Management
2	Class 1: any ocular muscle weakness, all other muscle strength normal Class 2: **mild** weakness affecting muscles other than ocular muscles	Permanently discontinue ICI Hospitalization Neurology consultation Start pyridostigmine 30 mg/3 times daily Consider starting prednisone 20 mg day. Increase by 5 mg every 3–5 days with a maximum dosage l of 1.0 mg/kg/day
3	Class 3: **moderate** weakness affecting muscles other than ocular muscles	Permanently discontinue ICI Hospitalization with potential upgrade to ICU Frequent pulmonary assessments and pulmonology consultation if concern for respiratory failure Begin methylprednisolone 1.0–2.0 mg/kg/day Initiate IVIG 0.4 g/kg/day for 5 days or plasmapheresis If refractory to steroids and IVIG/plasmapheresis, consider further immunosuppression with rituximab (375 mg/m^2/week for 4 treatments or 500 mg/m^2/2 weeks for 2 treatments)
4	Class 4: **severe** weakness affecting muscles other than ocular muscles	

Adapted from NCCN management of ICI-related toxicities v 1 [13]
ICI immune checkpoint inhibitor, *IVIG* intravenous immunoglobulin

intravenous magnesium, fluoroquinolones, aminoglycosides, and macrolides [17]. While hospitalized, patients with MG may benefit from frequent pulmonary assessments, such as bedside pulmonary function tests, to monitor respiratory status and identify and prevent respiratory failure [13]. The resolution of MG may be slow and could require lifelong symptomatic treatment [13].

Ophthalmic irAEs: Uveitis

Ophthalmic irAEs are rare and comprise less than 1% of irAEs [63]. The low incidence of ocular irAEs may be in part due to the immune privilege of the eye, which normally prevents the invasion of both microorganisms and the immune system [64]. The most common ophthalmic irAEs include dry eye and uveitis, defined as intraocular inflammation involving the iris, ciliary body, or choroid; or both [63, 65]. Less common manifestations of ocular irAEs include inflammatory orbitopathy, blepharitis, choroidal neovascularization, retinal detachment, neuroretinitis, retinopathy, ocular myasthenia gravis, and keratitis [17]. This subsection focuses on the presentation, diagnosis, and management of uveitis.

Uveitis occurs in 1% of patients treated with ICIs and can occur in the anterior or posterior segment or panuveitis, inflammation in all the layers of the eye. The median time to onset is 2 months from ICI initiation [63]. As the incidence of uveitis is low, the majority of data regarding clinical presentation, management, and outcomes come from case reports and series [63, 66]. Comparatively, more cases of uveitis have been reported with ipilimumab than PD-1 therapies, which have reported more ocular irAEs than PD-L1 therapies [63, 66]. Uveitis has been reported to occur concurrently with other systemic irAEs, notably colitis [15, 63].

Patients may present with worsening vision, floaters, or conjunctival injection describes diffuse eye redness, which is consistent with the clinical presentation of ICI-uveitis [67]. Other presenting symptoms can include eye pain, change in color perception, blurry vision, and/or photophobia [68]. Other conditions, such as herpetic keratitis, preseptal cellulitis, and infectious uveitis, may mimic the presentation of uveitis [15]. A recent single-site case study by Kim et al. demonstrated bilateral eye involvement in 14 of 15 patients in the study [69].

The diagnosis of uveitis requires ophthalmic evaluation by or under the guidance of an ophthalmologist [65]. During the eye exam, the ophthalmologist may perform a visual acuity test, red reflex testing, slit-lamp examination to assess the anterior chamber, dilated fundus examination to assess the vitreous and posterior chambers, examination of the optic disk and retina, and fluorescein angiography to assess retinal venous leakage [15, 67].

The severity of ICI-associated uveitis is graded according to the CTCAE version 5 [3]. Management is detailed in Table 10.6. Ophthalmology guidance is appreciated for all grades of uveitis. Topical or systemic steroids prior to an eye evaluation should be avoided; they can worsen ocular eye infections [20]. Grade 1 uveitis does not require steroid therapy. ICIs may be restarted for grade 2 uveitis after the patient is no longer taking systemic corticosteroids for uveitis and has returned to grade 1 symptoms or less [17]. In the single-site case series by Kim et al. patients were typically

TABLE 10.6 Treatment by CTCAE grade for ICI-associated uveitis

Grade	Symptoms	Management
1	Asymptomatic	Continue ICI Supportive care, artificial tears Ophthalmology referral within 1 week
2	Vision 20/40 or better, anterior uveitis	Hold ICI Urgent ophthalmology consultation Ophthalmology guidance to treat with topical steroids with or without systemic prednisone or methylprednisone
3	Vision worse than 2/40, posterior or panuveitis	Permanently discontinue ICI Emergent ophthalmology consultation Ophthalmology guidance to treat with topical steroids with or without systemic prednisone or methylprednisone
4	Vision 20/200 or worse	

Adapted from Brahmer et al. JCO [17] and NCCN management of ICI-related toxicities v 1 [13]
ICI immune checkpoint inhibitor

treated with topical therapies (0.05% cyclosporine, 1% prednisolone acetate, 0.05% difluprednate and atropine) in combination with systemic corticosteroids: oral prednisone or IV methylprednisolone [17]. In the same case series, steroid-refractory cases of uveitis have been managed with IVIG and infliximab [70].

Pulmonary irAEs: Pneumonitis

Checkpoint inhibitor pneumonitis (CIP) is the most common respiratory irAE caused by PD-1/PD-L1 therapies [10]. This disease is defined by the presence of new pulmonary infiltrates on chest imaging, with new or worsening respiratory symptoms in the absence of infection, tumor progression, or cardiac dysfunction [10]. The incidence of CIP varies from 0 to 10% and has a median time to onset of 3 months from ICI initiation [10]. The incidence of CIP is higher with the use of PD-1/PD-L1 therapies as opposed to CTLA-4 therapies [71]. A recent meta-analysis of irAEs in NSCLC patients identified a 3.3 times higher risk of developing pneumonitis in patients treated with PD-1/PD-L1 therapies compared to patients treated with CTLA-4 therapies [72]. In a separate meta-analysis of patients with non-small-cell lung carcinoma (NSCLC) treated with PD-1/PD-L1 therapies, the overall incidence rate of CIP was 4.1%, high-grade (CTCAE grades 3+) was 1.8%, and CIP-related deaths was 0.4% [73]. Among patients hospitalized for irAEs, high-grade CIP was the most common admission diagnosis [74].

Risk factors for the development of CIP include use of combination ICI and adenocarcinoma tumor histology [75]. Patients treated with combination ICIs are also more likely to develop CIP earlier in their treatment course compared to those treated with ICI monotherapy, with a median time to onset of CIP of 2.8 months vs. 4.6 months [10]. Additionally, those treated with combination therapy are more likely to develop high-grade CIP compared to those treated with monotherapy [76]. Patients with NSCLC treated with PD-1/PD-L1 therapy had a higher incidence of all-grade pneumonitis development compared to melanoma (4.1% vs. 1.6%) [73]. Additionally, NSCLC is a risk factor for CIP-related deaths [77]. Interestingly, smoking status was not significantly associated with CIP development [77]. Certain risk factors, such as older age, oxygen administration, history of pulmonary surgery, lung radiation, decreased respiratory function, and pulmonary lesions, are associated with a predisposition toward drug-induced lung injury [73]. Currently, it is unknown if these risk factors contribute to an increased incidence of CIP [73].

The clinical presentation of CIP is varied, and mimics the symptoms associated with pulmonary metastases and respiratory infections [78]. Patients may present with unresolving dyspnea, non-productive cough, chest pain, or life-threatening respiratory compromise [79]. Physical examination may uncover a decreased oxygen saturation [17]. Laboratory studies and sputum cultures are unrevealing for CIP, as there are no identified biomarkers yet; however, they can be used to rule out other diagnoses. However, laboratory studies can rule out other infectious causes of pneumonia, which presents similarly to CIP. These studies can include nasal swab to identify viral pathogens, sputum culture, blood culture, and urine antigen tests for *Pneumococcus* and *Legionella* [13].

Diagnosing CIP begins with noninvasive imaging studies. CT scans are especially crucial for identifying CIP. All patients with a history of ICIs with new respiratory symptoms should undergo a contrast-enhanced high-resolution CT scan of the chest. Chest radiography fails to identify up to 25% of CIP cases [10]. The most common findings on CT scan are similar to cryptogenic organizing pneumonia with consolidative or ground-glass opacities (GGOs) in the peripheral or peribronchial distribution [77]. Additional CT findings of CIP resemble nonspecific interstitial pneumonia, with GGOs and reticular opacities in the lower lungs and periphery [10, 71, 80, 81]. CIP may also resemble acute interstitial pneumonia, acute respiratory distress syndrome, and hypersensitivity pneumonitis on CT imaging [81].

Pathological studies have not been widely used in the diagnosis of CIP [17]. However, if a bronchoscopy is performed, a bronchoalveolar lavage (BAL) demonstrating lymphocytosis greater than 20% is a hallmark of CIP [82]. Additionally, CIP BALs typically show an elevated CD4:CD8 lymphocyte ratio [82]. In a review article of 119 cases of pneumonitis, autopsies of patients who passed away from CIP reveal diffuse alveolar damage – which could be the underlying cause of death – in addition to granulomatous changes of the lung, similar to changes seen in sarcoidosis [77, 83].

Providers should have a healthy clinical suspicion of CIP in any patient recently treated with ICIs presenting with new respiratory symptoms [82]. Table 10.7 outlines the recommended treatment for each CTCAE grade of CIP. In general, asymptomatic CIP (grade 1) is found on imaging without needing to stop ICIs. These patients are reassessed within 1–2 weeks [13]. CT chest with contrast can be repeated in

Table 10.7 A quick reference schema of management of CIP by grade

Grade	Symptoms	Management
1	Asymptomatic with radiographical changes only	Consider holding ICI vs. continued with close monitoring Reassess in 1–2 weeks: evaluation of current symptoms and resting and ambulatory pulse oximetry Consider CT chest with contrast Can repeat CT chest in 4 weeks or as new symptoms develop
2	Mild new symptoms (dyspnea, non-productive cough) with radiographic changes	Hold ICI Consider pulmonology consultation Consider infectious workup If infection cannot be ruled out, consider initiating empiric antibiotics Consider initiating prednisone or methylprednisolone 1–2 mg/kg/day Monitor and reassess every 3–7 days: evaluation of current symptoms and pulse oximetry (resting and ambulatory)

TABLE 10.7 (continued)

Grade	Symptoms	Management
3	Worsening symptoms with new or higher oxygen requirements	Discontinue ICI permanently Hospitalization Pulmonology and infectious disease consultations Perform an infectious workup Bronchoscopy with BAL to rule out infection and malignant lung infiltration Commence methylprednisolone 1.0–2.0 mg/kg/day Assess response within 48 hours Additional immunosuppression if no improvement after 48 hours: Infliximab (5 mg/kg) IVIG (2 g/kg/day in divided doses over 2–5 days) Mycophenolate mofetil (1.0–1.5 g/ twice daily)
4	Life-threatening respiratory compromise	

Adapted from Balaji et al. Oncology [78] and NCCN management of ICI-related toxicities v 1.2019 [13]
ICI immune checkpoint inhibitor, *CT* computed tomography, *BAL* Bronchoalveolar lavage, *IVIG* intravenous immunoglobulin

4 weeks if there is no change in symptoms or repeated once symptoms change [13]. Grade 2 toxicities present with mild-to-moderate severity, changes on imaging, and may have worsening hypoxia. Practitioners may consider an infectious workup to rule out viral and bacterial causes of pneumonia. Radiologic imaging findings may take longer to improve compared to clinical symptomatology. Complete resolution may not be seen on CT chest until 2–8 weeks after initiating corticosteroid therapy [71]. Once symptoms return to a baseline, corticosteroids can be tapered over a minimum of 4–6 weeks; however, the median duration of corticosteroid use is 12 weeks [79]. If symptoms worsen or do not improve within 48–72 hours after starting corticosteroids, the CIP is treated as grade 3 and requires hospitalization [13].

High-grade CIP may progress toward life-threatening respiratory compromise if appropriate immunosuppressive therapy is not initiated quickly [82]. Pulmonology input and guidance is appreciated through a patient's hospitalization to aid in diagnosis and management of severe cases. Additional diagnostic studies, such as bronchoscopy with BAL assessment, may be considered to rule out other disease processes before starting high-dose corticosteroids or other immunosuppressive therapy in patients with concerning radiologic findings or symptomatic patients [82]. A multidisciplinary team may aid in the adjudication of these cases [84].

If symptoms do not improve or worsen within 48 hours, additional immunosuppression may be considered. Several case reports and series have successfully used mycophenolate mofetil, IVIG, infliximab, rituximab, and cyclophosphamide [78, 85]. While it has not yet been established which immunosuppressive management is superior, there are several ongoing prospective studies trying to elucidate optimal immunosuppressive management for corticosteroid-refractory cases of CIP. Importantly, treating clinicians should consider beginning prophylactic antimicrobials in patients treated with corticosteroids for extended periods of time in accordance with local guidelines, as well as additional follow-up CT scans to monitor resolution [78].

Gastrointestinal irAEs

Gastrointestinal irAEs, namely, diarrhea and colitis, are among the most common irAEs described in the literature. Diarrhea, which is defined as an increase in stool frequency, may occur in tandem with colitis, defined as an inflammation of the lining of the colon [17]. Among patients with melanoma in a phase III trial of CTLA-4 inhibitors, 27–31% experienced diarrhea [86]. A meta-analysis by Soularue et al. demonstrated that the incidence of colitis was 5.7–9.1% of patients treated with CTLA-4 inhibitors [87]. This same study highlighted the incidence of diarrhea was 12.1–13.7% and colitis was 0.7–1.6% in those treated with PD-1 inhibitors [87]. Those treated with combination CTLA-4 and PD-1 therapy have a 13.6% incidence of colitis [87]. When compared to combination CTLA-4 and PD-1 therapy, CTLA-4 inhibitors have a higher incidence of diarrhea [88, 89]. The median time to colitis onset was 11 days after starting CTLA-4 therapy [89, 90].

Immune-related (irAE-) hepatitis is another common manifestation of gastrointestinal irAEs. In patients who develop irAE-hepatitis, most patients manifest with elevations in liver markers, aspartate aminotransferase (AST) and alanine aminotransferase (ALT) and, rarely, elevations in bilirubin are seen [91]. In 1–5% of patients treated with ICIs, autoimmune hepatitis has been reported [92]. However, the incidence of irAE-hepatitis is even higher in combinations of chemotherapy and PD-1/PD-L1 therapy compared to PD-1/PD-L1 alone in NSCLC [93]. The typical time to onset is between 6 and12 weeks after initiating ICIs [94].

Immune-related (irAE-) pancreatitis is a relatively rare irAE in comparison to colitis and hepatitis. In a cohort study by Abu-Sbeih et al. of patients treated with either PD-1/PD-L1 or CTLA-4 monotherapy, 4% developed pancreatitis [95, 96]. In this same study, the incidence of irAE-pancreatitis was higher among the combination therapy treated group, 8% had developed IRAE-pancreatitis [95]. There is a notable increased risk of developing irAE-pancreatitis in those treated with combination CTLA-4 and PD-1 therapy [97]. The median time to development was 69 days with CTLA-4 monotherapy and 146 days with PD-1/PD-L1 monotherapy in the cohort study by Abu-Sbeih [95]. Interestingly, gastrointestinal irAE constitutes 25% of patients hospitalized for irAE management [74]. Of all confirmed hospitalized irAEs, 17% had colitis, 4% had irAE-hepatitis, and 4% had irAE-pancreatitis [74].

Further information about disease-specific diagnosis and management is detailed below for colitis, irAE-hepatitis, and irAE-pancreatitis.

Colitis

Colitis represents a majority of irAE-related deaths in those treated with CTLA-4 and combination immunotherapy [16]. In a meta-analysis of 613 fatal irAEs occurring in melanoma and NSCLC, the irAEs that proved most fatal were colitis from CTLA-4 monotherapy (70% of fatal irAEs) [16]. Colitis accounted for 17% of irAE-related deaths from PD-1/PD-L1 monotherapy and 37% from CTLA-4/PD-1 combination group [16]. While rare, in severe cases of colitis, bowel perforation has been reported [90]. Identified risk factors for developing colitis include a history of pre-existing bowel disease, such as Crohn's disease and ulcerative colitis [98], microbiome composition (higher *Bacteroides* compared to *Firmicutes*) [99], and treatment with CTLA-4 inhibitors, either monotherapy or in combination with PD-1 therapy [88].

Common clinical presentations of colitis include abdominal pain, nausea, cramping, diarrhea (with or without blood, mucus, or both), fever, constipation, and abdominal distension [12]. As is the case with many irAEs, colitis is a diagnosis of exclusion. Other common causes of colitis are found in Table 10.8 [100].

Initial recommended laboratory studies include a CBC, CMP, erythrocyte sedimentation rate (ESR), and CRP [12]. Stool cultures should be taken to identify possible bacterial,

Table 10.8 Differential diagnosis of colitis [100]

Diagnoses to exclude: Common causes of colitis
Clostridioides difficile infection
Other bacterial causes (*Salmonella*, *Campylobacter*, *Shigella*, and *E. coli* O157:H7)
CMV-associated colitis
Parasitic diarrhea: *Giardia, Cryptosporidium,* and intestinal amebiasis, microsporidia, *Cyclospora/isospora*
Neutropenic enterocolitis
Undiagnosed inflammatory bowel disease (Crohn's disease or ulcerative colitis)

viral, or parasitic pathogens, as well as *C. difficile* [17]. Additional stool calprotectin and/or lactoferrin are recommended as these may represent noninvasive measures of bowel inflammation that correlate with the presence of ulceration of endoscopy [17].

In patients with colitis after treatment with CTLA-4 inhibitors, a CT abdomen may demonstrate mesenteric vessel engorgement, bowel wall thickening, or pericolic fat stranding [101]. Pneumatosis, halo, target signs, or signs suggesting bowel obstruction or wall edema were radiologic findings not seen in colitis [101].

Colonoscopy is used in either cases of severe colitis or when the etiology of colitis is uncertain. Findings suggestive of colitis include diffuse erosions, ulcerations, inflammation, pseudopolyps, exudate, and friability [102, 103]. Colitis occurs more often in the descending colon compared to the ascending colon [103]. Endoscopic biopsies demonstrate increased cellularity in the lamina propria, neutrophilic inflammation with crypt abscesses, intraepithelial lymphocytosis, and apoptotic cells in the crypt epithelium [103].

Once the diagnosis of colitis is established, treatment follows the CTCAE version 5 severity grading system (Table 10.9) [3]. Patients who develop grade 1 colitis can be treated symptomatically with anti-diarrheal medications [13]. If there is no improvement in symptoms within 2 days of starting medication, consider a stool evaluation to rule out infectious causes of diarrhea [13]. Supportive care, including increased fluid intake and dietary changes, are

Table 10.9 Treatment algorithm for immune-mediated colitis

Grade	Symptoms	Management
1	Asymptomatic	Consider holding ICI Close clinical monitoring of symptoms (every 2–3 days) Oral rehydration Anti-diarrheal medication: Loperamide or diphenoxylate/atropine for 2–3 days

(continued)

Table 10.9 (continued)

Grade	Symptoms	Management
2	Mild new symptoms (abdominal pain, mucus +/– blood in the stool)	Hold ICI Gastroenterology consultation Initiate prednisone/methylprednisolone 1.0–2.0 mg/kg/day Consider testing stool lactoferrin and calprotectin to assess colonic inflammation Consider colonoscopy or flexible sigmoidoscopy
3	Moderate new symptoms (severe abdominal pain with peritoneal signs, mucus +/– blood in the stool, fever)	Discontinue CTLA-4 inhibitors permanently Temporarily stop PD-1/PD-L1 inhibitors Hospitalization and aggressive rehydration Gastroenterology consultation Consider colonoscopy to monitor disease and exclude other causes of colitis Commence methylprednisolone 1.0–2.0 mg/kg/day If no response to corticosteroids within 48 hours, regrade and start infliximab (5–10 mg/kg) or vedolizumab
4	Life-threatening consequences; potential bowel perforation, ischemia, necrosis, toxic megacolon	Discontinue ICI permanently Hospitalization and aggressive rehydration Gastroenterology consultation Consider colonoscopy to monitor disease and exclude other causes of colitis Commence methylprednisolone 1.0–2.0 mg/kg/day If no response to corticosteroids within 48 hours, start infliximab (5–10 mg/kg) or vedolizumab

Adapted from Brahmer et al. JCO [17] and NCCN management of ICI-related toxicities v 1 [13]
ICI immune checkpoint inhibitor

recommended. An example of a recommended dietary change is dietary change is the BRAT diet (bananas, rice, applesauce, and toast) to provide bowel rest [104]. Gastroenterology input and guidance is recommended for grade 2 and higher cases of colitis [90]. Patients treated with CTLA-4 inhibitors may consider permanently discontinuing therapy [90]. For patients with symptomatic colitis (grade 2+), corticosteroids (e.g., prednisone or methylprednisolone at a dose of 1 mg/kg/day) and supportive care [13] are recommended. If symptoms improve within 48–72 hours, corticosteroids can be tapered over 4–6 weeks [13].

If symptoms do not improve or worsen, the colitis will be regraded and additional immunosuppression may be warranted. Providers may use infliximab (5–10 mg/kg) or vedolizumab in cases of corticosteroid-refractory colitis. Vedolizumab, initially approved in the treatment of Crohn's disease and ulcerative colitis, is a humanized monoclonal IgG antibody against α4β7 integrin [105]. This integrin is expressed on a subset of CD4 lymphocytes and mediates their movement to the gastrointestinal (GI) tract. Vedolizumab specifically targets the GI tract and has been used effectively in cases of corticosteroid-refractory colitis, as reported in a case series by Bergqvist et al. [105]. For high grade of colitis, colonoscopy can help locate areas of active inflammation and guide the intensity and length of immunosuppressive therapy needed [95]. If patients develop corticosteroid- or nonsteroidal immunosuppression-refractory colitis, consider colonoscopy or flexible sigmoidoscopy to identify other causes of colitis.

Resumption of ICIs is not recommended for grade 3 or higher toxicities if a CTLA-4 inhibitor was the inciting agent of the colitis [17]. Providers may consider restarting PD-1/PD-L1 inhibitors for toxicities grade 3 or below if the patient's colitis returns to a grade 1 toxicity or less [17]. A recent study by Abu-Sbeih et al. demonstrated that one-third of patients who resumed therapy after colitis had a recrudescence of their colitis, although the recurrence occurred less with PD-1/PD-L1 inhibitors as compared to CTLA-4 inhibitors [95]. Colonoscopy is often warranted in patients who may have their ICIs restarted to ensure complete resolution of their colitis [95].

Immune-Related Hepatitis

Immune-related hepatitis is a common cause of irAE-associated death in those treated with ICIs. A meta-analysis of irAE-related deaths by Wang et al. demonstrated that of all irAE-related deaths, 16% in the CTLA-4 group, 35% in the PD-1/PD-L1 group, and 22% in the combination therapy group were attributable to irAE-hepatitis [16]. CTLA-4 and PD-1 combination therapies (specifically of nivolumab and ipilimumab) have a higher risk of hepatitis development – 20% in patients treated with combined therapy [106] compared to 5% in clinical trials of monotherapy [107]. It is unclear whether previous liver injury: alcohol-related cirrhosis, hepatitis C infection, or non-alcoholic fatty liver disease are risk factors for the development of irAE-hepatitis [106, 108, 109].

Typically, irAE-hepatitis presents silently, with large elevations in aspartate aminotransferase (AST) and alanine aminotransferase (ALT) on routine laboratory studies. The elevation of AST and ALT tends to occur in tandem [106]. Patients may present with nonspecific symptoms, such as generalized weakness, nausea, abdominal pain, yellowing of the skin, eyes, and mucous membranes, dark urine, and fever. Elevations in AST and ALT are markedly higher among symptomatic patients [106]. irAE-hepatitis may become fulminant liver failure, with alterations in albumin and PT-INR levels and can result in death [106].

Diagnosis begins with initial laboratory testing, which should include CBC, CMP, serology panel for viral hepatitis, acetaminophen levels, and autoimmune hepatitis antibodies (ANCA, smooth muscle antibody, mitochondrial antibody, F-actin, and anti-LKM-1) to rule out other causes of drug-related or viral hepatitis or disease-related hepatic dysfunction [107]. Through the course of ICI therapy, patients' AST and ALT levels should be routinely monitored to identify changes from baseline [15].

Radiologic imaging is often used to rule out hepatic metastasis and extrahepatic cholestasis, which are more common causes of liver injury than irAE-hepatitis [110]. CT abdomen imaging resembles patterns similar to acute hepatitis: mild hepatomegaly, periportal edema, and periportal lymphadenopathy [111]. Ultrasound may also be used to identify irAE-hepatitis, and studies show prominent echogenicity of the portal vein, periportal edema, and edema of the gallbladder wall [111]. MRI of the liver is less commonly used but can reveal periportal edema through increased T2 hyperintensity of the periportal vein and space [111].

Liver biopsy is not routinely completed to diagnose irAE-hepatitis initially, but can be a useful tool in cases of corticosteroid-refractory hepatitis [112]. However, in a case series by Zen et al. histopathological samples from ten patients with irAE-hepatitis revealed infiltrating lymphocytes, lobular hepatitis, mild portal inflammation, and, less commonly, fibrin ring granulomas [113]. The patterns observed in irAE-hepatitis are similar to other causes of acute liver injury: viral hepatitis, acute alcoholic hepatitis, and drug-induced liver injury. irAE-hepatitis is not similar to patterns of injury seen in either cirrhosis or chronic liver injury [106].

Treatment for irAE-hepatitis should begin once AST and ALT levels are elevated between 2 and 5 times the upper-limit of normal (ULN). The grading and management schema is reported in Table 10.10 [3].

Grade 1 toxicities do not warrant stopping ICIs. These patients require close clinical monitoring with biweekly laboratory investigations and are managed supportively [13]. For grade 2 toxicities, ICIs are held. However, ICIs can be restarted if patients return to grade 1 toxicity or less [13]. After 3–5 days of initial corticosteroid therapy, if symptoms improve, corticosteroids can be tapered over 4–6 weeks. If patients do not show improvement after 3–5 days, consider regrading the toxicity and increasing corticosteroid dosage [13].

TABLE 10.10 Treatment algorithm by CTCAE grade for IR-hepatitis

Grade	Symptoms	Management
1	Asymptomatic AST +/− ALT up to 3× ULN Total bilirubin up to 1.5× ULN	Continue ICI Consider holding ICI if trends of AST/ALT increase Close clinical monitoring of symptoms and reassess AST/ALT and total bilirubin laboratory values every 2–3 days
2	Asymptomatic AST +/− ALT 3–5× ULN Total bilirubin 1.5–3× ULN	Hold ICI Monitor AST, ALT, and total bilirubin levels every 3–5 days Consider starting prednisone 0.5–1.0 mg/kg/day
3	Symptomatic liver dysfunction AST +/− ALT 5–20× ULN Total bilirubin 3–10× ULN	Discontinue ICI permanently Hospitalization and hepatology consultation Monitor AST/ALT and total bilirubin levels every 1–2 days Initiate prednisone 1–2 mg/kg/day If no improvement within 3 days, consider non-steroidal immunosuppression (mycophenolate mofetil)
4	Liver failure AST +/− ALT >20× ULN Total bilirubin >10× ULN	Discontinue ICI permanently Hospitalization and hepatology consultation Monitor AST/ALT and total bilirubin levels daily Commence prednisone/methylprednisolone 2 mg/kg/day Consider liver biopsy if no contraindications If no improvement, consider non-steroidal immunosuppression (mycophenolate mofetil)

Adapted from Brahmer et al. JCO [17] and NCCN management of ICI-related toxicities v 1 [13]

ICI immune checkpoint inhibitor, *AST* aspartate aminotransferase, *ALT* alanine aminotransferase, *ULN* upper limit of normal

Hepatology input is valuable for grades 3+ toxicities for treatment guidance and determining whether a liver biopsy may aid in diagnosis. For either grade 3 or 4 toxicities, if no improvement occurs within 3 days, consider using non-steroidal immunosuppression. In corticosteroid-refractory cases, infliximab is not recommended due to its reported hepatotoxic side effects [17, 114]. Case studies have shown successful use of mycophenolate mofetil, tacrolimus, azathioprine, and antithymocyte globulin for corticosteroid-refractory irAE-hepatitis [2, 17, 115, 116]. However, mycophenolate mofetil is the current recommended standard for corticosteroid-refractory cases of irAE-hepatitis [13]. If patients' symptoms return to baseline, corticosteroids may be tapered over a 4–6 week course [17, 116].

Immune-Related Pancreatitis

While death from irAE-pancreatitis is infrequent, patients may develop long-term complications affecting the exocrine and endocrine pancreas, such as the development of insulin-dependent diabetes mellitus and pancreatic atrophy [95, 96].

In a literature review by Friedman et al., it was identified that patients with a prior history of pancreatitis are at an increased risk of irAE-pancreatitis from ICIs [117]. In this review, the risk factors for developing long-term complications of irAE-pancreatitis, such as insulin-dependent diabetes mellitus and pancreatic atrophy, included smoking history and hyperlipidemia [117].

Patients may be asymptomatic or present with a variety of symptoms that include epigastric pain, nausea, vomiting, fever, and diarrhea [12, 118, 119]. Like traditional, acute pancreatitis, irAE-pancreatitis may be detected by identifying elevated lipase or amylase levels on laboratory testing; however, this abnormality is often nonspecific and may be found incidentally [95].

In addition to a physical examination and patient history, initial laboratory testing should include CBC, CMP, amylase, lipase, and elastase [120]. Common causes of acute pancreatitis, such as gallstones and alcohol intoxication, should be ruled out prior to initiating treatment for irAE-pancreatitis. CT abdomen scans are commonly used to evaluate irAE-pancreatitis. In cases of irAE-pancreatitis, radiologic imaging can reveal inflammation, segmental hypoenhancement, peri-pancreatic fat stranding, pancreatic enlargement, similar to traditional, acute pancreatitis [95, 120]. However, in grades 1–2 irAE-pancreatitis, radiologic imaging may not show evidence of inflammation [121]. Further imaging, such as cholangiopancreatography or MRCP, can be considered if CT abdomen scans are unrevealing [85].

Treatments stratified by CTCAE grade is shown in Table 10.11 [3]. Because the incidence of irAE-pancreatitis is

TABLE 10.11 Treatment guidelines for immune-mediated pancreatitis

Grade	Symptoms	Management
1	Asymptomatic elevations of serum lipase ≤ 3× ULN amylase and/or ≤ 3× ULN lipase	If isolated elevation of pancreatic enzymes, continue ICI Evaluate for pancreatitis Intravenous hydration Consider gastroenterology referral
2	Moderate >3–5× ULN amylase and/or > 3–5× ULN lipase	Hold ICI Intravenous hydration Start prednisone or methylprednisolone 0.5–1.0 mg/kg/day Gastroenterology consultation
3 4	Severe >5× ULN amylase and/or > 5× ULN lipase	Discontinue ICI permanently Aggressive intravenous hydration Hospitalization and gastroenterology consultation Start prednisone or methylprednisolone 1.0–2.0 mg/kg/day

Adapted from NCCN Guidelines version 1 [13]
ICI immune checkpoint inhibitor

rare, and the presentation is variable, current management guidelines are limited. Gastroenterology specialist input is appreciated for grade 2 toxicities and beyond. Grade 3 and 4 toxicities are managed similarly. New data suggest that corticosteroid use may not be recommended for irAE-pancreatitis, instead, focusing on aggressive intravenous hydration [95].

Hematologic irAEs: Immune-Related Thrombocytopenia

Cytopenias (grades 2+) from ICIs are reported in less than 0.5% of patients treated with PD-1/PD-L1 inhibitors; however, no significant difference in incidence rates were seen between types of ICIs in large reported cohort studies [117, 121]. The spectrum of hematological irAEs includes hemolytic anemias, neutropenia, thrombocytopenia, and pancytopenia/ immune aplastic anemia [122–124]. Of these adverse events, immune-related (irAE) thrombocytopenia is one of the most common hematological irAEs. In a study of cytopenias from PD-1/PD-L1 inhibitors, irAE-thrombocytopenia accounted for 26% of cases [122]. Generally, the median time of onset for irAE-thrombocytopenia is 12 weeks from ICI initiation [122]. Risk factors for the development of irAE-thrombocytopenia include psoriasis, vitiligo, idiopathic thrombocytic purpura, and Hashimoto's thyroiditis and concurrent use of other thrombocytopenia-inducing drugs such as quinine, sulfonylurea, glitazone, metformin, and colchicine [122, 125].

Diagnosis is challenging as irAE-thrombocytopenia has no identified biomarkers that can distinguish between immune-related causes and other causes. Common causes of thrombocytopenia to consider include acquired thrombotic thrombocytopenia, hemolytic uremic syndrome, bone marrow metastases, myelodysplastic syndrome, immune thrombocytopenic purpura (ITP), heparin-induced thrombocytopenia, and disseminated intravascular coagulation [17]. A thorough patient history can provide vital information about drug and toxin exposures [17]. Physical examination may reveal areas of petechiae, purpura, and hepatosplenomegaly [126]. Initial laboratory testing should include a CBC, CMP, peripheral blood smear, direct Coombs test, reticulocyte count, and viral serology panel (HIV and HCV) [17, 126]. Bone marrow biopsies can be helpful in diagnosing irAE-thrombocytopenia and can show areas of hypercellularity with increased megakaryocytes, consistent with a picture of ITP [122, 126, 127].

Table 10.12 illustrates the current treatment guidelines by CTCAE grading [3] of irAE-thrombocytopenia. Hematology consultations are useful in cases where guideline-based man-

Table 10.12 A guideline for immune-related thrombocytopenia by CTCAE grade

Grade	Platelet count	Management
1	< 100 K platelets/μL	Continue ICI Close clinical and laboratory monitoring of symptoms
2	< 75 K platelets/μL	Hold ICI, can restart if symptoms return to grade 1 or less Begin prednisone 1.0 mg/kg/day; taper for 4–6 weeks Consider using IVIG in conjunction to steroids
3	< 50 K platelets/μL	Hold ICI, can restart if symptoms return to grade 1 or less Hospitalization and hematology consultation
4	< 25 K platelets/μL	Consider platelet transfusion Begin prednisone 1.0–2.0 mg/kg/day; taper for 4–6 weeks Consider one dose of IVIG 1 g/kg, repeat as necessary Additional immunosuppression: Rituximab, mycophenolate mofetil, cyclophosphamide, cyclosporine, thrombopoietin receptor agonists

Adapted from Brahmer et al. JCO [17]
ICI immune checkpoint inhibitor, *IVIG* intravenous immunoglobulin

agement does not result in improvement. In addition to corticosteroids, a one-time dose of IVIG (1 g/kg) may be used in patients with more severe irAE-thrombocytopenia or for faster improvement in patients with lower grades of irAE-thrombocytopenia [17]. Intravenous immunoglobulin may be re-dosed as necessary. Providers may consider platelet infusions for extremely low platelet counts, typically less than 10,000 platelets per μL [125]. If irAE-thrombocytopenia remains refractory to steroids and IVIG, the successful use of rituximab, cyclosporine, cyclophosphamide, mycophenolate mofetil, and thrombopoietin receptor agonists have been reported in the literature as case reports and series [12, 17, 121, 122].

Cardiovascular irAEs: Myocarditis and Pericarditis

Cardiovascular irAEs are more difficult to identify relative to the spectrum of organ system irAEs, and constitute less than 1% of documented irAEs by current reports [128]. However, cardiac irAEs can lead to significant morbidity and mortality [129, 130] and are likely more prevalent than previously reported due to historical under-recognition of these toxicities. The most common cardiac toxicity is myocarditis, followed by pericarditis [131, 132]; these two toxicities will be the focus of this chapter. Cases of conduction abnormalities, vasculitis, and Takotsubo cardiomyopathy secondary to ICI therapy have also been reported [133, 134].

Patients with cardiac irAEs can present with a wide spectrum of symptoms ranging from fatigue and myalgias to more specific symptoms, such as chest pain, dyspnea, palpitations, and syncope [130, 135]. Postmortem assessment of cardiac biopsies from patients who died of fulminant myocarditis demonstrated lymphocytic infiltrate with a predominance of CD8-positive cells in the myocardium [136], suggesting a T-cell-mediated mechanism for this irAE. The mechanism underlying ICI-induced pericarditis is unknown. Likewise, there are no known risk factors for the development of myocarditis, pericarditis, or other the rarer cardiac irAEs.

The prevalence and frequency of myocarditis is higher, and the severity greater, in patients with melanoma treated with ipilimumab/ nivolumab combination therapy compared to patients on either monotherapy [128]. Myocarditis is typically diagnosed at a median 17–30 days after initial exposure to therapy [128, 129], but cases of fatal fulminant myocarditis have been reported as early as 12–15 days after the first dose of ICI therapy [130]. Patient presentation may range from asymptomatic to acute decompensated heart failure, cardiogenic shock, pulmonary edema, or ventricular arrhythmias [135]. Initial diagnostic evaluation for all cardiac irAEs includes electrocardiogram (EKG), cardiac biomarkers, and cardiac imaging (either echocardiogram or cardiac MRI) [135]. Cardiac MRI specifically can be helpful to differentiate drug-induced myocarditis from other potential etiologies [132]. Endomyocardial biopsy may be indicated when the noninvasive workup has yielded equivocal results [12, 135].

Changes indicative of myocarditis include elevated cardiac enzymes (CK-MB, troponin, pro-BNP) and new EKG changes [12, 135]. The most commonly reported EKG changes in myocarditis include new nonspecific T-wave changes, new arrhythmias, heart block, and ischemic changes mimicking recent myocardial infarction [135]. EKG changes specific to checkpoint inhibitor myocarditis are currently unknown. Echocardiograms may show a new reduced ejection fraction [12]. Pericarditis can be severe enough to present with hypoxemia and may present on echocardiogram or on a CT of the chest with or without an associated pericardial effusion [134]. EKG changes consistent with pericarditis include diffuse ST segment elevations and PR segment depressions, but these changes are not specific to checkpoint inhibitor pericarditis.

Cardiac toxicities of all types and all grades should be managed with a tripartite approach that includes cessation of ICI therapy, immunosuppression, and cardiology consultation [12]. Treatment of myocarditis and pericarditis depends on the severity of the toxicity, but typically involves initiation of intravenous methylprednisolone 500–1000 mg daily until a patient achieves clinical stability, followed by oral prednisone starting at 1 mg/kg and tapered as tolerated [12] (Table 10.13). Glucocorticoid therapy for

Table 10.13 A guideline for checkpoint inhibitor cardiovascular toxicities by CTCAE grade

Grade	Description	Management
1	Abnormal cardiac biomarker testing, including abnormal ECG	Baseline EEG and cardiac biomarker assessment (BNP, troponin) to establish if there is a notable change with therapy Mild abnormalities should be observed closely during therapy
2	Abnormal screening tests with mild symptoms	Control cardiac diseases optimally Control cardiac disease risk factors proactively (hypertension, hyperlipidemia, smoking, diabetes)
3	Moderately abnormal testing or symptoms with mild activity	BNP > 500 pg/ml, troponin >99% institutional normal, new ECG findings Consider withholding ICI; if a period of stabilization is achieved, it may be reasonable to re-challenge the patient with ICI with close monitoring If confirmed cardiac injury or decompensation, hold ICI until stabilized Consider corticosteroids if myocarditis suspected Patients with confirmed myocarditis should receive emergent high-dose corticosteroids (1 mg/kg intravenous methylprednisolone for at least several days) until improved to grade ≤ 1; after that, consider at least 4–5 weeks of tapering doses

(continued)

Table 10.13 (continued)

Grade	Description	Management
4	Moderate to severe decompensation, intravenous medication or intervention required, life-threatening conditions	Permanently discontinue ICI If myocarditis is identified, consider high-dose corticosteroids Add additional immunosuppressive agents in severe refractory cases Give additional supportive treatments, including appropriate treatment of heart failure

Adapted from Puzanov et al. [15]
ICI immune checkpoint inhibitor, *ECG* electrocardiogram, *BNP* brain natriuretic peptide

checkpoint inhibitor cardiac toxicity has been shown to improve left ventricular ejection fraction by 50% [131]. Cases that do not respond to glucocorticoid therapy should be advanced to alternate immunosuppressive options, such as mycophenolate, infliximab, or intravenous immunoglobulin (IVIG), based on published guidelines. Patients presenting with new arrhythmias or heart blocks should be evaluated by electrophysiology for consideration of cardiac device insertion [12].

The gaps in our understanding of cardiac irAEs include knowledge of risk factors, optimal early detection strategies, and optimization of management. One proposed strategy for risk stratification involves a baseline cardiac evaluation, including EKG, cardiac biomarkers, and routine surveillance for patients with pre-existing cardiac risk factors, such as hypertension, coronary artery disease, diabetes mellitus, obesity, smoking history, or notable family history [137]. Prospective studies comparing additional immunosuppression and their outcomes for cases refractory to glucocorticoids could help elucidate an optimal immunosuppression algorithm for these patients.

Dermatologic irAEs: Maculopapular Dermatitis and Pruritus

Dermatologic toxicities are the most commonly reported irAE among all checkpoint inhibitor therapies, with incidence ranging from 30 to 40% of patients receiving PD-1/PD-L1 inhibitors and as high as 50% of patients receiving ipilimumab [138]. However, the vast majority of these cases are low grade (CTCAE ≤2), and < 3% of cases of cutaneous toxicity are grade 3+ in severity [86]. The most common cutaneous toxicities include maculopapular rash and pruritus [86]. Other possible dermatologic irAEs include lichenoid dermatitis, vitiligo, and bullous dermatoses, such as bullous pemphigoid [86]. Vitiligo in particular is a common toxicity among patients with melanoma [91]. Cases of severe adverse drug reactions, such as Stevens-Johnson syndrome/toxic epidermal necrolysis (SJS/TEN) and drug rash with eosinophilia and systemic symptoms (DRESS) have been reported and are rare but important irAEs in this patient population [139]. Studies are ongoing to identify patient biomarkers that herald increased risk for cutaneous irAEs, and one identified risk factor for dermatologic toxicity is combination ICI therapy [140]. A wide spectrum exists for time to onset of toxicity, ranging from 2 weeks after dose one to several months after start of therapy [141].

Diagnostic evaluation for patients with a new rash or pruritus begins with a thorough patient history and physical examination that includes the skin and mucous membranes, lymph nodes, testing for positive Nikolsky sign, and evaluation of the total body surface area (BSA) affected [12]. Focusing on the presence of alarm signs and symptoms, such as more than 30% BSA affected, positive Nikolsky sign, or mucous membrane involvement, as well as duration of symptoms can help determine the need for further workup [12]. Biopsy is recommended for patients with any of the above signs, and serologies for bullous toxicities and pemphigus vulgaris could be helpful if biopsy is not possible [12].

Management of maculopapular rash is determined by the percent total BSA affected as well as the morbidity associated with the rash, as delineated in the CTCAE criteria (Table 10.14). Grade 1 or 2 rash does not necessitate discontinuation of ICI and typically responds well to a combination of oral antihistamines and topical corticosteroids (class I, such as clobetasol for body, class V/VI, such as hydrocortisone 2.5% for face) [138]. Oral corticosteroid therapy can be

Table 10.14 A guideline for checkpoint inhibitor maculopapular rash/dermatitis by CTCAE grade

Grade	Description	Management
1	Macules/papules covering <10% BSA with or without symptoms (e.g., pruritus, burning, tightness)	Continue ICI Oral antihistamines Cetirizine/loratidine 10 mg daily (non-sedating); hydroxyzine 10–25 mg QID, or at bedtime Topical corticosteroids Class I topical corticosteroid (clobetasol propionate, halobetasol propionate, betamethasone dipropionate cream or ointment) for body; class V/VI corticosteroid (aclometasone, desonide, hydrocortisone 2.5% cream) for face
2	Macules/papules covering 10–30% BSA with or without symptoms (e.g., pruritus, burning, tightness); limiting instrumental ADL	Continue ICI Non-urgent dermatology referral Oral antihistamines Cetirizine/loratidine 10 mg daily (non-sedating); hydroxyzine 10–25 mg QID, or at bedtime Topical corticosteroids (see grade 1) As above Cetirizine/loratidine 10 mg daily (non-sedating); hydroxyzine 10–25 mg QID, or at bedtime

Table 10.14 (continued)

Grade	Description	Management
3	Macules/papules covering >30% BSA with or without associated symptoms; limiting self-care ADL	Hold ICI Same-day dermatology consult Rule out systemic hypersensitivity: CBC with differential, CMP Oral antihistamines Cetirizine/loratidine 10 mg daily (non-sedating); hydroxyzine 10–25 mg QID, or at bedtime Systemic corticosteroids Prednisone 0.5–1 mg/kg/day (or equivalent dose of methylprednisolone) until rash resolves to ≤ grade 1

Adapted from Puzanov et al. 2017 [15]
ICI immune checkpoint inhibitor, *CMP*: complete metabolic panel, QID: four times daily

considered for symptomatic patients with grade 2 rash [138]. Dermatology referral is encouraged for both grade 2+ cases. Additionally, patients with grade 3 rash should temporarily cease ICI with consideration to permanently discontinue therapy depending on the degree of morbidity. Patients with grade 3 rash are typically treated with systemic corticosteroids and require a skin biopsy to evaluate the features of rash and more specific immunosuppressive choices.

Grade 1 and 2 pruritus management, similar to maculopapular rash, consists of oral antihistamines and topical corticosteroids (Table 10.15). Grade 2 pruritus cases should also receive oral corticosteroids, prednisone 0.5–1 mg/kg/day, tapered over 2 weeks, and receive a dermatology referral [138]. Methylprednisolone equivalent is sufficient if oral steroids are not possible. Grade 3 pruritus necessitates all of the above therapies as well as a dermatology referral. GABA agonists, such as pregabalin or gabapentin 100–300 mg three times daily, can be used for refractory grade 3 pruritus [138]. NK-1 ago-

TABLE 10.15 A guideline for checkpoint inhibitor pruritus by CTCAE grade

Grade	Description	Management
1	Mild or localized; topical intervention indicated	Emollients with cream or ointment based, fragrance-free products Class I topical corticosteroid (clobetasol propionate, halobetasol propionate, betamethasone dipropionate) for body; class V/VI corticosteroid (aclometasone, desonide, hydrocortisone 2.5%) for face, *and* oral antihistamines (e.g., cetirizine/loratidine 10 mg daily, hydroxyzine 10–25 mg QID, or at bedtime
2	Intense or widespread; intermittent; skin changes from scratching (e.g., edema, papulation, excoriation, lichenification, oozing/crusts); oral intervention indicated; limiting instrumental ADL	Dermatology referral Class I topical steroid (clobetasol propionate, halobetasol propionate, betamethasone dipropionate) for body; class V/VI steroid (aclometasone, desonide, hydrocortisone 2.5%) for face, and oral antihistamines (e.g., cetirizine/loratidine 10 mg daily, hydroxyzine 10–25 mg QID, or at bedtime Oral corticosteroids Prednisone 0.51 mg/kg/day (or equivalent of methylprednisolone) tapered over 2 weeks
3	Intense or widespread; constant; limiting self-care ADL or sleep; oral corticosteroid or immunosuppressive therapy indicated	Dermatology referral GABA agonist (pregabalin, gabapentin 100–300 mg TID) Oral corticosteroid Prednisone 0.5–1 mg/kg/day (or equivalent of methylprednisolone) tapered over 2 weeks

Adapted from Puzanov et al. [15]
TID three times daily, *QID* four times daily

nists, such as aprepitant, have also shown promise in drastically improving checkpoint inhibitor pruritus refractory to corticosteroid therapy [142].

Although the rate of high-grade dermatologic toxicities is very low, the overall incidence of these events is high, and they have a significant impact on quality-of-life. Avenues for future study include understanding the pathogenesis of severe dermatoses and identifying risk factors and biomarkers to identify patients who are at risk for specific irAEs.

Renal irAEs

Initial data on checkpoint inhibitor nephrotoxicity showed an incidence rate of 2% for monotherapy and 5% for combination therapy [143]. However, recent data from cohort studies has shown that renal toxicity is much more common than previously reported, with incidence rates ranging from 9.9 to 29% based on reported ICI clinical trials across tumor types [143, 144]. Interstitial nephritis is the most common renal toxicity from ICIs, but cases of glomerulonephritis, lupus nephritis, and granulomatous nephritis have also been reported [143, 145, 146]. An important risk factor for renal toxicity is combination therapy, particularly ICI combined with chemotherapy [93]. Time of onset varies by ICI, with CTLA-4-associated toxicity occurring at a range of 2–3 months from start of therapy and PD-1-associated toxicity occurring much later at a range of 3–10 months after start of therapy [143].

Most patients with renal toxicities are asymptomatic and are only detected through laboratory testing or surveillance [12]. Symptoms of renal toxicity include altered mental status, nausea, vomiting, oliguria, or dyspnea [12]. Diagnostic evaluation should include urinalysis, serum creatinine, and serum electrolytes, and renal ultrasound can be considered to evaluate for structural pathologies [12]. An elevated serum creatinine above baseline, pyuria, hematuria, and eosinophilia are consistent with renal toxicity, although laboratory values specific for ICI-nephrotoxicity have not yet been identified [144, 147]. Renal biopsy is not necessary for diagnosis, but can show a lymphocytic infiltrate with plasma cells and eosinophils as well as granulomatous changes [144]. Notably, complement levels and immunofluorescence staining are typically normal in these cases [144].

Nephritis is graded and managed according to CTCAE guidelines (Table 10.16). Patients with grade 1 nephritis can

Table 10.16 A guideline for checkpoint inhibitor nephritis by CTCAE grade

Grade	Description	Management
1	Creatinine level increase of >0.3 mg/dL; creatinine 1.5–2.0× above baseline	Continue ICI but initiate workup to evaluate possible causes and monitor closely
2	Creatinine 2–3× above baseline	Hold ICI Resume when creatinine decreased to ≤grade 1 Consider timing of event and response to treatment when making a decision Start corticosteroids Discontinue ICI for persistent or recurrent elevation
3	Creatinine >3× baseline or > 4.0 mg/dL; hospitalization indicated	Hold ICI Consider resuming treatment if grade 3 resolves and cause of event is confirmed. Timing of event and response to treatment should be considered in making a decision Start corticosteroids Discontinue ICI for persistent or recurrent elevation
4	Life-threatening consequences; dialysis indicated	Permanently discontinue ICI Start corticosteroids

Adapted from Puzanov et al. [15]
ICI immune checkpoint inhibitor

continue to receive ICIs, but should be monitored and evaluated for other potential etiologies [15]. Patients with grade 2 and 3 cases are advised to withhold ICI therapy and start on corticosteroid therapy [15]; patients typically start on prednisone 1 mg/kg/day, which is tapered once the serum creatinine improves to grade 1 [12, 15]. Patients with grade 4 nephritis may require dialysis and nephrology consultation in addition to corticosteroids [15]. ICI therapy may be restarted once serum creatinine normalizes to baseline, but therapy should be discontinued if patients present with persistent or recurrent creatinine elevations [15]. Additional immunosuppression with mycophenolate mofetil can be considered in steroid-refractory cases of nephritis, based on a large case series [12].

There is much still to learn regarding the mechanism of injury in checkpoint inhibitor nephrotoxicity. Further studies exploring this pathophysiology may shed light on why there is a discrepancy in time to injury between CTLA-4 inhibitors and PD-1 inhibitors.

Endocrine irAEs: Hypophysitis, Hypothyroidism, and Type 1 Diabetes Mellitus

The incidence of common endocrine toxicities, such as hypophysitis and thyroid dysfunction, is reported at approximately 10% [148]. However, endocrinopathies are difficult to diagnose due to their nonspecific symptomatology; thus, the true incidence may be higher than reported [148]. The organs most often affected by ICI therapy are the thyroid gland, pituitary gland, pancreas, and adrenal glands, but parathyroid involvement has been reported as well [149]. The most common ICI endocrine toxicities are hypothyroidism and hypophysitis [149]. Hyperthyroidism and thyroiditis are also frequently seen in this patient population [149]. Type 1 diabetes mellitus, while a relatively rare endocrine toxicity, is an event of interest due to its chronicity. Combination checkpoint inhibitor therapy is a risk factor for developing endocrine toxicities [149]. This section will discuss the diagnostic evaluation and management of checkpoint inhibitor hypophysitis, hypothyroidism, and type 1 diabetes mellitus.

Evaluation should begin with a history and physical examination, with particular attention to visual fields to evaluate for hypophysitis, as well as a thyroid exam to evaluate for goiter and assessment of deep tendon reflexes [12]. Diagnostic studies that examine the hypothalamic-pituitary-adrenal and hypothalamic-pituitary-gonadal axes are important for distinguishing between primary and secondary endocrinopathies. These studies include Thyroid stimulating hormone (TSH), free T4, Luteinizing hormone (LH), Follicle-stimulating hormone (FSH), Adrenocorticotropic hormone (ACTH), cortisol, and serum electrolytes [12]. Evaluation for type 1 diabetes mellitus includes urinalysis and serum electrolytes, as well as a fasting C-peptide, glutamic acid decarboxylase (GAD) antibody, insulinoma-associated protein 2 (IAP2) protein antibody, and zinc transporter (Zt8) antibody [150]. A low fasting C-peptide and elevated antibody markers suggest autoimmune diabetes mellitus and would help to differentiate this diagnosis from new type II diabetes mellitus, but these findings are not always identified [150].

Management of hypophysitis, hypothyroidism, and autoimmune diabetes mellitus is performed according to CTCAE grading criteria. Intervention is not indicated for grade 1 hypophysitis or hypothyroidism (Table 10.17) [15]. All patients with grade 2 or higher endocrine toxicity should be referred to an endocrinologist [15]. Patients with hypophysitis resulting in central adrenal insufficiency can be treated with physiologic steroid replacement using hydrocortisone, those with central hypothyroidism can be treated with levothyroxine 1 mcg/kg, and those with central hypogonadism can consider hormone replacement therapy or testosterone provided that it does not conflict with their cancer type [15]. Patients should be monitored every 3 months for the first

TABLE 10.17 A guideline for checkpoint inhibitor hypophysitis by CTCAE grade

Grade	Description	Management
1	Asymptomatic or mild symptoms; clinical or diagnostic observations only; intervention not indicated	Hold ICI if ≥ grade 2 irAE until workup is completed and appropriate hormone replacement is started If central adrenal insufficiency: start physiologic steroid replacement: Hydrocortisone ~10 mg/m² (HC 15 mg am, 5 mg at 3 pm) Periodic assessment (e.g., every 3 months in the first year, every 6 months thereafter): clinical monitoring and repeat hormone levels (am cortisol and ACTH and/or low-dose cosyntropin stimulation test) to assess recovery If central hypothyroidism: start thyroid hormone (levothyroxine 1mcg/kg) Repeat thyroid function testing 6–8 weeks after initiation of thyroid hormone and then periodically (e.g., every 3 months in the first year and every 6 months thereafter) to assess recovery If central hypogonadism, repeat hormone levels in 2–3 months and consider testosterone in men or HRT in women if appropriate for cancer type
2	Moderate; minimal, local or noninvasive intervention indicated; limiting age-appropriate instrumental ADL	
3	Severe or medically significant but not immediately life-threatening; hospitalization or prolongation of existing hospitalization indicated; disabling; limiting self-care ADL	For severe/life-threatening symptoms such as adrenal crisis, severe headache, visual field deficiency: Hospitalize as appropriate. High-dose corticosteroid (prednisone 1 mg/kg/day) (or equivalent dose of methylprednisolone) in the acute phase, followed by taper over 1 month. Adrenal crisis should be managed per standard guidelines. If central hypothyroidism, replace thyroid hormone (see above) after corticosteroids have been initiated
4	Life-threatening consequences; urgent intervention indicated	

Adapted from Puzanov et al. [15]
ICI immune checkpoint inhibitor, *HRT* hormone replacement therapy

year, with repeat thyroid hormone testing in the first 6–8 weeks after the start of therapy, and monitored every 6 months thereafter [15]. ICI therapy should be held for cases grade 2 or higher until appropriate hormone repletion has begun [15] (Table 10.17).

It is crucial to recognize that hypophysitis can cause secondary adrenal insufficiency and hypothyroidism, as replacing thyroid hormone prior to cortisol replacement can precipitate adrenal crisis [15]. Patients with severe symptoms, such as severe headache, visual field defects, or adrenal crisis, require hospitalization and prompt intervention with standard adrenal crisis management and corticosteroids (prednisone 1 mg/kg/day tapered over 1 month after stabilization) [15]. Patients in adrenal crisis with resulting central hypothyroidism should receive thyroid replacement only after corticosteroids have been initiated [15].

Checkpoint inhibitor-induced hypothyroidism can be treated with standard thyroid hormone replacement therapy [15]. These patients should be monitored every 3 months for the first year, and every 6 months thereafter, with repeat thyroid function testing 6–8 weeks after the start of therapy [15]. ICI should be held for cases grade 3 or higher and can be continued once symptoms resolve to grade 2 or better [15] (Table 10.18).

The majority of cases of autoimmune type I diabetes mellitus present in diabetic ketoacidosis, and these patients should be hospitalized and treated according to standard guidelines [15] (Table 10.19). These patients should be educated on lifestyle changes and blood glucose monitoring, and treated with insulin per standard guidelines [15]. In contrast to standard management of checkpoint inhibitor toxicities, there is little benefit in using corticosteroids for managing hyperglycemia [150].

While treatment for checkpoint inhibitor endocrine toxicities is very similar to standard treatment guidelines, there is a paucity of data identifying autoimmune risk factors for developing these sequelae, and this could be a promising

Table 10.18 A guideline for checkpoint inhibitor hypothyroidism by CTCAE grade

Grade	Description	Management
1	Asymptomatic; clinical or diagnostic observations only; intervention not indicated	Hold ICI for ≥grade 3 irAEs ICI can be continued after resolution of symptoms to grade 2 or better Start standard thyroid replacement therapy: initial dose can be the full dose (1.6 mcg/kg) in young, healthy patients, but a reduced dose of 25–50mcg should be initiated in elderly patients with known cardiovascular disease
2	Symptomatic; thyroid replacement indicated; limiting instrumental ADL	Repeat TSH and free T4 testing after 6–8 weeks and adjust thyroid hormone dose accordingly. If TSH is above reference range, increase thyroid hormone dose by 12.5 mcg to 25 mcg
3	Severe symptoms; limiting self-care ADL; hospitalization indicated	After identification of the appropriate maintenance dose, further evaluation is required every year, or sooner if patient's status changes
4	Life-threatening consequences; urgent intervention indicated	After identification of the appropriate maintenance dose, further evaluation is required every year, or sooner if patient's status changes

Adapted from Puzanov et al. [15]
ICI immune checkpoint inhibitor, *ADL* activities of daily living

area of future study. Notably, certain HLA subtypes have been associated with autoimmune type 1 diabetes mellitus secondary to ICI therapy [150, 151]. Once high-risk patients are identified, prevention and screening protocols should be developed to reduce the overall risk of developing these toxicities.

TABLE 10.19 A guideline for checkpoint inhibitor hyperglycemia by CTCAE grade

Grade	CTCAE description	Management
1	Fasting glucose > ULN – 160 mg/dL (>ULN – 8.9 mmol/L)	Type 1 DM with diabetic ketoacidosis: Hold ICI; hospitalize and initiate treatment per standard guidelines Type 1 DM without diabetic ketoacidosis: Hold ICI for hyperglycemia ≥ grade 3. Treat with insulin and continue ICI when patient recovers to grade 1 Treat with insulin per standard guidelines and restart ICI when patient recovers to grade 1 Provide patient education on diet and lifestyle modification, and blood glucose testing
2	Fasting glucose >160–250 mg/dL (>8.9–13.9 mmol/L)	
3	Fasting glucose >250–500 mg/dL (>13.9–27.8 mmol/L); hospitalization indicated	
4	Fasting glucose >500 mg/dL (>27.8 mmol/L); life-threatening consequences	

Adapted from Puzanov et al. [15]
ICI immune checkpoint inhibitor

Conclusions and Future Directions

Immune checkpoint inhibitors are associated with toxicities that can affect almost any organ system in the body, with a highly variable time to onset. The underlying mechanisms of checkpoint inhibitor toxicity may shed light regarding why different irAEs occur at different time points. Although different toxicities may have different mechanisms, it is known that CTLA-4 has a widespread effect on inhibition of the immune response, whereas PD-1 performs its inhibitory effects at a later stage of the immune response [1]. Patients who receive anti-CTLA-4 therapy tend to experience interstitial nephritis earlier in their treatment course, about 2–3 months from start of treatment, compared to patients who receive anti-PD-1 therapy, who experience nephritis about 3–10 months from start of treatment [143]. This may be due to the narrower target effects of PD-1 inhibition compared to CTLA-4 inhibition, though the complete explanation for this time disparity remains an active area for further study. Vitiligo is a dermatologic toxicity specific to patients with melanoma who receive ICI therapy, a phenomenon partially explained by identical antigens that are present on melanocytes and melanoma tumor cells [152]. Checkpoint inhibitor toxicities have been associated with different mechanisms depending on the irAE in question. Associations have been found between type I diabetes and particular HLA phenotypes, checkpoint inhibitor colitis and alterations in the gut microbiome, myocarditis and T-cell infiltration, vitiligo and shared antigens between tumor and target tissues, and, finally, endocrinopathies and autoantibody formation [1]. Clarifying the mechanism of action may also explain why certain organs have a propensity to experience toxicity in particular tumor types.

Recent studies have identified an association between the development of irAEs and efficacy of ICI therapy. Patients with advanced non-small-cell lung cancer treated with nivolumab experienced a survival benefit when they experienced two or more irAEs [7]. Similar associations have been observed in melanoma, renal cell carcinoma, urothelial cell carcinoma, gastrointestinal cancers, and head and neck squamous cell cancer treated with ICI [153]. The exact connection between these two entities is not entirely understood, but may also be subject to a lead-time bias, as those more likely to respond to treatment may receive more ICI therapy, and subsequently develop irAEs.

Future research in the field of irAEs will focus on identifying risk factors for the development of specific irAEs. Although pre-existing autoimmune disease increases the risk of immunotherapy toxicity, these patients may derive similar anti-tumor effects from ICIs and can now receive immunotherapy in FDA-approved indications [154]. Genetic parameters, such as HLA haplotype, and tumor characteristics, such as histology, may also predispose certain populations to develop irAEs [155, 156]. Immunotherapy is steadily becoming commonplace in the community, and so developing comprehensive screening and surveillance protocols to find and monitor patients predisposed to developing particular toxicities is an active area of development. One group has posited a surveillance strategy to detect and potentially prevent life-threatening cardiotoxicity in patients with cardiac risk factors [137]. Further understanding of mechanisms and risk factors, as well as advancements in preventative approaches, will be the next frontier of irAE research.

References

1. Postow MA, Sidlow R, Hellmann MD. Immune-related adverse events associated with immune checkpoint blockade. N Engl J Med. 2018;378(2):158–68.
2. Haanen JB, Carbonnel F, Robert C, Kerr KM, Peters S, Larkin J, Jordan K. Management of toxicities from immunotherapy: ESMO clinical practice guidelines for diagnosis, treatment and follow-up. Ann Oncol. 2017;28(suppl_4):iv119–42.
3. US Dept of Health and Human Services. Common terminology criteria for adverse events (CTCAE). Version 5.0. US Dept of Health and Human Services. 2017. https://ctep.cancer.gov/protocoldevelopment/electronic_applications/docs/CTCAE_v5_Quick_Reference_5x7.pdf
4. Eggermont AM, Chiarion-Sileni V, Grob JJ, Dummer R, Wolchok JD, Schmidt H. Prolonged survival in stage III melanoma with Ipilimumab adjuvant therapy. N Engl J Med. 2016;375(19):1845–55.
5. Hodi FS, O'Day SJ, McDermott DF, Weber RW, Sosman JA, Haanen JB, et al. Improved survival with Ipilimumab in patients with metastatic melanoma. N Engl J Med. 2010;363(8):711–23.
6. Xing P, Zhang F, Wang G, Xu Y, Li C, Wang S, Guo Y, Cai S, Wang Y, Li J. Incidence rates of immune-related adverse events and their correlation with response in advanced solid tumours treated with NIVO or NIVO+ IPI: a systematic review and meta-analysis. J Immunother Cancer. 2019;7(1):341.

7. Carlino MS, Long GV. Ipilimumab combined with Nivolumab: a standard of Care for the Treatment of advanced melanoma? Clin Cancer Res. 2016;22(16):3992–8.
8. Wolchok JD, Kluger H, Callahan MK, Postow MA, Rizvi NA, Lesokhin AM, et al. Nivolumab plus ipilimumab in advanced melanoma. N Engl J Med. 2013;369:122–33.
9. Morganstein DL, Lai Z, Spain L, Diem S, Levine D, Mace C, et al. Thyroid abnormalities following the use of cytotoxic T-lymphocyte antigen-4 and programmed death receptor protein-1 inhibitors in the treatment of melanoma. Clin Endocrinol. 2017;86(4):614–20.
10. Naidoo J, Wang X, Woo KM, Iyriboz T, Halpenny D, Cunningham J, et al. Pneumonitis in patients treated with anti–programmed Death-1/programmed death ligand 1 therapy. J Clin Oncol. 2017;35(7):709–17.
11. Abdel-Rahman O, El Halawani H, Fouad M. Risk of endocrine complications in cancer patients treated with immune check point inhibitors: a meta-analysis. Future Oncol. 2016;12(3):413–25.
12. Connolly C, Bambhania K, Naidoo J. Immune-related adverse events: a case-based approach. Front Oncol. 2019;9(530):1–15
13. Thompson JA, Schneider BJ, Brahmer J, Andrews S, Armand P, Bhatia S, et al. Management of immunotherapy-related toxicities, version 1.2019, NCCN clinical practice guidelines in oncology. J Natl Compr Cancer Netw. 2019;17(3):255–89.
14. Haanen JBAG, Carbonnel F, Robert C, Kerr KM, Peters S, Larkin J, et al. Management of toxicities from immunotherapy: ESMO clinical practice guidelines for diagnosis, treatment and follow-up. Ann Oncol. 2018;29(Supplement_4):iv264–6.
15. Puzanov I, Diab A, Abdallah K, Bingham CO, Brogdon C, Dadu R, et al. Managing toxicities associated with immune checkpoint inhibitors: consensus recommendations from the Society for Immunotherapy of Cancer (SITC) Toxicity Management Working Group. J Immunother Cancer. 2017;5(1):95.
16. Wang DY, Salem JE, Cohen JV, Chandra S, Menzer C, Ye F, Zhao S, Das S, Beckermann KE, Ha L, Rathmell WK. Fatal toxic effects associated with immune checkpoint inhibitors: a systematic review and meta-analysis. JAMA Oncol. 2018;4(12):1721–8.
17. Brahmer JR, Lacchetti C, Schneider BJ, Atkins MB, Brassil KJ, Caterino JM, et al. Management of immune-related adverse events in patients treated with immune checkpoint inhibitor therapy: American Society of Clinical Oncology Clinical

Practice Guideline. J Clin Oncol Off J Am Soc Clin Oncol. 2018;36(17):1714–68.
18. Aarli JA. The immune system and the nervous system. Sur Prog. 1983;229:137–54.
19. Larkin J, Chmielowski B, Lao CD, Hodi FS, Sharfman W, Weber J, et al. Neurologic serious adverse events associated with Nivolumab plus Ipilimumab or Nivolumab alone in advanced melanoma, including a case series of encephalitis. Oncologist. 2017;22(6):709–18.
20. Kamath SD, Kumthekar PU. Immune checkpoint inhibitors for the treatment of central nervous system (CNS) metastatic disease. Frontiers in oncology. 2018;8(414):1–7.
21. Bot I, Blank CU, Boogerd W, Brandsma D. Neurological immune-related adverse events of ipilimumab. Pract Neurol. 2013;13(4):278–80.
22. Cuzzubbo S, Javeri F, Tissier M, Roumi A, Barlog C, Doridam J, et al. Neurological adverse events associated with immune checkpoint inhibitors: review of the literature. Eur J Cancer. 2017;73:1–8.
23. Nguyen BH, Kuo J, Budiman A, Christie H, Ali S. Two cases of clinical myasthenia gravis associated with pembrolizumab use in responding melanoma patients. Melanoma Res. 2017;27(2):152–4.
24. Hottinger AF. Neurologic complications of immune checkpoint inhibitors. Curr Opin Neurol. 2016;29(6):806–12.
25. Wick W, Hertenstein A, Platten M. Neurological sequelae of cancer immunotherapies and targeted therapies. Lancet Oncol. 2016;17(12):e529–41.
26. Cuzzubbo S, Tissier M. Neurological adverse events associated with the immune checkpoint inhibitors: review of the literature and characterization of the neurological patterns. Neuro-Oncology. 2016;18(suppl_4):iv25–6.
27. Fellner A, Makranz C, Lotem M, Bokstein F, Taliansky A, Rosenberg S, et al. Neurologic complications of immune checkpoint inhibitors. J Neuro-Oncol. 2018;137(3):601–9.
28. Dubey D, David W, Amato A, Reynolds K, Clement N, Chute D, et al. Varied phenotypes and management of immune checkpoint inhibitor-associated neuropathies. Neurology. 2019;93(11):e1093–103.
29. Blackmon JT, Viator TM, Conry RM. Central nervous system toxicities of anti-cancer immune checkpoint blockade. J Neurol Neuromed. 2016;1(4):39–45.

30. Mandel JJ, Olar A, Aldape KD, Tremont-Lukats IW. Lambrolizumab induced central nervous system (CNS) toxicity. J Neurol Sci. 2014;344(0):229–31.
31. Feng S, Coward J, McCaffrey E, Coucher J, Kalokerinos P, O'Bryne K. Pembrolizumab-induced encephalopathy: a review of neurological toxicities with immune checkpoint inhibitors. J Thorac Oncol. 2017;12(11):1626–35.
32. Liao B, Shroff S, Kamiya-Matsuoka C, Tummala S. Atypical neurological complications of ipilimumab therapy in patients with metastatic melanoma. Neuro-Oncology. 2014;16(4):589–93.
33. Lancaster E. The diagnosis and treatment of autoimmune encephalitis. J Clin Neurol. 2016;12(1):1–13.
34. Shah S, Dunn-Pirio A, Luedke M, Morgenlander J, Skeen M, Eckstein C. Nivolumab-induced autoimmune encephalitis in two patients with lung adenocarcinoma. Case Rep Neurolog Med. 2018:1–4.
35. Zafar Z, Vogler C, Hudali T, Bhattarai M. Nivolumab-associated acute demyelinating encephalitis: a case report and literature review. Clin Med Res. 2019;17(1–2):29–33.
36. Segreti J, Harris AA. Acute bacterial meningitis. Infect Dis Clin N Am. 1996;10(4):797–809.
37. Logan SA, MacMahon E. Viral meningitis. BMJ. 2008;336(7634):36–40.
38. Dubey D, Pittock SJ, Kelly CR, McKeon A, Lopez-Chiriboga AS, Lennon VA, Gadoth A, Smith CY, Bryant SC, Klein CJ, Aksamit AJ. Autoimmune encephalitis epidemiology and a comparison to infectious encephalitis. Ann Neurol. 2018;83(1):166–77.
39. Williams TJ, Benavides DR, Patrice K, Dalmau JO, Ávila d, Ribeiro AL, Le DT, et al. Association of Autoimmune Encephalitis with Combined Immune Checkpoint Inhibitor Treatment for metastatic Cancer. JAMA Neurol. 2016;73(8):928–33.
40. Johnson DB, Manouchehri A, Haugh AM, Quach HT, Balko JM, Lebrun-Vignes B, et al. Neurologic toxicity associated with immune checkpoint inhibitors: a pharmacovigilance study. J Immunother Cancer. 2019;7(1):134.
41. Gaudy-Marqueste C, Monestier S, Franques J, Cantais E, Richard M, Grob J. A severe case of ipilimumab-induced guillain-barré syndrome revealed by an occlusive enteric neuropathy: a differential diagnosis for ipilimumab-induced colitis. J Immunother. 2013;36(1):77–8.
42. Sepúlveda M, Martinez-Hernandez E, Gaba L, Victoria I, Sola-Valls N, Falgàs N, et al. Motor polyradiculopathy during pem-

brolizumab treatment of metastatic melanoma. Muscle Nerve. 2017;56(6):E162–7.

43. Mansoukis G, Koch J, Sommerville RB, EL-Dokla A, Harms MB, AL-Lozi MT, et al. Multifocal radiculopathy during Ipilimumab treatment of melanoma. Muscle Nerve. 2013;48:440–4.
44. Supakornnumporn S, Katirji B. Guillain-Barre syndrome triggered by immune checkpoint inhibitors: a case report and literature review. J Clin Neuromuscul Dis. 2017;19(2):80–3.
45. Spain L, Tippu Z, Larkin JM, Carr A, Turajlic S. How we treat neurological toxicity from immune checkpoint inhibitors. ESMO open. 2019;4(Suppl 4):1–5.
46. Thaipisuttikul I, Chapman P, Avila E. Peripheral neuropathy associated with Ipilimumab: a report of two cases. J Immunother. (Hagerstown, Md.: 1997). 2015;38(2):77.
47. Chen X, Haggiagi A, Tzatha E, DeAngelis LM, Santomasso B. Electrophysiological findings in immune checkpoint inhibitor-related peripheral neuropathy. Clin Neurophysiol. 2019;130(8):1440–5.
48. Wijdicks EF, Klein CJ. Guillain-barre syndrome. In: Mayo Clinic Proceedings 1 Mar 2017, vol. 92, no. 3. Elsevier. p. 467–79.
49. Dalakas MC. Neurological complications of immune checkpoint inhibitors: what happens when you 'take the brakes off'the immune system. Therapeutic advances in neurological disorders. 2018;11:1–9.
50. Suzuki S, Ishikawa N, Konoeda F, Seki N, Fukushima S, Takahashi K, et al. Nivolumab-related myasthenia gravis with myositis and myocarditis in Japan. Neurology. 2017;89(11):1127–34.
51. Makarious D, Horwood K, Coward JIG. Myasthenia gravis: an emerging toxicity of immune checkpoint inhibitors. Eur J Cancer. 2017;82:128–36.
52. Garcia CA, El-Ali A, Rath TJ, Contis LC, Gorantla V, Drappatz J, Davar D. Neurologic immune-related adverse events associated with adjuvant ipilimumab: report of two cases. J Immunother Cancer. 2018;6(1):83.
53. Fukasawa Y, Sasaki K, Natsume M, Nakashima M, Ota S, Watanabe K, Takahashi Y, Kondo F, Kozuma K, Seki N. Nivolumab-induced myocarditis concomitant with myasthenia gravis. Case Rep Oncol. 2017;10:809–12.
54. Gonzalez NL, Puwanant A, Lu A, Marks SM, Živković SA. Myasthenia triggered by immune checkpoint inhibitors: new case and literature review. Neuromuscul Disord. 2017;27(3):266–8.

55. Johnson DB, et al. Myasthenia gravis induced by Ipilimumab in patients with metastatic melanoma. J Clin Oncol. 2015;33(33):e122–4.
56. Chen JH, et al. Coexisting myasthenia gravis, myositis, and polyneuropathy induced by ipilimumab and nivolumab in a patient with non-small-cell lung cancer: a case report and literature review. Medicine (Baltimore). 2017;96(50):e9262.
57. Becquart O, Lacotte J, Malissart P, Nadal J, Lesage C, Guillot B, et al. Myasthenia gravis induced by immune checkpoint inhibitors. J Immunother. 2019;42(8):309–12.
58. Bennett DLH, Mills KR, Riordan-Eva P, Barnes PRJ, Rose MR. Anti-MuSK antibodies in a case of ocular myasthenia gravis. J Neurol Neurosurg Psychiatry. 2006;77(4):564–5.
59. Montes V, Sousa S, Pita F, Guerreiro R, Carmona C. Myasthenia gravis induced by ipilimumab in a patient with metastatic melanoma. Frontiers in neurology. 2018;9(150)1–3.
60. Romi F. Thymoma in myasthenia gravis: from diagnosis to treatment. Autoimmun Dis. 2011:1–5.
61. Trouth AJ, Dabi A, Solieman N, Kurukumbi M, Kalyanam J. Myasthenia gravis: a review. Autoimmun Dis. 2012:1–10.
62. Maggi L, Mantegazza R. Treatment of myasthenia gravis. Clin Drug Investig. 2011;31(10):691–701.
63. Dalvin LA, Shields CL, Orloff M, Sato T, Shields JA. Checkpoint inhibitor immune therapy: systemic indications and ophthalmic side effects. Retina. 2018;38(6):1063–78.
64. de Andrade FA, Fiorot SH, El B, Provenzano J, Martins VJ, Levy RA. The autoimmune diseases of the eyes. Autoimmun Rev. 2016;15(3):258–71.
65. Chang CJ, Chen SJ, Hwang DK, Liu CJ. Bilateral anterior uveitis after immunotherapy for malignant melanoma. Taiwan J Ophthalmol. 2018;8(3):173–5. https://doi.org/10.4103/tjo.tjo_88_17.
66. Fang T, Marberley DA, Ethminan M. Ocular adverse events with immune checkpoint inhibitors. J Curr Ophthalmol. 2019;31:319–22.
67. Conrady C, Conrady C, Larochelle M, Larochelle M, Pecen P, Pecen P, et al. Checkpoint inhibitor-induced uveitis: a case series. Graefes Arch Clin Exp Ophthalmol. 2018;256(1):187–91.
68. Aaberg MT, Aaberg TM. Pembrolizumab administration associated with posterior uveitis. Retinal Cases Brief Rep. 2016;11(4):1–351.

69. Kim JM, Materin MA, Sznol M, Kluger HM, Weiss S, Chow J, et al. Ophthalmic immune-related adverse events of immunotherapy: a single-site case series. Ophthalmology. 2019;126(7):1058–62.
70. Pasadhika S, Rosenbaum JT. Update on the use of systemic biologic agents in the treatment of non-infectious uveitis. BTT. 2014;8:67–81.
71. Friedman CF, Proverbs-Singh TA, Postow MA. Treatment of the immune-related adverse effects of immune checkpoint inhibitors: a review. JAMA Oncol. 2016;2(10):1346–53.
72. Cadranel J, Canellas A, Matton L, Darrason M, Parrot A, Naccache JM, Lavolé A, Ruppert AM, Fallet V. Pulmonary complications of immune checkpoint inhibitors in patients with nonsmall cell lung cancer. Eur Respir Rev. 2019;28(153): 190058.
73. Nishino M, Giobbie-Hurder A, Hatabu H, Ramaiya NH, Hodi FS. Incidence of programmed cell death 1 inhibitor–related pneumonitis in patients with advanced Cancer: a systematic review and meta-analysis. JAMA Oncol. 2016;2(12):1607–16.
74. Balaji A, Zhang J, Wills B, Marrone KA, Elmariah H, Yarchoan M, et al. Immune-related adverse events requiring hospitalization: Spectrum of toxicity, treatment, and outcomes. J Oncol Pract. 2019;15(9):e825–34.
75. Suresh K, Psoter KJ, Voong KR, Shankar B, Forde PM, Ettinger DS, et al. Impact of checkpoint inhibitor pneumonitis on survival in NSCLC patients receiving immune checkpoint immunotherapy. J Thorac Oncol. 14(3):494–502.
76. Postow MA, Chesney J, Pavlick AC, Robert C, Grossmann K, McDermott D, et al. Nivolumab and Ipilimumab versus Ipilimumab in untreated melanoma. N Engl J Med. 2015;372(21):2006–17.
77. Chuzi S, Tavora F, Cruz M, Costa R, Chae YK, Carneiro BA, et al. Clinical features, diagnostic challenges, and management strategies in checkpoint inhibitor-related pneumonitis. Cancer Manag Res. 2017;9:207–13.
78. Balaji A, Verde F, Suresh K, Naidoo J. Pneumonitis from anti–PD-1/PD-L1 therapy. Cancer Netw. 2017;31(10):739–46.
79. Rashdan S, Minna JD, Gerber DE. Diagnosis and management of pulmonary toxicity associated with cancer immunotherapy. Lancet Respir Med. 2018;6(6):472–8.
80. Barjaktarevic IZ, Qadir N, Suri A, Santamauro JT, Stover D. Organizing pneumonia as a side effect of Ipilimumab treatment of melanoma. Chest. 2013;143(3):858–61.

81. Tirumani SH, Ramaiya NH, Keraliya A, Bailey ND, Ott PA, Hodi FS, et al. Radiographic profiling of immune-related adverse events in advanced melanoma patients treated with Ipilimumab. Cancer Immunol Res. 2015;3(10):1185–92.
82. Suresh K, Naidoo J, Zhong Q, Xiong Y, Mammen J, de Flores MV, et al. The alveolar immune cell landscape is dysregulated in checkpoint inhibitor pneumonitis. J Clin Investig. 2019;129(10):4305–15.
83. Koelzer VH, Rothschild SI, Zihler D, Wicki A, Willi B, Willi N, et al. Systemic inflammation in a melanoma patient treated with immune checkpoint inhibitors—an autopsy study. J Immunother Cancer. 2016;4(1):13.
84. Naidoo J, Cappelli L, Lipson EJ, Forde PM, Sharfman WH, Zhang J, Mammen J, Moseley K, Suresh K, Mehta S, Sander I. A multidisciplinary toxicity team for cancer immunotherapy-related adverse events. J Natl Compr Cancer Netw. 2019;17(6):712–20.
85. Trinh S, Le A, Gowani S, La-Beck NM. Management of immune-related adverse events associated with immune checkpoint inhibitor therapy: a Minireview of current clinical guidelines. Asia Pac J Oncol Nurs. 2019;6(2):154–60.
86. Hodi FS, O'Day SJ, McDermott DF, Weber RW, Sosman JA, Haanen JB, Gonzalez R, Robert C, Schadendorf D, Hassel JC, Akerley W. Improved survival with ipilimumab in patients with metastatic melanoma. N Engl J Med. 2010;363(8):711–23.
87. Soularue E, Lepage P, Colombel JF, Coutzac C, Faleck D, Marthey L, Collins M, Chaput N, Robert C, Carbonnel F. Enterocolitis due to immune checkpoint inhibitors: a systematic review. Gut. 2018;67(11):2056–67.
88. Cabanillas G. Immune related adverse events and their treatment in melanoma patients receiving ipilimumab. JCO. 2017;35(15_suppl):e14598-e14598.
89. Gupta A, De Felice KM, Loftus EV, Khanna S. Systematic review: colitis associated with anti-CTLA-4 therapy. Aliment Pharmacol Ther. 2015;42(4):406–17.
90. Reddy HG, Schneider BJ, Tai AW. Immune checkpoint inhibitor-associated colitis and hepatitis. Clin Transl Gastroenterol. 2018;9:9.
91. Weber JS. Practical management of immune-related adverse events from immune checkpoint protein antibodies for the oncologist. Am Soc Clin Oncol Educ Book. 2012:174–7.

92. Zeimer M, Koukoulioti E, Simon JC, Berg T. Managing immune checkpoint-inhibitor-induced severe autoimmune-like hepatitis by liver-directed topical steroids. J Hepatol. 2017;66(3):657–9.
93. Gandhi L, Rodríguez-Abreu D, Gadgeel S, Esteban E, Felip E, De Angelis F, Domine M, Clingan P, Hochmair MJ, Powell SF, Cheng SY. Pembrolizumab plus chemotherapy in metastatic non–small-cell lung cancer. N Engl J Med. 2018;378(22):2078–92.
94. Kähler KC, Hassel JC, Heinzerling L, Loquai C, Mössner R, Ugurel S, et al. Management of side effects of immune checkpoint blockade by anti-CTLA-4 and anti-PD-1 antibodies in metastatic melanoma. J Dtsch Dermatol Ges. 2016;14(7):662–81.
95. Abu-Sbeih H, Tang T, Lu Y, Thirumurthi S, Altan M, Jazaeri AA, et al. Clinical characteristics and outcomes of immune checkpoint inhibitor-induced pancreatic injury. J Immunother Cancer. 2019;7(1):31.
96. George J, Bajaj D, Sankaramangalam K, Yoo JW, Joshi NS, Gettinger S, et al. Incidence of pancreatitis with the use of immune checkpoint inhibitors (ICI) in advanced cancers: a systematic review and meta-analysis. Pancreatology. 2019;19(4):587–94.
97. Su Q, Zhang X, Zhang C, Hou Y, Yao Y, Cao B. Risk of immune-related pancreatitis in patients with solid tumors treated with immune checkpoint inhibitors: systematic assessment with meta-analysis. J Immunol Res. 2018:e1027323.
98. Abu-Sbeih H, Faleck DM, Ricciuti B, Mendelsohn RB, Naqash AR, Cohen JV, et al. Immune checkpoint inhibitor therapy in patients with preexisting inflammatory bowel disease. J Clin Oncol. 2019:JCO1901674.
99. Dubin K, Callahan MK, Ren B, Khanin R, Viale A, Ling L, et al. Intestinal microbiome analyses identify melanoma patients at risk for checkpoint-blockade-induced colitis. Nat Commun. 2016;7(1):1–8.
100. Papaconstantinou HT, Thomas JS. Bacterial colitis. Clin Colon Rectal Surg. 2007;20(1):18–27.
101. Kim KW, Ramaiya NH, Krajewski KM, Shinagare AB, Howard SA, Jagannathan JP, et al. Ipilimumab-associated colitis: CT findings. AJR Am J Roentgenol. 2013;200(5):W468–74.
102. Cramer P, Bresalier R. Gastrointestinal and hepatic complications of immune checkpoint inhibitors. Curr Gastroenterol Rep. 2017;19(1):1–9.

103. Geukes Foppen MH, Rozeman EA, van Wilpe S, Postma C, Snaebjornsson P, van Thienen JV, et al. Immune checkpoint inhibition-related colitis: symptoms, endoscopic features, histology and response to management. ESMO Open. 2018;3(1):e000278.
104. Grover S, Rahma OE, Hashemi N, Lim RM. Gastrointestinal and hepatic toxicities of checkpoint inhibitors: algorithms for management. Am Soc Clin Oncol Educ Book. 2018;(38):13–19.
105. Bergqvist V, Hertervig E, Gedeon P, Kopljar M, Griph H, Kinhult S, Carneiro A, Marsal J. Vedolizumab treatment for immune checkpoint inhibitor-induced enterocolitis. Cancer Immunol Immunother. 2017;66(5):581–92.
106. Cheung V, Gupta T, Payne M, Middleton MR, Collier JD, Simmons A, et al. Immunotherapy-related hepatitis: real-world experience from a tertiary Centre. Frontline Gastroenterol. 2019;10(4):364–71.
107. Wolchok JD, Hoos A, O'Day S, Weber JS, Hamid O, Lebbé C, Maio M, Binder M, Bohnsack O, Nichol G, Humphrey R, Hodi FS. Guidelines for the evaluation of immune therapy activity in solid tumors: immune-related response criteria. Clin Cancer Res. 2009;15:7412–20.
108. Gauci M, Baroudjian B, Zeboulon C, Pages C, Poté N, Roux O, et al. Immune-related hepatitis with immunotherapy: are corticosteroids always needed? J Hepatol. 2018;69(2):548–50.
109. Suzman DL, Pelosof L, Rosenberg A, Avigan MI. Hepatotoxicity of immune checkpoint inhibitors: an evolving picture of risk associated with a vital class of immunotherapy agents. Liver Int. 2018;38(6):976–87.
110. Tsung I, Dolan R, Lao CD, Fecher L, Riggenbach K, Yeboah-Korang A, et al. Liver injury is most commonly due to hepatic metastases rather than drug hepatotoxicity during pembrolizumab immunotherapy. Aliment Pharmacol Ther. 2019;50(7):800–8.
111. Widmann G, Nguyen VA, Plaickner J, Jaschke W. Imaging features of toxicities by immune checkpoint inhibitors in Cancer therapy. Curr Radiol Rep. 2017;5(11):1–10.
112. Hsu C, Marshall JL, He AR. Workup and Management of Immune-Mediated Hepatobiliary Pancreatic Toxicities That Develop During Immune Checkpoint Inhibitor Treatment. The oncologist. 2020;25(2):105–111.
113. Zen Y, Yeh MM. Hepatotoxicity of immune checkpoint inhibitors: a histology study of seven cases in comparison with auto-

immune hepatitis and idiosyncratic drug-induced liver injury. Mod Pathol. 2018;31(6):965–73.
114. Zhang HC, Luo W, Wang Y. Acute liver injury in the context of immune checkpoint inhibitor-related colitis treated with infliximab. J Immunother Cancer. 2019;7(1):47.
115. Chmiel KD, Suan D, Liddle C, Nankivell B, Ibrahim R, Bautista C, et al. Resolution of severe ipilimumab-induced hepatitis after antithymocyte globulin therapy. J Clin Oncol. 2011;29(9):237.
116. Sanjeevaiah A, Kerr T, Beg MS. Approach and management of checkpoint inhibitor-related immune hepatitis. J Gastrointest Oncol. 2018;9(1):220–4.
117. Delanoy N, Michot J, Comont T, Kramkimel N, Lazarovici J, Dupont R, et al. Haematological immune-related adverse events induced by anti-PD-1 or anti-PD-L1 immunotherapy: a descriptive observational study. Lancet Haematol. 2019;6(1):e48–57.
118. Kohlmann J, Wagenknecht D, Simon J, Ziemer M. Immune-related pancreatitis associated with checkpoint blockade in melanoma. Melanoma Res. 2019;29(5):549–52.
119. Friedman CF, Clark V, Raikhel AV, Barz T, Shoushtari AN, Momtaz P, et al. Thinking critically about classifying adverse events: incidence of pancreatitis in patients treated with Nivolumab + Ipilimumab. J Natl Cancer Inst. 2017;109(4):1–3.
120. Saito H, Ono K. Nivolumab-induced pancreatitis: an immune-related adverse event. Radiology. 2019;293(3):521.
121. Shiuan E, Beckermann KE, Ozgun A, Kelly C, McKean M, McQuade J, et al. Thrombocytopenia in patients with melanoma receiving immune checkpoint inhibitor therapy. J Immunother Cancer. 2017;5(1):8.
122. Calvo R. Hematological side effects of immune checkpoint inhibitors: the example of immune-related thrombocytopenia. Front Pharmacol. 2019;10:454.
123. Tanios GE, Doley PB, Munker R. Autoimmune hemolytic anemia associated with the use of immune checkpoint inhibitors for cancer: 68 cases from the Food and Drug Administration database and review. Eur J Haematol. 2019;102:157–62.
124. Michot JM, Lazarovici J, Tier A, Champiat S, Voisin AL, Ebbo M, et al. Haematological immune-related adverse events with immune checkpoint inhibitos, how to manage? Eur J Cancer. 2019;122:72–90.

125. Papazafiropoulou A, Papanas N, Pappas S, Maltezos E, Mikhailidis DP. Effects of oral hypoglycemic agents on platelet function. J Diabetes Complicat. 2015;29(6):846–51.
126. Karakas Y, Yuce D, Kılıckap S. Immune thrombocytopenia induced by Nivolumab in a metastatic non-small cell lung Cancer patient. Oncol Res Treat. 2017;40(10):621–2.
127. Neunert C, Lim W, Crowther M, Cohen A, Solberg L, Crowther MA. The American Society of Hematology 2011 evidence-based practice guideline for immune thrombocytopenia. Blood. 2011;117(16):4190–207.
128. Varricchi G, Galdiero M, Marone G, Criscuolo G, Triassi M, Bonaduce D, et al. Cardiotoxicity of immune checkpoint inhibitors. ESMO Open. 2017;2:e000247. https://doi.org/10.1136/esmoopen-2017-000247.
129. Salem J, Manouchehri A, Moey M, Lebrun-Vignes B, Bastarache L, Pariente A, et al. Cardiovascular toxicities associated with immune checkpoint inhibitors: an observational, retrospective, pharmacovigilance study. Lancet Oncol. 2018;19:1579–89. https://doi.org/10.1016/S1470-2045(18)30608-9.
130. Johnson DB, Balko JM, Compton ML, Chalkias S, Gorham J, Xu Y, et al. Fulminant myocarditis with combination immune checkpoint blockade. N Engl J Med. 2016;375:1749–55. https://doi.org/10.1056/NEJMoa1609214.
131. Yang S, Asnani A. Cardiotoxicities associated with immune checkpoint inhibitors. Curr Probl Cancer. 2018;42:422–32.
132. Semper H, Muehlberg F, Schulz-Menger J, Allewelt M, Grohé C. Drug-induced myocarditis after nivolumab treatment in a patient with PDL1- negative squamous cell carcinoma of the lung. Lung Cancer. 2016;99:117–9.
133. Geisler BP, Raad RA, Esaian D, Sharon E, Schwartz DR Apical ballooning and cardiomyopathy in a melanoma patient treated with ipilimumab: a case of takotsubo-like syndrome.
134. de Almeida DVP, Gomes JR, Haddad FJ, Buzaid AC. Immune-mediated pericarditis with pericardial tamponade during nivolumab therapy. J Immunother. 2018;41:329–31.
135. Upadhrasta S, Elias H, Patel K, Zheng L. Managing cardiotoxicity associated with immune checkpoint inhibitors. Chronic Dis Transl Med. 2019;5(1):6–14.
136. Läubli H, Balmelli C, Bossard M, Pfister O, Glatz K, Zippelius A. Acute heart failure due to autoimmune myocarditis

under pembrolizumab treatment for metastatic melanoma. J Immunother Cancer. 2015;3:11.
137. Lyon AR, Yousaf N, Battisti NM, Moslehi J, Larkin J. Immune checkpoint inhibitors and cardiovascular toxicity. Lancet Oncol. 2018;19(9):e447–58.
138. Villadolid J, Amin A. Immune checkpoint inhibitors in clinical practice: update on management of immune-related toxicities. Transl Lung Cancer Res. 2015;4(5):560–75.
139. Spain L, Diem S, Larkin J. Management of toxicities of immune checkpoint inhibitors. Cancer Treat Rev. 2016;44:51–60.
140. Larkin J, et al. Combined Nivolumab and Ipilimumab or monotherapy in untreated melanoma. N Engl J Med. 2015;373(1):23–34.
141. Robert C, Schachter J, Long G, Arance A, Grob J, Mortier L, et al. Pembrolizumab versus ipilimumab in advanced melanoma. N Engl J Med. 2015;372:2521–32. https://doi.org/10.1056/NEJMoa1503093.
142. Ito J, Fujimoto D, Nakamura A, Nagano T, Uehara K, Imai Y, Tomii K. Aprepitant for refractory nivolumab-induced pruritus. Lung Cancer. 2017;109:58–61.
143. Cortazar FB, et al. Clinicopathological features of acute kidney injury associated with immune checkpoint inhibitors. Kidney Int. 2016;90(3):638–47.
144. Wanchoo R, Karam S, Uppal NN, Barta VS, Deray G, Devoe C, et al. Adverse renal effects of immune checkpoint inhibitors: a narrative review. Am J Nephrol. 2017;45(2):160–9.
145. Fadel F, El Karoui K, Knebelmann B. Anti-CTLA4 antibody-induced lupus nephritis. N Engl J Med. 2009;361(2):211–2.
146. Thajudeen B, et al. Ipilimumab granulomatous interstitial nephritis. Am J Ther. 2015;22(3):e84–7.
147. Shirali A, Perazella M, Gettinger S. Association of acute interstitial nephritis with programmed cell death 1 inhibitor therapy in lung cancer patients. Am J Kidney Dis. 2016;68:287–91. https://doi.org/10.1053/j.ajkd.2016.02.057.
148. El Majzoub I, Qdaisat A, Thein K, Win M, Han M, Jacobson K, et al. Adverse effects of immune checkpoint therapy in cancer patients visiting the emergency department of a comprehensive cancer center. Ann Emerg Med. 2019;73:79–87. https://doi.org/10.1016/j.annemergmed.2018.04.019.
149. Barroso-Sousa R, Barry WT, Garrido-Castro AC, Hodi FS, Min L, Krop IE, Tolaney SM. Incidence of endocrine dysfunction following the use of different immune checkpoint inhibitor

regimens: a systematic review and meta-analysis. JAMA Oncol. 2018;4(2):173–82.
150. Kapke J, Shaheen Z, Kilari D, Knudson P, Wong S. Immune checkpoint inhibitor-associated type 1 diabetes mellitus: case series, review of the literature, and optimal management. Case Rep Oncol. 2017;10(3):897–909.
151. Usui Y, Udagawa H, Matsomoto S, Imai K, Ohashi K, Ishibashi M, et al. Association of serum anti-GAD antibody and HLA haplotypes with type 1 diabetes mellitus triggered by Nivolumab in patients with non-small cell lung cancer. J Thorac Oncol. 2017;12:e41–3.
152. Larsabal M, Marti A, Jacquemin C, Rambert J, Thiolat D, Dousset L, et al. Vitiligo-like lesions occurring in patients receiving anti-programmed cell death–1 therapies are clinically and biologically distinct from vitiligo. J Am Acad Dermatol. 2017;76:863–70. https://doi.org/10.1016/j.jaad.2016.10.044.
153. Das S, Johnson DB. Immune-related adverse events and anti-tumor efficacy of immune checkpoint inhibitors. J Immunother Cancer. 2019;7:1–11.
154. Johnson D, Sullivan R, Menzies A. Immune checkpoint inhibitors in challenging populations. Cancer. 2017;123:1904–11. https://doi.org/10.1002/cncr.30642.
155. Cappelli L, Dorak M, Bettinotti M, Bingham C, Shah A. Association of HLA-DRB1 shared epitope alleles and immune checkpoint inhibitor induced inflammatory arthritis. Rheumatology. 2018;58:476–80. https://doi.org/10.1093/rheumatology/key358.
156. Suresh K, Voong K, Shankar B, Forde P, Ettinger D, Marrone K, et al. Pneumonitis in non–small cell lung cancer patients receiving immune checkpoint immunotherapy: incidence and risk factors. J Thorac Oncol. 2018;13:1930–9. https://doi.org/10.1016/j.jtho.2018.08.2035.

Chapter 11
Immune-Related Adverse Events with Other Cancer Immunotherapies

Sebastian Bruera and Cerena K. Leung

In addition to immune-checkpoint inhibitors, other forms of immunotherapy and immunomodulation have been developed for the treatment of cancer. The most promising therapies include chimeric antigen receptor T-cell (CAR-T) therapy, cytokines (such as interleukin-2 and interferon), and therapeutic vaccines. There are several other cytokines, vaccines, and cellular engineering techniques involving cells of the immune system that are currently being studied in animal models and phase 1 randomized control trials. This chapter will provide an overview of some of the more commonly used non-immune-checkpoint inhibitor immunotherapies along with immune-related adverse events that may occur with their use.

S. Bruera (✉)
Department of Medicine, Section of Immunology, Allergy, and Rheumatology, Baylor College of Medicine, Houston, TX, USA
e-mail: bruera@bcm.edu

C. K. Leung
Department of General Internal Medicine, The University of Texas MD Anderson Cancer Center, Houston, TX, USA
e-mail: ckleung2@mdanderson.org

M. E. Suarez-Almazor, L. H. Calabrese (eds.), *Rheumatic Diseases and Syndromes Induced by Cancer Immunotherapy*,
https://doi.org/10.1007/978-3-030-56824-5_11

Adoptive Cell Therapies: Chimeric Antigen Receptor T-Cell (CAR-T) Therapy

Adoptive cell therapy, or cellular immunotherapy, uses immune cells to target tumors. Within this field, chimeric antigen receptor T-cell (CAR-T) therapy is rapidly emerging as a highly effective treatment for various hematologic malignancies. Chimeric antigen receptor T-cell therapy utilizes a patient's own T-cells, which are engineered to target tumor antigens and are expected to initiate a long-lasting immune response against the patient's tumor.

Presently, CAR-T-cells are manufactured from autologous T-cells. A patient's T-cells are harvested via leukapheresis. Genes encoding a chimeric antigen receptor (CAR) specific to a cancer, such as CD19 present in CD19+ acute lymphoblastic leukemia, are transduced into the T-cell genetic code. T-cells subsequently express the CAR on their cell surface. The CAR-T-cells are infused into the patient after lymphodepletion. They bind to the extracellular antigen that is expressed on the cancer cell, resulting in increased cytokine release, CAR-T-cell proliferation, and tumor cell death [1].

Chimeric antigen receptor T-cell therapy has resulted in high rates of remission in otherwise fatal malignancies, such as acute lymphoblastic leukemia. However, there are also unique toxicities associated with this therapy. Two of the most worrisome adverse events from CAR-T therapy are cytokine release syndrome (CRS) and immune effector cell-associated neurotoxicity syndrome (ICANS.)

Cytokine Release Syndrome

Cytokine release syndrome is an inflammatory state that results from the binding of CAR-T-cells to their targeted antigen [2]. After binding to tumor cell antigens, the CAR-T-cells release cytokines that activate endothelial cells and antigen presenting cells, the most prominent of which is macrophages. Occasionally, a massive inflammatory response occurs, causing CRS. Interleukins (IL) released by macrophages and endothelial cells, such as IL-1 and IL-6, are central to the pathogenesis of CRS, though many other cytokines, including interferon-gamma (IFNg), IL-15, IL-8, and IL-10, have also been implicated. The hyperinflammatory response and activation of the innate immune system are responsible for many of the signs and symptoms of CRS, including fever, hypotension, and hypoxia that can result from capillary leaks.

The incidence of CRS varies, depending on the grade of severity of CRS, the specific chimeric antigen receptor (e.g., CD19 or CD22), and the malignancy that is being treated. Significant CRS requiring treatment may occur in 20–50% of patients [3]. Factors that increase the risk of developing CRS include higher tumor burden, lymphodepletion therapy with fludarabine, older age, comorbidities, and increased baseline levels of IL-6. Other biomarkers, including gp130, IFN-g, and von Willebrand factor, are currently being investigated to determine their value as a prognostic biomarker for the development of CRS during CAR-T therapy as well as a diagnostic tool.

Initial clinical manifestations of CRS include fever and flu-like symptoms. While most cases are mild, the syndrome can progress to shock with multi-organ failure, hypoxic respiratory failure, and disseminated intravascular coagulation. The onset of CRS usually occurs within 24 to 72 hours after CAR-T infusion and can persist for over one week. Both the American Society of Transplantation and Cellular Therapy (ASTCT) and the CAR-T-Cell Therapy-Associated Toxicity (CARTOX) group have developed a grading scale to determine the severity of CRS and to guide treatment as summarized in Table 11.1 [4, 5]. Trending c-reactive protein (CRP) and ferritin levels are helpful in determining response to interventions, though CRP typically falls dramatically after administration of tocilizumab.

The treatment of grade 1 and, in some cases, of grade 2 CRS is typically intravenous fluids and supportive care [6]. Severe CRS, defined as some cases of grade 2 (depending on physician's discretion), grade 3, and grade 4, is treated with

Table 11.1 American Society of Transplantation and Cellular Therapy and CARTOX grading scales for CRS [4, 5]

CRS Grade	ASTCT scale	CARTOX scale
Grade 1	Temperature ≥ 38.0 degrees Celsius without hypotension or hypoxia	Temperature ≥ 38.0 degrees Celsius Grade 1 organ toxicity
Grade 2	Temperature ≥ 38.0 degrees Celsius with hypotension not requiring vasopressors and/or hypoxia requiring the use of low-flow nasal cannula (≤6 L/minute)	Hypotension responding to intravenous fluids or low-dose vasopressors Hypoxia requiring $FiO_2 < 40\%$ Grade 2 organ toxicity
Grade 3	Temperature ≥ 38.0 degrees Celsius with hypotension requiring 1 vasopressor with or without vasopressin and/or hypoxia requiring high-flow nasal cannula (>6 L/minute), face-mask, nonrebreather mask, or Venturi mask	Hypotension needing high-dose or multiple vasopressors Hypoxia requiring $FiO_2 \geq 40\%$ Grade 3 organ toxicity or grade 4 transaminitis
Grade 4	Temperature ≥ 38.0 degrees Celsius with hypotension requiring multiple vasopressors (excluding vasopressin) and/or hypoxia requiring positive pressure	Life-threatening hypotension Needing ventilator support Grade 4 organ toxicity except for grade 4 transaminitis

intravenous tocilizumab at 8 mg/kg (not to exceed 800 mg). Treatment should be initiated immediately upon suspicion and can be repeated every six hours up to a total of four doses if there is inadequate response. Clinical improvement may be seen within hours. The use of tocilizumab in the treatment of CRS has not been shown to decrease tumor response rates to CAR-T therapy. In severe cases, corticosteroids may be used as an adjunct therapy, but this may irreversibly impair

CAR-T-cell efficacy. Steroid tapering should be done as rapidly as possible once the patient demonstrates a favorable response. Other potential therapies under investigation include siltuximab (anti-IL-6 antibody), ruxolitinib (JAK 1/2 inhibitor), anakinra (IL-1 receptor antagonist), etanercept (TNF-inhibitor), and dasatinib (lymphocyte-specific protein tyrosine kinase inhibitor) [7–9].

Preventive therapy with prophylactic tocilizumab in patients who are at high risk of developing CRS is currently being evaluated, both prior to and in conjunction with infusion of CAR-T-cells.

Immune Effector Cell-Associated Neurotoxicity Syndrome

Previously referred to as CAR-T-cell-related encephalopathy syndrome (CRES), immune effector cell-associated neurotoxicity syndrome (ICANS) typically occurs in conjunction with CRS. However, there have been cases where the onset of ICANS has occurred weeks after the infusion of CAR-T-cells. The pathophysiology of ICANS is not well understood but likely involves an increased permeability of the blood–brain barrier that results in the infiltration of immune cells and cytokines into the cerebrospinal fluid [10]. Risk factors for ICANS include neurologic comorbidities, high tumor burden, high CAR-T expansion, thrombocytopenia, and the use of fludarabine for lymphodepletion [11]. Ferritin levels positively correlate with disease severity.

The diagnosis of ICANS is clinical. Clinical manifestations include encephalopathy, seizures, dysphagia, tremors, headaches, depressed levels of consciousness, and cerebral edema that can be fatal [5]. Magnetic resonance imaging (MRI) may demonstrate vasogenic edema but is usually used to rule out other causes of similar symptoms, such as ischemia, malignancy, or infection. Often times, MRIs are unremarkable in patients with ICANS. The Immune Effector Cell-Associated Encephalopathy (ICE) score was developed

Table 11.2 Immune Effector Cell-Associated Encephalopathy (ICE) score [4, 5]

ICE
Orientation: To year, month, city, and hospital: *4 points*
Naming: Ability to name three objects (such as clock, book, and pen): *3 points*
Following commands: Ability to follow simple commands: *1 point*
Writing: Ability to write a sentence: *1 point*
Attention: Ability to count backward from 100 by 10: *1 point*

Score 7–9: Grade 1 ICANS
Score 3–6: Grade 2 ICANS
Score 0–2: Grade 3 ICANS
Score 0: Grade 4 ICANs

by the CARTOX and ASTCT working groups to grade severity of ICANS and to guide clinical treatment (Table 11.2).

Tocilizumab is not effective for the treatment of ICANS and is only utilized if there is concurrent cytokine release syndrome [5]. It is hypothesized that this may be due to the fact that tocilizumab does not cross the blood–brain barrier. The treatment largely consists of supportive management, such as anti-epileptics. Intravenous dexamethasone, 10 mg every six hours, is recommended for grade 2–3 ICANS as it can penetrate the brain, but high-dose methylprednisolone (1 g intravenously) is advised for grade 4 ICANS. Corticosteroids are continued until ICANS severity improves to grade 1 prior to being tapered. Other experimental options include siltuximab, as this directly inhibits IL-6 as opposed to the receptor, and anakinra.

Cytokines

Cytokines are small proteins that are critical in cell signaling and activation, and inactivation of various components of the immune system. To date, there are currently two cytokines that have received Food and Drug Administration (FDA) approval for the treatment of cancer: recombinant interferon (IFN)-α and IL-2. As mentioned in Chap. 1, there are various early clinical trials investigating the infusion or blocking of cytokines with or without checkpoint inhibitors.

Recombinant Interferon-Alpha

Interferons are cytokines produced by the innate immune system that are classically involved in combatting viral infections. There are three types of IFN: type 1, type 2, and type 3. Type 1 IFN largely consists of IFN-α. Interferon-α has been used to treat hepatitis B, hepatitis C, and various cancers [12]. Anti-tumor mechanisms of IFN-α include inhibition of tumor growth by causing apoptosis and preventing cell proliferation, and activation of immune cells such as natural killer cells that target cancer cells [13, 14]. The use of IFN therapy is important in regard to rheumatic diseases as high levels of IFN gene expression have been associated with the development of and the severity of autoimmune disorders, most notably systemic lupus erythematosus [15]. In fact, anti-interferon therapy has been used in the treatment of systemic lupus and is currently under investigation as a therapeutic option for rheumatoid arthritis [16].

Several IFN therapies have been used for the treatment of cancer, including IFNα-2a and IFNα-2b. These recombinant biologics are similar in structure and function. Interferon has been used to treat cancer for many years, including hairy cell leukemia, renal cell carcinoma, follicular lymphoma, melanoma, and Kaposi's sarcoma. However, the use of IFN has declined, as immune checkpoint inhibitors have become the first-line therapy for many of these malignancies.

There are various immune-related adverse effects with the use of IFNα. The use of IFNα in the treatment of hepatitis is associated with the formation of autoantibodies, especially antinuclear antibodies at high titers [17]. Although the formation of autoantibodies does not necessarily cause autoimmunity, there have been many reports of patients developing autoimmunity or flares of underlying autoimmune diseases after treatment with IFNα-, a phenomenon that has also been seen in cancer populations [18, 19]. Autoimmune diseases that have developed after treatment with IFN include thyroiditis, rheumatoid arthritis, lupus, sarcoidosis, psoriatic arthritis, adrenal insufficiency, pituitary dysfunction, and autoimmune diabetes.

Most available data for adverse events in patients with pre-existing rheumatic disease who received IFN therapy were published from the 1980s to the 2000s in the setting of treatment for viral hepatitis. This is largely because patients with underlying rheumatic diseases were eligible to undergo treatment, whereas a personal history of autoimmune disease is an exclusion criterion in most trials studying the use of interferon therapy within the cancer population [20–22]. The autoimmune diseases that most commonly flare after treatment with IFN are systemic lupus erythematosus and rheumatoid arthritis.

Patients should be closely monitored during therapy for the development of flaring autoimmune disease while on therapy. Some patients will have complete resolution with minimal systemic therapy and cessation of IFN therapy, but others may require lifelong treatment for the new underlying disease [21, 23]. Currently, there are no available prognostic data regarding underlying patient characteristics that may increase the risk of developing a flare or autoimmunity besides having pre existing autoimmune disease. Prophylactic therapy with hydroxychloroquine can be considered in patients with autoimmunity who are undergoing IFN therapy to prevent flares, though this has been poorly studied [24]. Interestingly, the development of autoimmune phenomena, while undergoing IFN therapy for melanoma, is associated with increases in relapse-free survival [25].

Recombinant Interleukin-2 Therapy

Aldesleukin (recombinant IL-2) has been used for the treatment of melanoma and renal cell carcinoma. Interleukin-2 causes proliferation of specific subsets of T-cells that target tumor cells and can potentially be an effective immunomodulator for the treatment of cancer [26]. On the other hand, IL-2 is critical for the development of self-tolerance; IL-2-knockout mouse models develop autoimmunity [27]. Therefore, although recombinant IL-2 has been effective for selected malignancies, high doses needed for treatment are associated with a variety of immune-related adverse events such as vascular leak syndrome, myocarditis, and cytokine storm [28].

Vascular Leak Syndrome

Vascular leak, or capillary leak syndrome, is characterized by the diffusion of intravascular fluid to interstitial spaces, causing "third spacing" or anasarca, pulmonary edema, low blood pressures, and, in severe cases, death [29]. This occurs in varying degrees in up to half of the patients who receive high-dose IL-2 therapy [30]. Interleukin-2 causes the release of other cytokines increasing endothelial permeability and allowing various proteins to enter the interstitial space. This leads to a decrease in intravascular volume which activates the renin and aldosterone system, ultimately resulting in sodium retention, fluid retention, and anasarca. Symptoms usually occur within 6 hours of IL-2 infusion. Infusions are typically administered in an inpatient setting and given in fractionated doses every 8 hours to monitor for adverse effects. In hypotensive patients, the most important treatment is adequate resuscitation with crystalline fluids and vasopressor support as needed. Colloid solutions can extravasate to the extravascular space. Some patients may also require renal replacement therapy and noninvasive or invasive means of oxygen supplementation.

Myocarditis

Myocarditis, albeit rarely, has been reported with IL-2 infusions [31–33]. Patients with myocarditis will typically present with chest pain and elevated troponins. Acute myocardial infarction is important to consider, as IL-2 infusions can cause decreased blood pressure and subsequent demand ischemia that can cause infarction. In the case of myocarditis, a cardiac catheterization will reveal unobstructed coronary arteries, and cardiac magnetic resonance imaging may help confirm the diagnosis. The treatment consists of withholding IL-2 and supportive care, though symptoms may persist for days after IL-2 discontinuation. Some providers have also administered corticosteroids in treating severe cases.

Given the aforementioned toxicities and novel treatment options, high-dose recombinant IL-2 therapy has largely fallen out of favor as a primary treatment option for melanoma and renal cell carcinoma. Nonetheless, alternative administrations of IL-2 are currently being explored. For example, aerosolized IL-2 is being evaluated as there may be theoretical improvement in managing pulmonary metastases with possibly a more favorable toxicity profile (NCT:01590069 on ClinicalTrials.gov). Interleukin-2 is also being studied as an adjunct therapy with CAR T-cell infusions (NCT:01955460 on ClinicalTrials.gov).

Vaccines

The use of therapeutic vaccines for the treatment of various cancers has been an important area of investigation, but, to date, only Sipuleucel-T has been approved by the FDA.

Sipuleucel-T

Sipuleucel-T is a therapeutic vaccine used for the treatment of metastatic castration-resistant prostate cancer. Autologous antigen-presenting cells (dendritic cells) are isolated via leukapheresis. The dendritic cells are exposed to prostatic acid phosphate and granulocyte-macrophage colony-stimulating factor (GM-CSF). Dendritic cells presenting these antigens on their surface are then reinfused into patients every two weeks. The dendritic cells activate T-cells to target prostate cancer cells that express these antigens. Sipuleucel-T has modest effects on overall patient survival [34]. It is well tolerated and has not been associated with the development of immune-related adverse events to date [35]. Acute infusion reactions can cause a flu-like illness that self-resolves within 48 hours.

Mycobacterium bovis Bacillus Calmette-Guérin (BCG)

The *Mycobacterium bovis* BCG species was initially discovered as a potential vaccine for tuberculosis. It was subsequently found to be useful in the treatment of bladder cancer. As an irrigant, BCG can promote immune responses that improve survival in the treatment of bladder cancer and has remained a standard of care for many decades. Irrigation with BCG causes a response in both the adaptive and innate immune systems that target bladder tumor cells, as evidenced by positive purified protein derivative skin testing [36]. Adverse events with this therapy are typically divided into early and late. Early complications are usually local and consist of cystitis, hematuria, and fevers without evidence of sepsis. Late complications include chronic cystitis, granulomatous infections along the urinary tract, and, very rarely, BCG infections of the lungs, bones, joints, or aorta [37]. In addition, BCG treatment has occasionally been associated with the development of inflammatory arthritis, which is thought to be a reactive arthritis similar to what occurs with other infections [38]. A case series of 89 patients has described the reactive arthritis that occurs with BCG [39]. It typically occurs, on average, after six instillations and two weeks after the last instillation. The presentation can be polyarthritis or oligoarthritis, and symmetric or asymmetric. After the diagnosis is confirmed, the treatment is typically with nonsteroidal anti-inflammatory drugs, and corticosteroids if there is no response. If symptoms persist, patients may require disease-modifying anti-rheumatic drugs (DMARDs).

Conclusions and Future Directions

Although immunotherapy has been utilized for cancer treatment for decades, the discovery of checkpoint inhibitors and CAR-T therapy has transformed the field of oncology, leading to overall increased survival in previously fatal malignancies. Several new therapeutic options in animal models and early clinical trials are being explored (see Chap. 1). As these treatments develop, new immune-related adverse events will likely arise, and it is the knowledge and experiences from previous and current therapies that will be critical in learning how to address them.

References

1. Benmebarek MR, et al. Killing mechanisms of chimeric antigen receptor (CAR) T cells. Int J Mol Sci. 2019;20(6):1–21.
2. Frey N, Porter D. Cytokine release syndrome with chimeric antigen receptor T cell therapy. Biol Blood Marrow Transplant. 2019;25(4):e123–7.
3. Cao G, Lei L, Zhu X. Efficiency and safety of autologous chimeric antigen receptor T-cells therapy used for patients with lymphoma: a systematic review and meta-analysis. Medicine (Baltimore). 2019;98(42):e17506.
4. Lee DW, et al. ASTCT consensus grading for cytokine release syndrome and neurologic toxicity associated with immune effector cells. Biol Blood Marrow Transplant. 2019;25(4):625–38.
5. Neelapu SS, et al. Chimeric antigen receptor T-cell therapy – assessment and management of toxicities. Nat Rev Clin Oncol. 2018;15(1):47–62.
6. Brudno JN, Kochenderfer JN. Toxicities of chimeric antigen receptor T cells: recognition and management. Blood. 2016;127(26):3321–30.
7. Mestermann K, G.T., Weber J, Rydzek J, Frenz S, Nerreter T, Mades A, Sadelain M, Einsele H, Hudecek M, The tyrosine

kinase inhibitor dasatinib acts as a pharmacologic on/off switch for CAR-T cells. Sci Transl Med. 2019;11(499):1–11.
8. Murthy H, et al. Cytokine release syndrome: current perspectives. Immunotargets Ther. 2019;8:43–52.
9. Giavridis T, et al. CAR-T cell-induced cytokine release syndrome is mediated by macrophages and abated by IL-1 blockade. Nat Med. 2018;24(6):731–8.
10. Gust J, et al. Endothelial activation and blood-brain barrier disruption in neurotoxicity after adoptive immunotherapy with CD19 CAR-T cells. Cancer Discov. 2017;7(12):1404–19.
11. Gauthier J, Turtle CJ. Insights into cytokine release syndrome and neurotoxicity after CD19-specific CAR-T cell therapy. Curr Res Transl Med. 2018;66(2):50–2.
12. Kirkwood J. Cancer immunotherapy: the interferon-alpha experience. Semin Oncol. 2002;29(3) Suppl 7:18–26.
13. Muller L, Aigner P, Stoiber D, Type I. Interferons and natural killer cell regulation in cancer. Front Immunol. 2017;8:304.
14. Kotredes KP, Gamero AM. Interferons as inducers of apoptosis in malignant cells. J Interf Cytokine Res. 2013;33(4):162–70.
15. Petri M, et al. Association between changes in gene signatures expression and disease activity among patients with systemic lupus erythematosus. BMC Med Genet. 2019;12(1):4.
16. Morand EF, et al. Trial of anifrolumab in active systemic lupus erythematosus. N Engl J Med. 2020;382(3):211–21.
17. Noda K, et al. Induction of antinuclear antibody after interferon therapy in patients with type-C chronic hepatitis: its relation to the efficacy of therapy. Scand J Gastroenterol. 1996;31(7):716–22.
18. Ronnblom LE, Alm G, Oberg KE. Autoimmunity after alpha-interferon therapy for malignant carcinoid tumors. Ann Intern Med. 1991;115(3):178–83.
19. Gota C, Calabrese L. Induction of clinical autoimmune disease by therapeutic interferon-alpha. Autoimmunity. 2003;36(8):511–8.
20. Conlon KC, Urba W, Smith JW II, Steis RG, Longo DL, Clark JW. Exacerbation of symptoms of autoimmune disease in patients receiving alpha-interferon therapy. Cancer. 1990;65(10):2237–42.
21. Niewold TB, Swedler WI. Systemic lupus erythematosus arising during interferon-alpha therapy for cryoglobulinemic vasculitis associated with hepatitis C. Clin Rheumatol. 2005;24(2):178–81.
22. Dumoulin FL, Leifeld L, Sauerbruch T, Spengler U. Autoimmunity induced by interferon-alpha therapy for chronic viral hepaitis. Biomed Pharmacother. 1999;53:242–54.

23. Ho V, McLean A, Terry S. Severe systemic lupus erythematosus induced by antiviral treatment for hepatitis C. J Clin Rheumatol. 2008;14(3):166–8.
24. Nesher G, Ruchlemer R. Alpha-interferon-induced arthritis: clinical presentation, treatment, and prevention. Semin Arthritis Rheum. 1998;27(6):360–5.
25. Stuckert JJS II, et al. Interferon alfa-induced autoimmunity and serum S100 levels as predictive and prognostic biomarkers in high-risk melanoma in the ECOG-intergroup phase II trial E2696. J Clin Oncol. 2007;25(18_suppl):8506.
26. Skrombolas D, Frelinger JG. Challenges and developing solutions for increasing the benefits of IL-2 treatment in tumor therapy. Expert Rev Clin Immunol. 2014;10(2):207–17.
27. Horak I. Immunodeficiency in IL-2-knockout mice. Clin Immunol Immunopathol. 1995;76:S172–S173.
28. Marabondo S, Kaufman HL. High-dose interleukin-2 (IL-2) for the treatment of melanoma: safety considerations and future directions. Expert Opin Drug Saf. 2017;16(12):1347–57.
29. Siddall E, Khatri M, Radhakrishnan J. Capillary leak syndrome: etiologies, pathophysiology, and management. Kidney Int. 2017;92(1):37–46.
30. Jeong GH, et al. Incidence of capillary leak syndrome as an adverse effect of drugs in cancer patients: a systematic review and meta-analysis. J Clin Med. 2019;8:2.
31. Kragel AH, William T, Feinberg L, Pittaluga S, Striker LM, Roberts WC, Lotze MT, Yang JJ, Rosenberg SA. Pathologic findings associated with interleukin-2-based immunotherapy for cancer: a postmortem study of 19 patients. Hum Pathol. 1990;21(5):493–502.
32. Thavendiranathan P, et al. Fulminant myocarditis owing to high-dose interleukin-2 therapy for metastatic melanoma. Br J Radiol. 2011;84(1001):e99–e102.
33. Eisner RM, Husain A, Clark JI. Case report and brief review: IL-2-induced myocarditis. Cancer Investig. 2004;22(3):401–4.
34. Kawalec P, et al. Sipuleucel-T immunotherapy for castration-resistant prostate cancer. A systematic review and meta-analysis. Arch Med Sci. 2012;8(5):767–75.
35. Dores GM, B.-G.M., Perez-Vilar S, Adverse events associated with the use of sipuleucel-T reported to the US Food and Drug Administration's Adverse Event Reporting System, 2010–2017. JAMA Netw Open. 2019;2(8):1–14.

36. Pettenati C, Ingersoll MA. Mechanisms of BCG immunotherapy and its outlook for bladder cancer. Nat Rev Urol. 2018;15(10):615–25.
37. Liu Y, et al. Clinical Spectrum of complications induced by Intravesical immunotherapy of Bacillus Calmette-Guerin for bladder Cancer. J Oncol. 2019;2019:6230409.
38. Shoenfeld Y, et al. Bcg and autoimmunity: another two-edged sword. J Autoimmun. 2001;16(3):235–40.
39. Bernini L, et al. Reactive arthritis induced by intravesical BCG therapy for bladder cancer: our clinical experience and systematic review of the literature. Autoimmun Rev. 2013;12(12):1150–9.

Part III
Cancer Immunotherapy in Patients with Pre-existing Rheumatic Diseases

Chapter 12
Cancer Immunotherapy in Patients with Preexisting Inflammatory Arthritis

Uma Thanarajasingam and Noha Abdel-Wahab

Introduction

Immune checkpoint inhibitors (ICI) novel immunotherapeutic agents, are increasingly being considered as a standard of care for numerous cancers including in the adjuvant setting significantly increasing the population of patients exposed to these agents [1–9]. Despite therapeutic benefits, ICI can frequently cause off-target inflammation and autoimmunity in various organs, which can sometimes be life-threatening [10–13]. Therefore, patients with a dual diagnosis of cancer

U. Thanarajasingam (✉)
Mayo Clinic, Rochester, MN, USA
e-mail: Thanarajasingam.Uma@mayo.edu

N. Abdel-Wahab
The University of Texas MD Anderson Cancer Center, Houston, TX, USA

Assiut University Hospital, Faculty of Medicine, Assiut, Egypt
e-mail: nahassan@mdanderson.org

M. E. Suarez-Almazor, L. H. Calabrese (eds.), *Rheumatic Diseases and Syndromes Induced by Cancer Immunotherapy*,
https://doi.org/10.1007/978-3-030-56824-5_12

and autoimmune disease have been systematically excluded from ICI trials owing to concerns about exacerbation of their underlying autoimmunity and increasing their risk for immunotoxicity [14]. To date, our knowledge of the safety and efficacy of ICI in this patient population is limited to case reports, series, and observational studies. A recent systematic review and meta-analysis of observational studies reporting on ICI use in patients with cancer and autoimmune disease found that the pooled prevalence rate was 55% (95% confidence interval [CI] 44–66%) for any immune-related adverse events (irAEs), 29% (95% CI 11–49%) for autoimmune disease flares, and 30% (95% CI 24–35%) for de novo irAEs, and the mortality rate was 31% (95% CI 11–56%), but none attributed to autoimmune disease flares [15].

In this chapter, we will focus primarily on patients with preexisting inflammatory arthritis treated with ICI. We will summarize the available epidemiologic data, highlight specific elements of pathogenesis, and discuss an illustrative case of a rheumatoid arthritis (RA) patient treated with ICI for concomitant melanoma. In view of this case, we will then review the management strategy based on current guidelines and available evidence, in an effort to guide rheumatologists through the challenges we encounter during management of these patients until more robust prospective longitudinal studies become available.

Epidemiology

Rheumatoid Arthritis

Eight observational studies provided data on 86 patients with preexisting RA/inflammatory arthritis who had received ICI therapy, of whom 48 patients (56%) developed an arthritis flare following ICI initiation [16–23]. The largest cohort is a single-center, retrospective study which described 22 patients with RA and reported flares in 55% and de novo irAEs in 32% after ICI initiation [22]. In a multicenter French study, another 20 patients with RA were reported; 65% were receiving maintenance therapy for RA at ICI initiation (7 on methotrexate, 6 on corticosteroids at a dose ≤15 mg/day, and 1 each on hydroxychloroquine and rituximab). Flares occurred in 75% of patients with active RA and 60% of those receiving maintenance therapy (five on methotrexate and one on hydroxychloroquine) [18]. Corticosteroids were required for managing flares in 83% and increasing methotrexate dosage was needed in one patient. Discontinuation of ICI was required in 15% because of immunotoxicity and death was reported in 25%, but none was related to immunotoxicity.

In addition, a total of 38 patients with RA/inflammatory arthritis who have received ICI have been published in case reports and retrospective series which provided detailed description of each reported patient [14, 16, 24–40]. Median age was 66 (39–87) years, 52% were male, 92% had melanoma, 63% received ipilimumab, 68% (17 out of 25) had active joint symptoms, and 48% (11 out of 23) were receiving immunosuppressant therapies at ICI initiation; 10 were receiving corticosteroids, and 9 were receiving disease-modifying anti-rheumatic drugs (DMARDs) including 6 on hydroxychloroquine, and 1 each on methotrexate, sulfasalazine, leflunomide, and etanercept. Adverse events occurred in 82% after a median of 3 (0.1–8) weeks of ICI initiation; 61% had arthritis flares and 45% had de novo irAEs, while 18% tolerated treatment without incident. Arthritis flares occurred more frequently among patients who had active symptoms at ICI initiation compared to patients who did not have any symptoms (71% versus 31%) and occurred less frequently among patients who were maintained on immunosuppressant therapies at ICI initiation compared to those who were not (45% compared to 58%). As for de novo irAEs, the frequency and phenotype were similar to what has been reported in ICI trials, with colitis and hypophysitis being the most frequent, but other irAEs have also been reported including thyroiditis, hepatitis, nephritis, dermatitis, neuritis, encephalitis, cardiomyopathy, myositis, myasthenia gravis, and sicca symptoms. Arthritis flares and de novo irAEs required management with corticosteroids (up to 2 mg/kg/day) in 94% of patients, and 23% required additional disease-modifying anti-rheumatic medications or DMARDs (i.e., methotrexate, hydroxychloroquine, sulfasalazine, infliximab, and etanercept). Flares and de novo irAEs improved in all patients, but only one patient continued to have chronic arthritis symptoms. Discontinuation of ICI was reported in 56% (15 out of 27), primarily because of adverse events in 12 patients. Re-induction of ICI was reported in two patients who switched from ipilimumab to pembrolizumab: one had an arthritis flare and the other had de novo irAE after ICI rechallenge [28, 38]. In melanoma patients, the disease control rate was 60%. No treatment-related mortality was reported.

Spondyloarthritis

Six observational studies provided data on 18 patients with preexisting spondyloarthritis (SPA) treated with ICI [16–21, 23], and data of additional 20 patients have been published in case reports and retrospective series with detailed description of each patient [24, 25, 29, 30, 34, 40–45]. Overall, patients with different types of SPA were reported (14 psoriatic arthritis, 6 ankylosing spondylitis, 1 reactive arthritis, and 17 unspecified SPA). Their age ranged from 38 to 81 years, 60% were male, 67% had melanoma, 63% received anti-PD-1/PD-L1 agents, 33% (8 out of 24) had active joint symptoms, and 24% (5 out of 21) were receiving immunosuppressant therapies at ICI initiation; 4 were receiving corticosteroids and 3 were receiving DMARDs including 3 on methotrexate and 2 on etanercept. Adverse events occurred in 70% after a median of 2.8 (10–53.7) weeks of ICI initiation; 47% had flares and 38% had de novo irAEs, while 30% tolerated treatment without incident. More flares were observed among patients who had active symptoms at ICI initiation compared with patients who did not have any symptoms (50% versus 36%), while those receiving immunosuppressant therapies at ICI initiation seemed to have less flares than those without treatment (25% versus 50%); however, numbers were small. De novo irAEs included predominantly colitis and thyroiditis; two had sicca symptoms and one each had hypophysitis, hepatitis, dermatitis, uveitis, polymyalgia rheumatica, and multiple irAEs. Flares and de novo irAEs required corticosteroids in 63% (up to 2 mg/kg/day in a patient with psoriatic arthritis), and one patient each required methotrexate and apremilast leading to improvement in all patients. Discontinuation of ICI was reported in 19% (4 out of 21), and an additional patient required temporary ICI withhold until resolution of symptoms and did not have any adverse events upon treatment rechallenge.

Pathogenesis

What is happening immunologically in cancer patients who have preexisting autoimmune disease when treated with ICI remains an intriguing question that needs to be elucidated. Enhanced T helper 1 (Th1) and T helper 17 (Th17) immune responses and subsequent production of pro-inflammatory cytokines resulting from ICI therapy could play a role in the exacerbation of inflammation and autoimmunity in patients with preexisting autoimmune disease [46–50]. Of note, an altered regulatory T cell (Treg)/Th17 axis plays a role in the development of autoimmune diseases such as ankylosing spondylitis, psoriasis and psoriatic arthritis, and several others [51–56] and also plays a role in the pathogenesis of colitis-irAE in patients treated with ICI [57]. IL-17, a potent inflammatory cytokine primarily produced by Th17 cells, plays a key role in the pathogenesis of autoimmune arthritis including RA, SPA, and juvenile idiopathic arthritis; Th17 cells are expanded in peripheral blood of these patients during disease flares [58–61]. Notably, biologic agents targeting the development and survival of Th17 cells have shown therapeutic efficacy, especially in patients with SPA [58].

As IL-6 is a critical cytokine for induction of Th17 cells from naïve CD4+ T cells, and for inhibition of transforming growth factor beta-dependent Treg differentiation [62], IL-6 inhibition could rebalance the altered Treg/Th17 axis and control autoimmunity without dampening antitumor immune response. In patients with arthritis-irAE following ICI therapy, clinical presentation is often similar to patients with primary RA or SPA; however, only few were found to have positive rheumatoid factor (RF), antibodies against citric citrullinated peptide (anti-CCP), or antinuclear antibodies (ANA), raising a question about the role of B cells in the pathogenesis of arthritis-irAEs [63–65]. In fact, two out of three patients who presented with seropositive RA-like arthritis following ICI therapy were found to have anti-CCP antibodies in retrospective blood samples that were drawn before treatment initiation, suggesting a pre-RA status that manifested clinically only after ICI [66]. Antitumor necrosis factor alpha (TNFα) therapies were found to be effective for the management of arthritis-irAE and other irAEs, possibly through a direct effect on Th1 immune response or indirectly by decreasing IL-6 and subsequently Th17 activation [64, 67]. Although limited to retrospective case series, tocilizumab (an anti-IL-6 receptor antibody) was also found to be effective for the management of arthritis-irAEs without altering the tumor response to ICI therapy [63–65, 68, 69].

A growing evidence supports the fact that the genetic background of the host could plausibly play a role in susceptibility to de novo irAEs and to exacerbation of underlying autoimmunity following treatment with ICI. In cytotoxic T-lymphocyte-associated protein 4 (CTLA-4)-deficient mice, massive lymphoproliferative disorders occurred leading to death, while in programmed death-1 (PD-1)-/programmed death-ligand-1 (PD-L1)-knockout mice, a higher risk of inflammatory and autoimmune diseases was reported but was compatible with life [70–73]. In humans, single-nucleotide polymorphisms (SNPs) in CTLA-4 and PD-1 alleles have been linked to various autoimmune diseases including RA, ankylosing spondylitis, and systemic lupus erythematosus [71, 74–80]. Recently, 30 variants/SNPs were suggested as possible genetic markers of irAEs in patients receiving ICI therapy; few of these SNPs were mapped to genes that were previously thought to be associated with autoimmune diseases [81], yet larger studies are still warranted to validate these findings and establish the potential functional relevance of the identified SNPs.

Case Study

A 59-year-old Caucasian woman developed a left-sided jawline mass, which was biopsied and consistent with localized melanoma. She underwent wide local excision without additional therapy. Sentinel lymph node biopsy was not performed at the time. She had a history of seronegative, nonerosive RA diagnosed at age 50 primarily affecting the bilateral wrists and metacarpophalangeal (MCPs). She was initially treated with low-dose prednisone with excellent response and was then maintained on hydroxychloroquine monotherapy for 3 years, until she discontinued it on her own. She was lost to rheumatologic follow-up.

At age 67, after presenting urgently with nausea and abdominal pain, she was found to have multiple hepatic metastases. She was on no medications for her RA and had no joint symptoms at the time. She was started on ipilimumab and nivolumab. She tolerated the therapy well, with her only complaint being that of skin hypersensitivity. Three months later, she achieved a partial response to treatment and was transitioned to nivolumab monotherapy per protocol. Six months after starting immunotherapy, she developed mild arthralgias but did not seek treatment. However, over the subsequent 3 months, her symptoms progressed in severity and seemed to coincide and worsen with each nivolumab infusion. She developed over 3 h of morning stiffness and swelling in multiple joints including the bilateral wrists, knees, and ankles. Nine months after starting immunotherapy and approximately 3 months after arthritis symptoms significantly worsened, she was started on low-dose prednisone (10 mg daily for several weeks) by her local oncologist. Symptoms initially improved but recurred after prednisone was discontinued and subsequently worsened dramatically, causing profound functional impairment and pain requiring hospitalization. Nivolumab was discontinued 12 months after its initiation, and she reestablished rheumatologic care. She was started on prednisone 40 mg daily with only modest relief.

She was seen at a tertiary care center for a second opinion 2 months later. At that time, she had been off of nivolumab for 2 months and had remained on prednisone 40 mg daily. PET-CT demonstrated that her melanoma was in remission but did reveal symmetric uptake in several synovial joints including the shoulders, elbows, and wrists. Oncology recommended continuing to hold the nivolumab given that the melanoma was in remission. Per rheumatology, her presentation was consistent with highly active RA given her profound (>3 h) morning stiffness and physical exam demonstrating synovitis in multiple joints including the shoulders, wrists, MCPs, knees, ankles, and metatarsophalangeal (MTP) (CDAI score = 51.0). The patient was wheelchair bound. Review of systems was otherwise negative, specifically no Raynaud's disease, sicca, rash, serositis, or dysphagia. Additional workup revealed a normocytic anemia (hemoglobin 10.3 g/dL, normal range 11.6–15.0 g/dL), thrombocytosis (platelets 550, normal range 157–371 × 10^9/L), and elevated inflammatory markers (ESR 57 mm/1 h normal range 0–29 mm/1 h; C-reactive protein 57 mg/L, normal range <8 mg/L). The following serologic evaluation was negative or normal: antinuclear antibodies (ANA), rheumatoid factor, cytric citrullinated peptid (CCP), human leucocyte antigens (HLA)-B27, SS-A, SS-B, Smith, ribonucleoprotein (RNP), Jo-1, Scl-70, dsDNA, C3, and C4. At that time, little was known about the diagnosis or management of rheumatic irAEs and far less about patients with preexisting rheumatologic disease exposed to immunotherapy. While it was felt that the RA was likely being exacerbated by immunotherapy, concern was greater for prolonged exposure to high-dose prednisone and its impact on cancer progression. It was recommended that the patient should undergo intra-articular steroid injections to the most symptomatic joints (wrists), split the dose of prednisone to three times daily (in hopes of improving therapeutic response), and gradually attempt to taper the dose.

The patient was seen in follow-up 3 months later and had tapered to prednisone 10 mg daily. Her melanoma remained in complete remission, but inflammatory arthritis had progressed in severity (CADI = 66; see Fig. 12.1 for time course of inflammatory arthritis symptoms, treatment, response, and relevant laboratory and imaging findings). Plain X-rays of the hands, wrist, feet, ankles, and knees did not demonstrate any erosive disease. She required IV steroids followed by a gradual taper of high-dose oral steroids, and after discussion with oncology, methotrexate was added as a steroid-sparing agent, gradually uptitrated to a dose of 20 mg orally once weekly. Three months later, the patient endorsed some symptomatic and functional improvement, but the arthritis remained highly active (see Fig. 12.1; CDAI = 44.0). Methotrexate was uptitrated to 22.5 mg once weekly, and she underwent repeat intra-articular steroid injections to the wrists.

Unfortunately, she appreciated no response, and at follow-up 6 months after methotrexate had been initiated

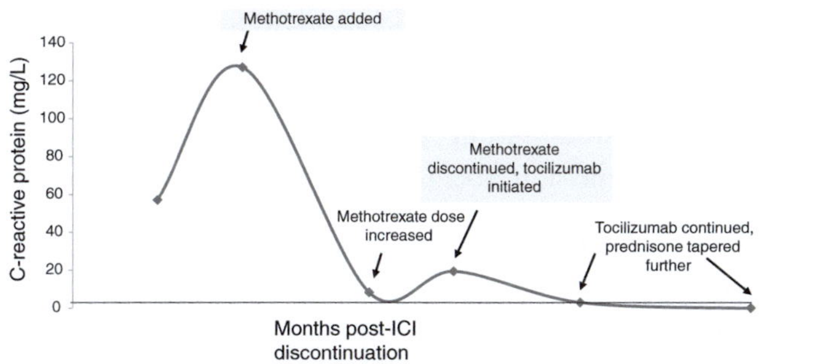

	2	4	7	9	12	16
Arthritis activity	High	High	High	High	Low	Remission
Melanoma status	Remission →					
MSK findings (PET-CT)	Synovitis bilateral shoulders, elbows, wrists, trochanteric bursa, knees, ankles			Synovitis bilateral shoulders, elbows, wrists, trochanteric bursa, knees, ankles		Mild synovitis bilateral wrists, knees, ankles *improved* from previous PET-CT

Figure 12.1 Overview of patient's clinical course, including cancer status, inflammatory arthritis disease activity, response to treatment, and associated imaging findings

(CDAI = 38), her arthritis remained highly active, and PET-CT showed no change in the previously noted synovial uptake. The melanoma remained in remission. Given the lack of response to methotrexate, rheumatology recommended switching to a TNF inhibitor, but oncology had concerns with this class of medications in the context of underlying melanoma. After discussion, it was felt that the theoretical risk for cancer recurrence might be less with tocilizumab. Methotrexate was discontinued, and the patient was started on tocilizumab 4 mg/kg by monthly infusion. The patient noted a marked subjective response to treatment after the third infusion and CRP normalized. As noted in Fig. 12.1, the patient continued to respond to tocilizumab and achieved a state of remission approximately 6 months after starting the therapy and was able to taper prednisone to below 5 mg daily. Attempts were made to discontinue the prednisone altogether, but the patient would have mild recurrence of her inflammatory arthritis. Given the persistence of symptoms over 18 months after discontinuation of all immunotherapy and the severity of her initial presentation, and given that the melanoma remained in remission, tocilizumab was continued monthly with sustained response.

This is a patient with preexisting seronegative RA whose symptoms had been subjectively very mild for many years and in remission at the time of metastatic melanoma diagnosis. RA symptoms recurred after 8 months on immunotherapy and rapidly progressed in severity. At the time, no specific guidelines for the management of rheumatic irAEs or irAEs in patients with preexisting autoimmune disease were available, contributing to the delay in recognition and treatment seen in this case. In addition, the patient's inflammatory arthritis became steroid refractory and persistent after ICI discontinuation, creating additional therapeutic challenges. Tocilizumab has been used successfully for other irAEs [68] as well as for ICI-induced inflammatory arthritis [63, 69] and was successful in this case without cancer recurrence.

Management

To date, the current treatment guidelines for patients with preexisting inflammatory arthritis who flare after ICI exposure are similar to those for patients who develop de novo inflammatory arthritis post-ICI (see Chap. 2.1). Overall, corticosteroids and withholding ICI therapy are mainstays for grade 2–4 toxicities, and addition of DMARDs is suggested for grade 3 and 4 toxicities that do not improve after 4 weeks of corticosteroids [82]. Recommended management of grade 1 toxicities is conservative (analgesia in the absence of corticosteroids and ICI continuation). Here, the authors would argue that patients with preexisting inflammatory arthritis may require more aggressive management of their toxicity to prevent further inflammatory arthritis progression and functional impairment (with the potential consequences illustrated in our case study) and would offer that treatment should be directed and escalated according to RA disease activity measures. In practice, most patients are treated with corticosteroids alone [3, 4], and DMARDs are added or reintroduced in only a minority of cases, largely because the data for the use, efficacy, and safety of conventional and biologic DMARDs (including TNF inhibitors and tocilizumab) in this patient population are very limited [18, 63, 68, 69]. Many as-yet unanswered questions regarding patients with preexisting inflammatory arthritis treated with ICI remain: Which patients can be exposed to ICI and when? What biomarkers can be used to identify patients at risk for irAEs in general and those with preexisting autoimmunity at greatest risk for disease flare and de novo irAEs? Should alternative non-ICI-based therapies be considered first? If quiescent, should baseline immunosuppression for inflammatory arthritis be discontinued prior to ICI treatment? When should ICI be discontinued when a patient's arthritis flares, and when can the ICI be reintroduced? If necessary for management, what steroid-sparing agents have the most favorable safety profile?

Currently, best practices would support a multidisciplinary approach and shared decision-making, early involvement by rheumatology (ideally prior to ICI therapy), and close clinical and laboratory monitoring.

References

1. KEYTRUDA-pembrolizumab [package insert]. County Cork IM, 2019. https://www.accessdata.fda.gov/drugsatfda_docs/label/2020/125514s067lbl.pdf.
2. YERVOY-ipilimumab [package insert]. Princeton NBS, 2019. https://www.accessdata.fda.gov/drugsatfda_docs/label/2019/125377s104lbl.pdf.
3. Opdivo-nivolumab [package insert]. Princeton NBMS, 2019. https://www.accessdata.fda.gov/drugsatfda_docs/label/2019/125554s075lbl.pdf.
4. Antonia SJ, Villegas A, Daniel D, Vicente D, Murakami S, Hui R, et al. Durvalumab after chemoradiotherapy in stage III non-small-cell lung cancer. N Engl J Med. 2017;377(20):1919–29.
5. Eggermont AM, Chiarion-Sileni V, Grob JJ, Dummer R, Wolchok JD, Schmidt H, et al. Adjuvant ipilimumab versus placebo after complete resection of high-risk stage III melanoma (EORTC 18071): a randomised, double-blind, phase 3 trial. Lancet Oncol. 2015;16(5):522–30.
6. Eggermont AMM, Blank CU, Mandala M, Long GV, Atkinson V, Dalle S, et al. Adjuvant pembrolizumab versus placebo in resected stage III melanoma. N Engl J Med. 2018;378(19):1789–801.
7. Weber J, Mandala M, Del Vecchio M, Gogas HJ, Arance AM, Cowey CL, et al. Adjuvant nivolumab versus ipilimumab in resected stage III or IV melanoma. N Engl J Med. 2017;377(19):1824–35.
8. Migden MR, Rischin D, Schmults CD, Guminski A, Hauschild A, Lewis KD, et al. PD-1 blockade with cemiplimab in advanced cutaneous squamous-cell carcinoma. N Engl J Med. 2018;379(4):341–51.
9. Rosenberg JE, Hoffman-Censits J, Powles T, van der Heijden MS, Balar AV, Necchi A, et al. Atezolizumab in patients with locally advanced and metastatic urothelial carcinoma who have progressed following treatment with platinum-based che-

motherapy: a single-arm, multicentre, phase 2 trial. Lancet. 2016;387(10031):1909–20.
10. Abdel-Wahab N, Shah M, Suarez-Almazor ME. Adverse events associated with immune checkpoint blockade in patients with cancer: a systematic review of case reports. PLoS One. 2016;11(7):e0160221.
11. Bertrand A, Kostine M, Barnetche T, Truchetet ME, Schaeverbeke T. Immune related adverse events associated with anti-CTLA-4 antibodies: systematic review and meta-analysis. BMC Med. 2015;13:211.
12. Wang Y, Zhou S, Yang F, Qi X, Wang X, Guan X, et al. Treatment-related adverse events of PD-1 and PD-L1 inhibitors in clinical trials: a systematic review and meta-analysis. JAMA Oncol. 2019;5(7):1008–19.
13. Wang P-F, Chen Y, Song S-Y, Wang T-J, Ji W-J, Li S-W, et al. Immune-related adverse events associated with anti-PD-1/PD-L1 treatment for malignancies: a meta-analysis. Front Pharmacol. 2017;8:730.
14. Abdel-Wahab N, Shah M, Lopez-Olivo MA, Suarez-Almazor ME. Use of immune checkpoint inhibitors in the treatment of patients with cancer and preexisting autoimmune disease: a systematic review. Ann Intern Med. 2018;168(2):121–30.
15. Lopez-Olivo MA, Abdel-Wahab N, Suárez-Almazor ME. A systematic review and meta-analysis of observational studies reporting on the use of checkpoint inhibitors in patients with cancer and pre-existing autoimmune disease. Arthritis Rheumatol (Suppl). 2019;71:10.
16. Richter MD, Pinkston O, Kottschade LA, Finnes HD, Markovic SN, Thanarajasingam U. Brief report: cancer immunotherapy in patients with preexisting rheumatic disease: the mayo clinic experience. Arthritis Rheumatol. 2018;70(3):356–60.
17. Menzies AM, Johnson DB, Ramanujam S, Atkinson VG, Wong AN, Park JJ, et al. Anti-PD-1 therapy in patients with advanced melanoma and preexisting autoimmune disorders or major toxicity with ipilimumab. Ann Oncol. 2017;28(2):368–76.
18. Tison A, Quere G, Misery L, Funck-Brentano E, Danlos FX, Routier E, et al. Safety and efficacy of immune checkpoint inhibitors in patients with cancer and preexisting autoimmune disease: a nationwide, Multicenter Cohort Study. Arthritis Rheumatol. 2019;71(12):2100–11.

19. Leonardi GC, Gainor JF, Altan M, Kravets S, Dahlberg SE, Gedmintas L, et al. Safety of programmed death-1 pathway inhibitors among patients with non-small-cell lung cancer and preexisting autoimmune disorders. J Clin Oncol. 2018;36(19):1905–12.
20. Liew DFL, Leung JLY, Liu B, Cebon J, Frauman AG, Buchanan RRC. Association of good oncological response to therapy with the development of rheumatic immune-related adverse events following PD-1 inhibitor therapy. Int J Rheum Dis. 2019;22(2):297–302.
21. Mooradian MJ, Nasrallah M, Gainor JF, Reynolds KL, Cohen JV, Lawrence DP, et al. Musculoskeletal rheumatic complications of immune checkpoint inhibitor therapy: a single center experience. Semin Arthritis Rheum. 2019;48(6):1127–32.
22. Efuni ECS, Boland P, Sandigursky S. Risk of immunotherapy related toxicity in patients with rheumatoid arthritis [abstract]. Arthritis Rheumatol. 2019;71:10.
23. Laaouad LRJ, Ennis D, Ye C, Al Jumaily K, Hudson M, Jamal S, Pope J, Nevskaya T, Saltman A, Himmel M, Fifi-Mah A, Tisseverasinghe A, Maltez N, Colmegna I, Hoa S. Preexisting autoimmune disease and rheumatic immune-related adverse events associated with cancer immunotherapy: a case series from the Canadian research group of rheumatology in immuno-oncology (CANRIO) [abstract]. Arthritis Rheumatol. 2019;71:10.
24. Mitchell EL, Lau PKH, Khoo C, Liew D, Leung J, Liu B, et al. Rheumatic immune-related adverse events secondary to anti-programmed death-1 antibodies and preliminary analysis on the impact of corticosteroids on anti-tumour response: a case series. Eur J Cancer. 2018;105:88–102.
25. Warner BM, Baer AN, Lipson EJ, Allen C, Hinrichs C, Rajan A, et al. Sicca syndrome associated with immune checkpoint inhibitor therapy. Oncologist. 2019;24(9):1259–69.
26. Zen Y, Yeh MM. Hepatotoxicity of immune checkpoint inhibitors: a histology study of seven cases in comparison with autoimmune hepatitis and idiosyncratic drug-induced liver injury. Mod Pathol. 2018;31(6):965–73.
27. Abdel-Wahab N, Safa H, Lopez-Olivo MA, Diab A, Suarez-Almazor M. Immune checkpoint inhibitors in patients with cancer and rheumatologic diseases: a systematic review of the literature. Ann Rheum Dis. 2019;78(Suppl 2):624.
28. Aya F, Ruiz-Esquide V, Viladot M, Font C, Prieto-Gonzalez S, Prat A, et al. Vasculitic neuropathy induced by pembrolizumab. Ann Oncol. 2017;28(2):433–4.

29. Calabrese C, Kirchner E, Kontzias A, Velcheti V, Calabrese LH. Rheumatic immune-related adverse events of checkpoint therapy for cancer: case series of a new nosological entity. RMD Open. 2017;3(1):e000412.
30. Gutzmer R, Koop A, Meier F, Hassel JC, Terheyden P, Zimmer L, et al. Programmed cell death protein-1 (PD-1) inhibitor therapy in patients with advanced melanoma and preexisting autoimmunity or ipilimumab-triggered autoimmunity. Eur J Cancer. 2017;75:24–32.
31. Hegde U, Chauhan A, Desai N. Myasthenic syndrome with pembrolizumab use. Neurology. 2017;88(16 Supplement):P6.75.
32. Johnson DB, Sullivan RJ, Ott PA, Carlino MS, Khushalani NI, Ye F, et al. Ipilimumab therapy in patients with advanced melanoma and preexisting autoimmune disorders. JAMA Oncol. 2015;2(2):234.
33. Kyi C, Carvajal RD, Wolchok JD, Postow MA. Ipilimumab in patients with melanoma and autoimmune disease. J Immunother Cancer. 2014;2(1):35.
34. Le Burel S, Champiat S, Routier E, Aspeslagh S, Albiges L, Szwebel TA, et al. Onset of connective tissue disease following anti-PD1/PD-L1 cancer immunotherapy. Ann Rheum Dis. 2017;77(3):468–9.
35. Lee B, Wong A, Kee D, Neeson P, Shackleton M, McArthur G, et al. The use of ipilimumab in patients with rheumatoid arthritis and metastatic melanoma. Ann Oncol. 2016;27(6):1174–7.
36. Puri A, Homsi J. The safety of pembrolizumab in metastatic melanoma and rheumatoid arthritis. Melanoma Res. 2017;27(5):519–23.
37. Zhu J, Li Y. Myasthenia gravis exacerbation associated with pembrolizumab. Muscle Nerve. 2016;54(3):506–7.
38. Benson Z, Gordon S, Nicolato P, Poklepovic A. Immunotherapy for metastatic melanoma with right atrial involvement in a patient with rheumatoid arthritis. Case Rep Oncol Med. 2017;2017:8095601.
39. Gandiga PC, Wang AR, Gonzalez-Rivera T, Sreih AG. Pembrolizumab-associated inflammatory myopathy. Rheumatology. 2018;57(2):397–8.
40. Kahler KC, Eigentler TK, Gesierich A, Heinzerling L, Loquai C, Meier F, et al. Ipilimumab in metastatic melanoma patients with pre-existing autoimmune disorders. Cancer Immunol Immunother. 2018;67(5):825–34.

41. Le Burel S, Champiat S, Mateus C, Marabelle A, Michot JM, Robert C, et al. Prevalence of immune-related systemic adverse events in patients treated with anti-programmed cell death 1/ anti-programmed cell death-ligand 1 agents: a single-centre pharmacovigilance database analysis. Eur J Cancer. 2017;82:34–44.
42. Johnson DB, Khushalani NI, Puzanov I, Mudigonda T, Kaufman H, Sosman JA, et al. Ipilimumab in metastatic melanoma patients with pre-existing autoimmune disorders. J Clin Oncol. 2015;33(15 Suppl. 1):9019.
43. Roche L, Murphy M, Power D. Treatment of Merkel cell carcinoma with pembrolizumab in a patient with psoriasis and psoriatic arthritis. Br J Dermatol. 2017;177(Suppl 1):143.
44. Phadke SD, Ghabour R, Swick BL, Swenson A, Milhem M, Zakharia Y. Pembrolizumab therapy triggering an exacerbation of preexisting autoimmune disease: a report of 2 patient cases. J Investig Med High Impact Case Rep. 2016;4(4):2324709616674316.
45. Kostine M, Rouxel L, Barnetche T, Veillon R, Martin F, Dutriaux C, et al. Rheumatic disorders associated with immune checkpoint inhibitors in patients with cancer-clinical aspects and relationship with tumour response: a single-centre prospective cohort study. Ann Rheum Dis. 2018;77(3):393–8.
46. Calabrese L, Velcheti V. Checkpoint immunotherapy: good for cancer therapy, bad for rheumatic diseases. Ann Rheum Dis. 2016;76(1):1–3.
47. Dulos J, Carven GJ, van Boxtel SJ, Evers S, Driessen-Engels LJ, Hobo W, et al. PD-1 blockade augments Th1 and Th17 and suppresses Th2 responses in peripheral blood from patients with prostate and advanced melanoma cancer. J Immunother. 2012;35(2):169–78.
48. von Euw E, Chodon T, Attar N, Jalil J, Koya RC, Comin-Anduix B, et al. CTLA4 blockade increases Th17 cells in patients with metastatic melanoma. J Transl Med. 2009;7:35.
49. Bailey SR, Nelson MH, Himes RA, Li Z, Mehrotra S, Paulos CM. Th17 cells in cancer: the ultimate identity crisis. Front Immunol. 2014;5:276.
50. Nelson M, Shirai K, Gupta R, Gilkeson G, Paulos CM. Understanding how immune checkpoint modulators alter pre-existing rheumatologic disorders in cancer patients. J Immunol. 2017;198(1 Supplement):120.7-.7.
51. Gracey E, Qaiyum Z, Almaghlouth I, Lawson D, Karki S, Avvaru N, et al. IL-7 primes IL-17 in mucosal-associated invariant T

(MAIT) cells, which contribute to the Th17-axis in ankylosing spondylitis. Ann Rheum Dis. 2016;75(12):2124–32.

52. Karczewski J, Dobrowolska A, Rychlewska-Hanczewska A, Adamski Z. New insights into the role of T cells in pathogenesis of psoriasis and psoriatic arthritis. Autoimmunity. 2016;49(7):435–50.
53. Kimura A, Kishimoto T. IL-6: regulator of Treg/Th17 balance. Eur J Immunol. 2010;40(7):1830–5.
54. Noack M, Miossec P. Th17 and regulatory T cell balance in autoimmune and inflammatory diseases. Autoimmun Rev. 2014;13(6):668–77.
55. Raychaudhuri SP, Raychaudhuri SK. IL-23/IL-17 axis in spondyloarthritis-bench to bedside. Clin Rheumatol. 2016;35(6):1437–41.
56. Yang J, Sundrud MS, Skepner J, Yamagata T. Targeting Th17 cells in autoimmune diseases. Trends Pharmacol Sci. 2014;35(10):493–500.
57. Callahan MK, Yang A, Tandon S, Xu Y, Subudhi SK, Roman RA, et al. Evaluation of serum IL-17 levels during ipilimumab therapy: correlation with colitis. J Clin Oncol. 2011;29(15):2505.
58. Lubberts E. The IL-23-IL-17 axis in inflammatory arthritis. Nat Rev Rheumatol. 2015;11(10):562.
59. Agarwal S, Misra R, Aggarwal A. Interleukin 17 levels are increased in juvenile idiopathic arthritis synovial fluid and induce synovial fibroblasts to produce proinflammatory cytokines and matrix metalloproteinases. J Rheumatol. 2008;35(3):515–9.
60. van Baarsen LG, Lebre MC, van der Coelen D, Aarrass S, Tang MW, Ramwadhdoebe TH, et al. Heterogeneous expression pattern of interleukin 17A (IL-17A), IL-17F and their receptors in synovium of rheumatoid arthritis, psoriatic arthritis and osteoarthritis: possible explanation for nonresponse to anti-IL-17 therapy? Arthritis Res Ther. 2014;16(4):426.
61. van Hamburg JP, Asmawidjaja PS, Davelaar N, Mus AM, Colin EM, Hazes JM, et al. Th17 cells, but not Th1 cells, from patients with early rheumatoid arthritis are potent inducers of matrix metalloproteinases and proinflammatory cytokines upon synovial fibroblast interaction, including autocrine interleukin-17A production. Arthritis Rheum. 2011;63(1):73–83.
62. Diehl S, Rincon M. The two faces of IL-6 on Th1/Th2 differentiation. Mol Immunol. 2002;39(9):531–6.

63. Abdel-Wahab N, Tayar JH, Diab A, Kim ST, Lu H, Suarez-Almazor ME. Inflammatory arthritis induced by the use of checkpoint inhibitors for immunotherapy of cancer. J Immuno Ther Cancer. 2017;5(2):687–99.
64. Cappelli LC, Gutierrez AK, Baer AN, Albayda J, Manno RL, Haque U, et al. Inflammatory arthritis and sicca syndrome induced by nivolumab and ipilimumab. Ann Rheum Dis. 2016;76(1):43–50.
65. Cappelli LC, Brahmer JR, Forde PM, Le DT, Lipson EJ, Naidoo J, et al. Clinical presentation of immune checkpoint inhibitor-induced inflammatory arthritis differs by immunotherapy regimen. Semin Arthritis Rheum. 2018;48(3):553–7.
66. Belkhir R, Burel SL, Dunogeant L, Marabelle A, Hollebecque A, Besse B, et al. Rheumatoid arthritis and polymyalgia rheumatica occurring after immune checkpoint inhibitor treatment. Ann Rheum Dis. 2017;76(10):1747–50.
67. Johnson DH, Zobniw CM, Trinh VA, Ma J, Bassett RL Jr, Abdel-Wahab N, et al. Infliximab associated with faster symptom resolution compared with corticosteroids alone for the management of immune-related enterocolitis. J Immunother Cancer. 2018;6(1):103.
68. Stroud CR, Hegde A, Cherry C, Naqash AR, Sharma N, Addepalli S, et al. Tocilizumab for the management of immune mediated adverse events secondary to PD-1 blockade. J Oncol Pharm Pract. 2019;25(3):551–7.
69. Kim ST, Tayar J, Trinh VA, Suarez-Almazor M, Garcia S, Hwu P, et al. Successful treatment of arthritis induced by checkpoint inhibitors with tocilizumab: a case series. Ann Rheum Dis. 2017;76(12):2061–4.
70. Okazaki T, Honjo T. The PD-1-PD-L pathway in immunological tolerance. Trends Immunol. 2006;27(4):195–201.
71. Scalapino KJ, Daikh DI. CTLA-4: a key regulatory point in the control of autoimmune disease. Immunol Rev. 2008;223:143–55.
72. Schildberg FA, Klein SR, Freeman GJ, Sharpe AH. Coinhibitory pathways in the B7-CD28 ligand-receptor family. Immunity. 2016;44(5):955–72.
73. Waterhouse P, Penninger JM, Timms E, Wakeham A, Shahinian A, Lee KP, et al. Lymphoproliferative disorders with early lethality in mice deficient in Ctla-4. Science. 1995;270(5238):985–8.
74. Barreto M, Santos E, Ferreira R, Fesel C, Fontes MF, Pereira C, et al. Evidence for CTLA4 as a susceptibility gene for systemic lupus erythematosus. Eur J Hum Genet. 2004;12(8):620–6.

75. Lee YH, Bae SC, Kim JH, Song GG. Meta-analysis of genetic polymorphisms in programmed cell death 1. Associations with rheumatoid arthritis, ankylosing spondylitis, and type 1 diabetes susceptibility. Z Rheumatol. 2015;74(3):230–9.
76. Lee YH, Kim JH, Seo YH, Choi SJ, Ji JD, Song GG. CTLA-4 polymorphisms and susceptibility to inflammatory bowel disease: a meta-analysis. Hum Immunol. 2014;75(5):414–21.
77. Lee YH, Woo JH, Choi SJ, Ji JD, Song GG. Association of programmed cell death 1 polymorphisms and systemic lupus erythematosus: a meta-analysis. Lupus. 2009;18(1):9–15.
78. Li G, Shi F, Liu J, Li Y. The effect of CTLA-4 A49G polymorphism on rheumatoid arthritis risk: a meta-analysis. Diagn Pathol. 2014;9:157.
79. Liu JL, Zhang FY, Liang YH, Xiao FL, Zhang SQ, Cheng YL, et al. Association between the PD1.3A/G polymorphism of the PDCD1 gene and systemic lupus erythematosus in European populations: a meta-analysis. JEADV. 2009;23(4):425–32.
80. Wu J, Zhang L, Zhou Y. The association between CTLA-4 (+49 A/G) polymorphism and susceptibility to ankylosing spondylitis: a meta-analysis. Int J Rheum Dis. 2015;19(12):1237–43.
81. Abdel-Wahab N, Yu RK, Diab A, Dadu R, Shannon V, Futreal A, et al. Genetic determinants of adverse events in cancer patients receiving immune checkpoint inhibitors. J Clin Oncol. 2019;37(15_suppl):2586.
82. Abdel-Wahab BC, Suarez-Almazor ME. Chapter 6: musculoskeletal and rheumatologic toxicities. In: Ernstoff M, Puzanov I, Robert C, Diab A, Hersey P, editors. SITC's guide to managing immunotherapy toxicity. 1st ed. New York: Demos Medical Publishing, an imprint of Springer Publishing Company, LLC; 2019. p. 171–84.

Chapter 13
Cancer Immunotherapy in Patients with Preexisting Rheumatic Diseases: Other Rheumatic Autoimmune Diseases

Marie Kostine and Alice Tison

Introduction

Blocking natural immune checkpoints is not only responsible for an enhancement of antitumoral immunity, but it may also lead to a break of self-tolerance, with the occurrence of immune-related adverse events (irAEs). Patients with preexisting inflammatory or autoimmune disease have been largely excluded from clinical trials assessing cancer immuno-

M. Kostine (✉)
Department of Rheumatology, Bordeaux University Hospital, Bordeaux, France
e-mail: marie.kostine@chu-bordeaux.fr

A. Tison
Department of Rheumatology, Brest University Hospital, Brest, France
e-mail: alice.tison@chu-brest.fr

M. E. Suarez-Almazor, L. H. Calabrese (eds.), *Rheumatic Diseases and Syndromes Induced by Cancer Immunotherapy*,
https://doi.org/10.1007/978-3-030-56824-5_13

therapy, due to the theoretical risk of worsening autoimmune manifestations. However, in clinical practice, the large efficacy of immune checkpoint inhibitors (ICIs) prompts clinicians to propose them to a wider population, such as patients with preexisting rheumatic autoimmune diseases. This chapter focuses on the use of ICIs in patients with preexisting rheumatic conditions other than inflammatory arthritis.

Epidemiology

The literature on the use of ICIs in patients with preexisting rheumatic autoimmune disease is growing, with reassuring safety data reported in numerous case reports and several retrospective series. Table 13.1 summarizes the main series assessing the safety of ICIs in patients with preexisting autoimmune diseases, all but one being retrospective [1–11].

Furthermore, a systematic review summarized original case reports, case series, and observational studies describing 123 patients with cancer and autoimmune disease who received ICIs [12]. The large majority of patients had metastatic melanoma (84%) and were treated either with anti-PD-1 (52%) or with ipilimumab (45%). A broad spectrum of preexisting autoimmune diseases was reported, including psoriasis and/or psoriatic arthritis, rheumatoid arthritis, autoimmune thyroid disease, ulcerative colitis, Crohn's disease, multiple sclerosis, myasthenia gravis, and sarcoidosis. Overall, half of the patients experienced a flare of their preexisting autoimmune disease, and 34% developed de novo irAEs.

So far, approximately 50 patients with preexisting rheumatic conditions other than inflammatory arthritis have been reported to be treated with ICIs, as described in Table 13.2.

Clinical Manifestations

Together, a flare of the preexisting inflammatory or autoimmune disease was observed in about half of myositis patients, 30% of SLE patients, 40% of Sjögren's patients, 25% of

Table 13.1 Main series assessing safety of immune checkpoint inhibitors in patients with preexisting autoimmune diseases

First author	Year	ICI(s)	N	Main autoimmune disease	Flare	irAE	Management
Johnson DB	2015	Ipilimumab	30	RA, psoriasis, MS, IBD, SLE, thyroiditis, sarcoidosis	27%	33%	GC, IFX ($n = 2$), 1 death (colitis)
Menzies AM	2016	Anti-PD-1	52	RA, psoriasis, IBD	38%	29%	ICI discontinuation for flare ($n = 2$) or irAE ($n = 4$)
Lee B	2016	Ipilimumab	8	RA	75%	50% (colitis)	NSAIDs ($n = 1$), GC, IFX ($n = 1$ for colitis), ICI discontinuation for 5 patients
Gutzmer R	2017	Anti-PD-1	19	Arthritis, myositis, vasculitis, PMR, sarcoidosis, psoriasis, IBD, MS, GB, thyroiditis	42%	16%	GC, IgIV for myositis

(continued)

Table 13.1 (continued)

First author	Year	ICI(s)	N	Main autoimmune disease	Flare	irAE	Management
Danlos FX	2018	Anti-PD-1	45	Vitiligo, psoriasis, thyroiditis, Sjögren, RA	24%	44%	GC, ICI continued for 75% of patients
Mitchell EL	2018	Anti-PD-1	12	PMR, PsA, RA, systemic sclerosis	83%	–	GC, HCQ, MTX, ICI discontinuation for 2 flares ($n = 2$)
Richter MD	2018	Ipilimumab anti-PD-1	16	RA, PMR, Sjögren, SLE, GCA	6%	38%	GC,and ICI discontinuation
Leonardi GC	2018	Anti-PD-(L)1	56	RA, PMR, psoriasis, IBD, thyroiditis	23%	38%	GC, ICI discontinuation for 14% of patients
Kähler KC	2018	Ipilimumab	41	Thyroiditis, RA, psoriasis, IBD	29%	29%	GC, HCQ, and SLZ ($n = 1$), IFX ($n = 1$ for colitis)
Cortellini A	2019	Anti-PD-1	85	Thyroiditis, psoriasis, IBD, RA, PMR, SLE, vasculitis	47% (10% for rheumatic diseases)	66%	ICI discontinuation for 7% of patients

Tison A	2019	All	112	Psoriasis, RA, IBD, SLE, PMR	47%	42%	GC, conventional synthetic disease-modifying antirheumatic drugs (csDMARDs) (MTX, AZA), TNFi ($n = 4$ for colitis), IgIV ($n = 2$), ICI discontinuation for 21% of patients

AZA azathioprine, *ICI* checkpoint inhibitor, *GB* Guillain-Barré syndrome, *GC* glucocorticoids, *GCA* giant cell arteritis, *HCQ* hydroxychloroquine, *IBD* inflammatory bowel disease, *IFX* infliximab, *IgIV* intravenous immunoglobulins, *irAE* immune-related adverse event, *MS* multiple sclerosis, *MTX* methotrexate, *NSAIDs* nonsteroidal anti-inflammatory drugs, *PMR* polymyalgia rheumatica, *PsA* psoriatic arthritis, *RA* rheumatoid arthritis, *SLE* systemic lupus erythematosus, *SLZ* sulfasalazine

Table 13.2 Observed risk of flare in preexisting rheumatic diseases other than inflammatory arthritis

Preexisting disease	*n*	Flare
Sarcoidosis	15	3 (20%)
SLE	13	4 (31%)
Systemic sclerosis	8	3 (25%)
Gougerot-Sjögren	7	3 (43%)
Myositis/dermatomyositis	2	1 (50%)
GPA	2	0
PAN	1	0
ANCA-associated vasculitis	1	0
EGPA	1	0
GCA	2	1 (50%)
Behçet	1	0

ANCA antineutrophil cytoplasmic antibodies, *EGPA* eosinophilic granulomatosis with polyangiitis, *GPA* granulomatosis with polyangiitis, *PAN* polyarteritis nodosa, *SLE* systemic lupus erythematosus

systemic sclerosis patients, and 20% of sarcoidosis patients, but less than 10% had to discontinue ICI therapy during a flare (Table 13.2). One patient with preexisting giant cell arteritis experienced a relapse. There was no flare reported for the few patients with other vasculitis and Behçet's disease. Furthermore, few patients experienced other irAEs, mainly colitis, hypophysitis, and thyroiditis. Among them, one Sjögren's patient developed interstitial pneumonitis, considered by the authors as an irAE rather than a flare of the preexisting autoimmune disease [7].

Diagnosis

Similar to irAEs, rheumatic diseases other than inflammatory arthritis, such as connective tissue diseases and vasculitis, may involve inflammation of various organs. Therefore, the differential diagnosis between a flare of the preexisting rheumatic disease and another unrelated irAE may be challenging.

There is no specific diagnostic workup. Usually, flare and/or irAE is diagnosed based on clinical symptoms, though all appropriate laboratory tests, imaging, and/or biopsy obtained to document and type organ inflammation will be useful for the diagnosis.

Furthermore, once a cancer patient with preexisting rheumatic disease receiving immunotherapy is referred for suspected flare, the rheumatologist should also always consider tumor progression or infection as differential diagnosis, usually already considered by the referring oncologist. Notably, the lack of improvement with glucocorticoids should raise this possibility before increasing immunosuppressive treatment.

Management

General Considerations

While there are several international guidelines for the management of irAEs in patients receiving ICIs [13–15], there are no dedicated guidelines regarding patients with preexisting rheumatic disease. A recent EULAR initiative assembled international experts primarily from rheumatology, immunology, and oncology fields who generated the first set of recommendations for the diagnosis and management of rheumatic irAEs arising as a direct consequence of ICI therapy [16].

Based on the available literature evidence and experts' opinion, the task force agreed that ICI therapy in patients with preexisting autoimmune rheumatic or connective tissue disease was not contraindicated, provided that the patient is well informed and closely monitored. Importantly, this remains a shared decision between the oncologist, rheumatologist, and the patient, and whether ICI will be used in a metastatic or adjuvant/neoadjuvant setting is a major aspect to be considered as the risk-benefit balance is different. For example, the use of adjuvant or neoadjuvant ICI seems to be too risky in patients with systemic sclerosis for whom high dose of glucocorticoids (required in case of severe irAE) is at risk of scleroderma renal crisis, while the benefit appears superior to the risk in a metastatic setting.

Baseline Evaluation and Immunosuppressive Regimen

A complete rheumatologic assessment should be performed in patients with preexisting rheumatic disease, both inflammatory arthritis and other rheumatic autoimmune conditions, before initiation of ICI therapy. This baseline evaluation will allow (1) patient education on the risk of autoimmune flare and/or other immune toxicities to prevent delay in diagnosis, (2) an accurate picture of the rheumatic disease activity, and (3) discussion regarding baseline immunosuppressive regimen.

Indeed, should we try to prevent flare and/or other irAEs by introducing or increasing immunosuppressive therapies? Or would the use of immunosuppressive therapies hamper the chance of antitumor response? There is no obvious answer. For example, the prophylactic use of budesonide has been tested to prevent ipilimumab-induced colitis in melanoma patients but did not improve tolerability [17]. Furthermore, recent preclinical and clinical data highlighted the deleterious impact of baseline glucocorticoids on ICI efficacy, when used at a dosage of greater than 10 mg/day [18–20]. Cautious interpretation is required as this was in patients treated with glucocorticoids for their cancer or cancer-related symptoms and not for autoimmune symptoms. There is scarce data regarding the management of csDMARDs at the initiation of ICIs. For example, we can imagine that hydroxychloroquine might have less impact than methotrexate on antitumor response, but this has to be demonstrated. Some series reported either shorter progression-free survival or lower response rate for patients receiving immunosuppressive therapies at ICI initiation [2, 11], while others did not [4, 8]. Owing to concerns regarding baseline immunosuppressive therapy, experts agreed on currently recommending the lowest immunosuppressive regimen possible at the start of ICI therapy, notably below 10 mg of prednisone per day if possible. Whether tapering baseline immunosuppressive treatment may lead to increased risk of flare and/or irAE is unknown, but it will likely be managed with glucocorticoids and/or DMARDs. Antitumor efficacy should remain a priority in the context of advanced cancer.

Recent data on 1250 patients from the Dutch Melanoma Treatment Registry (DMTR) revealed that patients experiencing a severe toxicity (n = 264) had a prolonged survival but abrogated for those who received TNF inhibitors [21]. Nevertheless, it has been demonstrated in mouse models that the prophylactic use of TNF inhibitors concomitantly with combined CTLA-4 and PD-1 immunotherapy ameliorated colitis and, in addition, improved antitumor efficacy [22]. These results suggest that TNF inhibition might dissociate efficacy and toxicity of combined ICIs therapies, noteworthy for patients with preexisting rheumatic autoimmune diseases. Of note, a phase I investigator-initiated trial (TICIMEL, NCT03293784) is currently testing the safety of such combined approach (double immunotherapy plus TNF inhibitor) in melanoma patients. The antitumor activity of tocilizumab administrated in combination with the double immunotherapy is also being tested in melanoma patients (NCT03999749). Therefore, future oncological data and prospective studies will probably challenge this recommendation of tapering immunosuppressive treatment over time.

Flare and/or irAE Management

In patients with preexisting rheumatic autoimmune disease other than inflammatory arthritis, flares of the underlying condition and other irAEs may occur under ICI therapy, requiring the use of glucocorticoids and/or DMARDs. While the use of DMARDs has been reported in patients with flare of preexisting inflammatory arthritis, it was very rarely required for patients with flare of preexisting rheumatic autoimmune disease other than inflammatory arthritis since systemic glucocorticoids were sufficient. ICI was discontinued in 8% of patients with preexisting autoimmune disease due to other irAEs, unrelated to their preexisting autoimmune disease.

Conclusion

The use of ICI in patients with preexisting rheumatic autoimmune disease other than inflammatory arthritis is possible but remains challenging, with a need for further prospective controlled studies and collaborative efforts to determine the optimal management of immunosuppressive treatment.

Case Study

A 66-year-old man was diagnosed in September 2019 with metastatic urothelial carcinoma and treated with gemcitabine and carboplatin as first-line treatment. After three cycles, CT scan showed evidence of disease progression with peritoneal carcinomatosis. After consideration of different options for systemic treatment with the patient, the oncologist aimed to start pembrolizumab, an anti-PD1-antibody, as second-line therapy.

However, he had a past history of systemic lupus erythematosus diagnosed 15 years ago, and he was still receiving hydroxychloroquine 200 mg twice a day and prednisone 5 mg/day. In that respect, he was referred to the department of rheumatology for baseline evaluation of this preexisting rheumatic disease before starting anti-PD-1 therapy. Initial evaluation at the time of the diagnosis was not available and requested to the other institution. Based on his personal medical documents, he presented initially with arthralgia and hematuria with normal kidney function, positive antinuclear antibodies (titer, 1/1280), and anti-dsDNA. There was no kidney biopsy performed. He was treated with hydroxychloroquine and prednisone (exact initial dosage unknown and then tapered to 5 mg/day), with no disease flare under this treatment and annual screening for hydroxychloroquine retinopathy.

In November 2019, he had no complains except abdominal pain related to peritoneal carcinomatosis, and physical examination did not reveal any potential organ inflammation of systemic lupus erythematosus. His estimated glomerular filtration rate (eGFR) was 60 ml/min/1.73 m^2 according to the Modification of Diet in Renal Disease (MDRD) formula, and urine protein-to-creatinine ratio was normal at 10 mg/mmol. Titer of antinuclear antibodies was 1:160, with negative anti-dsDNA (<10 UI/ml) and normal complement levels. Therefore, the preexisting systemic lupus erythematosus was considered inactive, and there was an interdisciplinary discussion regarding its ongoing treatment. According to current data and recommendations, prednisone dosage was below 10 mg/day, and since he was receiving 5 mg/day for several years, we decided to maintain such dosage. Further discussion regarding hydroxychloroquine treatment followed. While we can expect a possible preventive effect of disease flare under ICI treatment, the disease inactivity since several years was quite reassuring to allow treatment discontinuation. Finally, it was decided to discontinue hydroxychloroquine. The patient has been well informed of the possible risk of lupus flare and/or other immune toxicities and of any new symptoms.

He received six infusions of pembrolizumab without any flare or side effects, but unfortunately he experienced cancer progression.

References

1. Johnson DB, Sullivan RJ, Ott PA, Carlino MS, Khushalani NI, Ye F, et al. Ipilimumab therapy in patients with advanced melanoma and preexisting autoimmune disorders. JAMA Oncol. 2016;2(2):234–40.
2. Menzies AM, Johnson DB, Ramanujam S, Atkinson VG, Wong ANM, Park JJ, et al. Anti-PD-1 therapy in patients with advanced melanoma and preexisting autoimmune disorders or major toxicity with ipilimumab. Ann Oncol. 2017;28(2):368–76.
3. Lee B, Wong A, Kee D, Neeson P, Shackleton M, McArthur G, et al. The use of ipilimumab in patients with rheumatoid arthritis and metastatic melanoma. Ann Oncol. 2016;27(6):1174–7.
4. Gutzmer R, Koop A, Meier F, Hassel JC, Terheyden P, Zimmer L, et al. Programmed cell death protein-1 (PD-1) inhibitor therapy in patients with advanced melanoma and preexisting autoimmunity or ipilimumab-triggered autoimmunity. Eur J Cancer. 2017;75:24–32.
5. Danlos F-X, Voisin A-L, Dyevre V, Michot J-M, Routier E, Taillade L, et al. Safety and efficacy of anti-programmed death 1 antibodies in patients with cancer and pre-existing autoimmune or inflammatory disease. Eur J Cancer. 2018;91:21–9.
6. Mitchell EL, Lau PKH, Khoo C, Liew D, Leung J, Liu B, et al. Rheumatic immune-related adverse events secondary to anti-programmed death-1 antibodies and preliminary analysis on the impact of corticosteroids on anti-tumour response: a case series. Eur J Cancer. 2018;105:88–102.
7. Richter MD, Pinkston O, Kottschade LA, Finnes HD, Markovic SN, Thanarajasingam U. Cancer immunotherapy in patients with preexisting rheumatologic disease: the Mayo Clinic experience. In: Arthritis & rheumatology. New York: Wiley; 2018.
8. Leonardi GC, Gainor JF, Altan M, Kravets S, Dahlberg SE, Gedmintas L, et al. Safety of programmed death-1 pathway inhibitors among patients with non-small-cell lung cancer and preexisting autoimmune disorders. J Clin Oncol. 2018;36(19):1905.
9. Kähler KC, Eigentler TK, Gesierich A, Heinzerling L, Loquai C, Meier F, et al. Ipilimumab in metastatic melanoma patients with pre-existing autoimmune disorders. Cancer Immunol Immunother. 2018;67(5):825–34.
10. Cortellini A, Buti S, Santini D, Perrone F, Giusti R, Tiseo M, et al. Clinical outcomes of patients with advanced cancer

and pre-existing autoimmune diseases treated with anti-programmed death-1 immunotherapy: a real-world transverse study. Oncologist. 2019;24(6):e327.

11. Tison A, Quéré G, Misery L, Funck-Brentano E, Danlos F-X, Routier E, et al. Safety and efficacy of immune checkpoint inhibitors in patients with cancer and preexisting autoimmune disease: a nationwide multicenter cohort study. Arthritis Rheumatol. 2019;71(12):2100–11.
12. Abdel-Wahab N, Shah M, Lopez-Olivo MA, Suarez-Almazor ME. Use of immune checkpoint inhibitors in the treatment of patients with cancer and preexisting autoimmune disease: a systematic review. Ann Intern Med. 2018;168(2):121–30.
13. Haanen JB, Carbonnel F, Robert C, Kerr KM, Peters S, Larkin J, et al. Management of toxicities from immunotherapy: ESMO Clinical Practice Guidelines for diagnosis, treatment and follow-up. Ann Oncol. 2018;28(suppl_4):iv119–42.
14. Puzanov I, Diab A, Abdallah K, Bingham CO, Brogdon C, Dadu R, et al. Managing toxicities associated with immune checkpoint inhibitors: consensus recommendations from the Society for Immunotherapy of Cancer (SITC) Toxicity Management Working Group. J Immunother Cancer. 2017;5(1):95.
15. Brahmer JR, Lacchetti C, Schneider BJ, Atkins MB, Brassil KJ, Caterino JM, et al. Management of immune-related adverse events in patients treated with immune checkpoint inhibitor therapy: American society of clinical oncology clinical practice guideline. J Clin Oncol. 2018;36(17):1714–68.
16. Kostine M, Finckh A, Bingham CO, Visser K, Leipe J, Schulze-Koops H, et al. EULAR points to consider for the diagnosis and management of rheumatic immune-related adverse events due to cancer immunotherapy with checkpoint inhibitors. Ann Rheum Dis. 2020; https://doi.org/10.1136/annrheumdis-2020-217139.
17. Weber J, Thompson JA, Hamid O, Minor D, Amin A, Ron I, et al. A randomized, double-blind, placebo-controlled, phase II study comparing the tolerability and efficacy of ipilimumab administered with or without prophylactic budesonide in patients with unresectable stage III or IV melanoma. Clin Cancer Res. 2009;15(17):5591–8.
18. Arbour KC, Mezquita L, Long N, Rizvi H, Auclin E, Ni A, et al. Impact of baseline steroids on efficacy of programmed cell death-1 and programmed death-ligand 1 blockade in patients with non-small-cell lung cancer. J Clin Oncol. 2018;36(28):2872–8.

19. Tokunaga A, Sugiyama D, Maeda Y, Warner AB, Panageas KS, Ito S, et al. Selective inhibition of low-affinity memory CD8+ T cells by corticosteroids. J Exp Med. 2019;216(12):2701–13.
20. Draghi A, Borch TH, Radic HD, Chamberlain CA, Gokuldass A, Svane IM, et al. Differential effects of corticosteroids and anti-TNF on tumor-specific immune responses - implications for the management of irAEs. Int J Cancer. 2018;145(5):1408–13.
21. Verheijden RJ, May AM, Blank CU, Aarts MJB, van den Berkmortel FWPJ, van den Eertwegh AJM, et al. Association of anti-TNF with decreased survival in steroid refractory ipilimumab and anti-PD1 treated patients in the Dutch Melanoma Treatment Registry. Clin Cancer Res. 2020;26(9):2268–74.
22. Perez-Ruiz E, Minute L, Otano I, Alvarez M, Ochoa MC, Belsue V, et al. Prophylactic TNF blockade uncouples efficacy and toxicity in dual CTLA-4 and PD-1 immunotherapy. Nature. 2019;569(7756):428–32.

Part IV
General Principles of Management

Chapter 14
Management of Rheumatic Immune-Related Adverse Events (irAEs): General Principles

Alexa Simon Meara and Leonard H. Calabrese

Introduction

Immune-related adverse events (irAEs) are a consequence of immune checkpoint inhibitor (ICI) therapy. These irAEs result in the disruption of the immune system's normal checks and balances. ICIs are generally better tolerated compared to traditional cancer treatment such as cytotoxic chemotherapy. However, unlike traditional chemotherapy, adverse effects may be associated with the potential development of long-term multisystem chronic medical diseases,

A. S. Meara (✉)
The Ohio State University Wexner Medical Center, Division of Immunology and Rheumatology, Columbus, OH, USA
e-mail: Alexa.meara@osumc.edu

L. H. Calabrese
Department of Rheumatic and Immunologic Diseases, Cleveland Clinic Lerner College of Medicine of Case Western Reserve University, Cleveland, OH, USA
e-mail: calabrl@ccf.org

M. E. Suarez-Almazor, L. H. Calabrese (eds.), *Rheumatic Diseases and Syndromes Induced by Cancer Immunotherapy*,
https://doi.org/10.1007/978-3-030-56824-5_14

which may require medical management and physician subspecialist's care [1]. Thus, *irAEs can have long-term effects on patients and may be appreciated to varying degrees by treating clinicians, especially as their use disseminates from tertiary to community settings*. In addition, IrAEs can affect any organ and can be life-threatening (e.g., myocarditis or pneumonitis) or may be more amenable to treatment such as colitis, interstitial nephritis, inflammatory arthritis, polymyalgia rheumatica, vasculitis, or various skin changes [2]. ICIs gain new indications monthly and thus can be combined with other ICIs and with traditional chemotherapeutic agents. Understanding their side effects is imperative for personalized cancer care [3].

Guidelines

ICI adverse events are graded using the Common Terminology Criteria for Adverse Events (CTCAE) grading system (SERVICES., U.S.D.O.H.A.H., Common Terminology Criteria for Adverse Events (CTCAE) Version 4.03.2010), which ranges from grade 1 through grade 5 (grade 1, mild; grade 2, moderate (outpatient and inpatient care); grade 3, severe (hospitalization); grade 4, life-threatening; grade 5, death). Since irAEs are a relatively new concept, most rheumatic irAEs do not fit well into the existing CTCAE guidelines [4]. For example, severe inflammatory arthritis may not require a hospitalization or be life-threatening, but it can severely limit a patient's ability to function. This, along with the increasing number of ICIs being used and irAEs being reported, has resulted in rheumatic irAEs receiving more attention in the past 3 years. This has led to the addition of rheumatic irAEs to oncology guidelines and the development of guidelines for their management. The development of an appropriate grading system incorporating rheumatic irAEs may facilitate early referral to a rheumatologist to help improve recognition and treatment of irAEs in patients [5].

ASCO/SITC Guidelines

A general algorithm does not exist for rheumatic irAE diagnoses. Most guidelines are specific to the individual organ affected or symptoms caused by the irAE. In addition, each cancer organization (e.g., ASCO, SITC, and NCCN) has its own guidelines for irAEs [4, 6, 7] (see Figs. 14.1 and 14.2). Below is the NCCN guidelines summary page outlining immune chcckpoint inhibitor-related toxicities.

Some of these guidelines have attempted to provide specific recommendations for rheumatic irAEs. For example, the Society for Immunotherapy of Cancer (SITC) guidelines recommend referring any patient with CTCAE ≥ grade 2 inflammatory arthritis to a rheumatologist. In addition, patients whose symptoms persist beyond 6 weeks or require >20 mg of prednisone daily that cannot be tapered to <10 mg within 4 weeks should also be referred to a rheumatologist [6]. All patients with suspected myositis, vasculitis, and scleroderma should be referred to rheumatology irrelevant

National Comprehensive Cancer Network® NCCN

NCCN Guidelines Version 1.2019
Management of Immune Checkpoint Inhibitor-Related Toxicities

NCCN Guidelines Index
Table of Contents
Discussion

PRINCIPLES OF ROUTINE MONITORING

Baseline Assessment[a]	Monitoring Frequency[b]	Evaluation for Abnormal Findings/Symptoms
Clinical • Physical examination • Comprehensive patient history of any autoimmune/organ-specific disease, endocrinopathy, or infectious disease • Neurologic examination • Bowel habits (typical frequency/consistency)	Clinical exam at each visit with adverse event (AE) symptom assessment	Follow-up testing based on findings, symptoms
Imaging • CT imaging • Brain MRI if indicated	Periodic imaging as indicated	Follow-up testing as indicated based on imaging findings
General bloodwork • CBC with differential • Comprehensive metabolic panel • Infectious disease screening as indicated	Repeat every 2–3 weeks during immunotherapy, then in 6–12 weeks or as indicated	HbA1c for elevated glucose
Dermatologic (ICI_DERM-1) • Examination of skin and mucosa if history of immune-related skin disorder	Conduct/repeat as needed based on symptoms	Monitor affected BSA and lesion type; photographic documentation. Skin biopsy if indicated.
Pancreatic (ICI_ENDO-1) • Baseline testing is not required.	No routine monitoring needed if asymptomatic	Amylase, lipase, and consider abdominal imaging for suspected pancreatitis.
Thyroid (ICI_ENDO-2) • Thyroid-stimulating hormone (TSH), free thyroxine (T4)	Every 4–6 weeks during immunotherapy, then follow-up every 12 weeks as indicated	Total T3 if abnormal thyroid function suspected. TPO antibodies if TSH is high, TRAbs if TSH is low.
Adrenal/Pituitary (ICI_ENDO-3) • Adrenal: Serum cortisol • Pituitary: TSH, free T4	Every 2–3 weeks during immunotherapy, then follow-up every 6–12 weeks	Luteinizing hormone (LH), follicle-stimulating hormone (FSH), testosterone, adrenocorticotropic hormone (ACTH)
Pulmonary (ICI_PULM-1) • Oxygen saturation (resting and with ambulation) • Pulmonary function tests (PFTs) for high-risk patients	Repeat oxygen saturation tests based on symptoms	Chest CT to evaluate for pneumonitis, biopsy if needed to exclude other causes.
Cardiovascular (ICI_CARDIO-1) • Individualized assessment in consultation with cardiology as indicated	Consider periodic testing for those with abnormal baseline or symptoms	Individualized follow-up in consultation with cardiology as indicated
Musculoskeletal (ICI_MS-1) • Joint examination/functional assessment as needed for patients with pre-existing disease	No routine monitoring needed if asymptomatic	Consider rheumatology referral.

The James
The Ohio State University

Figure 14.1 NCCN example guidelines [7]

Recommendations from SITC: General Corticosteroid Recommendations

Grade of immune-related AE (CTCAE/equivalent)	Corticosteroid management	Additional notes
1	• Corticosteroids not usually indicated	• Continue immunotherapy
2	• If indicated, start oral prednisone 0.5-1 mg/kg/day if patient can take oral medication. • If IV required, start methylprednisolone 0.5-1 mg/kg/day IV • If no improvement in 2–3 days, increase corticosteroid dose to 2 mg/kg/day • Once improved to ≤grade 1 AE, start 4–6 week steroid taper	• Hold immunotherapy during corticosteroid use • Continue immunotherapy once resolved to ≤grade 1 and off corticosteroids • Start proton pump inhibitor for GI prophylaxis
3	• Start prednisone 1-2 mg/kg/day (or equivalent dose of methylprednisolone) • If no improvement in 2–3 days, add additional/alternative immune suppressant • Once improved to ≤ grade 1, start 4–6-week steroid taper • Provide supportive treatment as needed	• Hold immunotherapy; if symptoms do not improve in 4–6 weeks, discontinue immunotherapy • Consider intravenous corticosteroids • Start proton pump inhibitor for GI prophylaxis • Add PCP prophylaxis if more than 3 weeks of immunosuppression expected (>30 mg prednisone or equivalent/day)
4	• Start prednisone 1-2 mg/kg/day (or equivalent dose of methylprednisolone) • If no improvement in 2–3 days, add additional/alternative immune suppressant, e.g., infliximab • Provide supportive care as needed	• Discontinue immunotherapy • Continue intravenous corticosteroids • Start proton pump inhibitor for GI prophylaxis • Add PCP prophylaxis if more than 3 weeks of immunosuppression expected (>30 mg prednisone or equivalent/day)

Note: For steroid-refractory cases and/or when steroid sparing is desirable, management should be coordinated with disease specialists. AE, adverse event

The James

The Ohio State University

Figure 14.2 Society for Immunotherapy of Cancer (SITC) guidelines: an example of corticosteroid guideline [6]

of AE severity. Moreover, Naidoo et al. have proposed an inflammatory arthritis guideline similar to the SITC guideline [5]. These guidelines grade the severity of irAEs based on patients' symptoms and how they affect their daily lives.

General Principles of Immunosuppression for Rheumatic irAEs: Targeted Therapies

Choosing the right treatment for irAEs is a challenge that often requires multidisciplinary teams. Symptoms of irAEs should be adequately controlled with the overarching goal of not compromising the antitumor effect of ICIs. The current guidelines of irAEs are based on case reports and single academic institution populations as randomized controlled trials regarding irAEs are limited. However, as noted above, the recent cancer guidelines now include rheumatic irAEs for the first time. First-line treatment includes glucocorticoids with the ASCO and SITC guidelines recommending symptomatic irAEs be treated for at least a month with glucocorticoids [4, 6] (see Fig. 14.2). If glucocorticoid treatment is not sufficient after 4–6 weeks of therapy, disease-modifying antirheumatic drugs (DMARDs) or biologics should be included in the treatment regimen. However, robust data regarding the use of DMARDs and biologics are very limited, anecdotal, and highly subjective.

An underlying concern for the treatment of all irAEs is that effective immunosuppression for immune-mediated toxicities may blunt therapeutic effectiveness of ICIs. This is based on two sets of observations. First, there are growing data, especially for anti-CTLA-4-based therapy and also therapies targeting PD-1 pathways, that the presence of irAEs is associated with a beneficial effect on antitumoral effects of immunotherapy [8]. Implicit in this belief is the concept that the generation of irAE is a biomarker of effective immunoenhancement from immunotherapy. Also implicit in this concept is that excessive or overly robust immunosuppression for incident irAEs may theoretically blunt this antitumoral effect. This topic has just been elegantly reviewed in detail [9]. Finally, several studies now suggest that identification of irAEs combined with less glucocorticoid use may lead to a better prognosis [10–12]. This consideration is particularly important for the irAE of inflammatory arthritis, as a recent study has documented that up to 40% of such patients may have a chronic course even up to 2 years following discontinuation of ICI therapy [13]. Based on these considerations, clearly more work is needed in this area, and it begs for study of more targeted therapies. Please see Table 14.1 for summary of therapeutics.

Anti-TNF-Directed Therapies

Anti-TNF-directed therapies have been the most utilized therapy for all irAEs that have failed to resolve with glucocorticoids. Infliximab has been the anti-TNF of choice due to its use as an infusion and ease of hospital access compared to other injectable anti-TNFs that require insurance clearance before use [14, 26]. There has been a traditional belief in rheumatology that anti-TNFs should not be used

Table 14.1 Targeted therapy of rheumatic irAEs

Targeted therapy	Antitumor effect of the targeted therapy	Safety concerns for the targeted therapy	irAEs that have been treated by targeted therapy
TNF	Mixed data [14, 15]	Infections	Colitis [4] IA [5]
IL-6	May improve anti-PD-1 efficacy	Perforation Infections	IA [16] PMR [17] GCA [18]
IL-1	No data	Infection	MAS [19]
IL-17	Mixed data [20]	Infection [21] Unmask Colitis [21]	Spondyloarthropathy psoriasis
B cell	No data	Infections	Grade 4 irAEs [22]
JAKi	Mixed data [23]	Infections [24] Thrombosis	Unknown
Abatacept	No data	Infection	Myocarditis [25]

irAE immune-related adverse events, *TNF* tumor necrosis factor, *JAKi* janus kinase inhibitors, *IL* interleukin, *IA* inflammatory arthritis, *PMR* polymyalgia rheumatica, *GCA* giant cell arteritis, *MAS* macrophage activation syndrome

with patients who have had a diagnosis of melanoma or malignancy within 5 years based on large data studies [27]. ICIs and the subsequent explosion of irAEs have suggested that anti-TNFs can be used for these patients, but whether the antitumor effect persists remains controversial. Regardless, infliximab is the first-line treatment for colitis and inflammatory arthritis leading patients affected by those irAEs to do well on this therapy [14, 28]. However, more controlled human studies are needed. Interestingly, a recent study of mice with cancer treated by ICI that developed colitis and treated with anti-TNFs demonstrated decreased toxicity but preserved efficacy [5, 13, 29]. Another trial, adding to the controversy surrounding anti-TNFs, is a retrospective analysis of the Dutch Melanoma Registry which showed that despite improved survival, with severe irAEs, use of anti-TNFs may offset [15]. There needs to be more human prospective trials to truly understand these risks and to explain these benefits and harms to patients.

Anti-IL-6-Directed Therapies

Anti-IL-6 therapy is widely used in rheumatology for the treatment of various autoimmune conditions including inflammatory arthritis, vasculitis, and more recently polymyalgia rheumatica [2, 18]. Thus, using an anti-IL-6 agent for these rheumatic irAEs makes sense. As with anti-TNF therapy, however, there is a limited amount of reliable data with only case reports available of anti-IL-6 agents' use in the treatment of irAEs [18]. A single-center retrospective study of 34 patients showed that 27 patients improved after receiving the anti-IL-6 receptor antibody, tocilizumab, for various irAEs with no changes in survival [10, 16, 18]. Currently, a clinical trial (NCT03601611) is underway assessing the efficacy of tocilizumab in patients with irAE arthritis and irAE colitis after ICI use.

Anti-IL-1-Directed Therapies

There are no reported cases of the use of anti-IL-1-directed therapies for irAEs. However, anti-IL-1 therapy is used to treat pericarditis, cold autoimmune inflammatory disease, and macrophage activation syndrome [19]. Thus, it is plausible that there will be a need for anti-IL-1 therapy [19]. It is relatively unknown whether there are antitumor effects of IL-1 which will require further investigation.

Anti-IL-17-Directed Therapies

Anti-IL-17-directed therapies treat diverse autoimmune diseases that fall under the categories of spondyloarthropathies such as psoriasis, psoriatic arthritis, and ankylosing spondylitis [21]. There are case reports of anti-IL-17 used for spondyloarthropathy-like irAEs [30]. There is mixed data based on isolated case reports questioning whether anti-IL-17 promotes tumor growth. Therefore, both preclinical and human trials are required [20, 31].

Anti-B-Cell-Directed Therapies

The use of rituximab or other anti-B-cell agents is often the first-line treatment for most rheumatic diseases in patients with previous malignancy. Thus, there is a large body of data showing the efficacy, safety, and preservation of the antitumor effect in traditional chemotherapy when rituximab has been concomitantly provided. There are current cancer treatment guidelines of irAEs which cite rituximab as an option for severe (grade 4) and refractory irAEs such as myositis, myocarditis, and encephalitis [2, 3, 6]. However, the evidence within these guidelines is only empiric.

Janus Kinase Inhibitors (Jak-i)

Jak-i are used to treat a wide variety of rheumatic diseases and are attractive to patients because they are administered orally [24]. However, there is limited data on the use of Jak-i with irAEs and mixed data on the progression of tumor response using these drugs [23]. Thus, these drugs should be used sparingly and with caution until more data are developed. Patients on these drugs should be monitored closely.

Abatacept

Abatacept is a fusion protein composed of the Fc region of the immunoglobulin IgG1 fused to the extracellular domain of cytotoxic T-lymphocyte-associated protein 4 (CTLA-4) [32]. The CTLA-4 portion binds to CD80/86 located on antigen-presenting cells competing with CD28, thus inhibiting T-cell activation [32]. The ICI, ipilimumab, is a monoclonal antibody to CTLA-4, disabling the CTLA-4's ability to turn off the T cell and downregulate the immune system [33]. Thus, there is a great theoretic concern as these two drugs are in direct competition of each other. The concern of using abatacept is that there would be a reversal of the antitumor effect produced by the ICI. There are few reports of the use of such therapies, but recently clinical experiences with abatacept have been reported [18]. Therefore, loss of effective antitumoral response is of great concern. A brief report using abatacept successfully treated myocarditis with no ill effects on tumoral responses [25, 30].

The other questions include when to stop ICI based on irAEs. In general, these guidelines recommend holding ICIs for grade 4 irAEs. The recommendations for grade 3 irAEs depend on its type [6].

There are many other targeted therapeutics not described here, including agents such as vedolizumab (integrin inhibitor used for colitis), IL-12/-23 inhibitors, and calcineurin antagonists that require further consideration and investigation [10]. As the use of ICIs grows, so will the number of irAEs patients' experience. Understanding the treatments for irAEs that control the symptoms and preserve the antitumor effect is key. More human studies are needed in addition to a multidisciplinary approach to these complex patients.

Conclusions

We are only at the beginning of the era of immunotherapy to treat cancer, and there remain many unanswered questions and challenges surrounding the management and treatment of irAEs. While rheumatic irAEs are not the most commonly encountered irAEs, they are distinctive in their chronicity and can be severe and difficult to manage with concomitant cancer diagnosis. There are numerous other targeted therapy options that may have a role in the treatment of rheumatic irAEs, by extrapolating knowledge from their use in de novo immune-mediated diseases, including janus kinase inhibitors, calcineurin antagonists, rapamycin inhibitors, and therapies directed against IL-1, IL-17, and IL-12/-23. Recent calls for more intense immunopathophysiologic investigations of individual patients with severe irAEs and creating a more personalized approach to therapy incorporating such agents are moving ever closer [34]. Please see Table 14.1 for summary of therapeutics.

There is a need and opportunity for rheumatologists to participate as central figures in the evolving clinical trials of treatment of irAEs. Rheumatologists will be increasingly called upon to manage both rheumatic irAEs and those occurring in patients with preexisting rheumatic diseases receiving immunotherapy. At this point in time, it is crucial that rheumatologists stay informed of this new field and work inter-professionally to accurately diagnose and manage these disorders in collaboration with treating oncologists.

References

1. Calabrese L, Mariette X. The evolving role of the rheumatologist in the management of immune-related adverse events (irAEs) caused by cancer immunotherapy. Ann Rheum Dis. 2018;77(2):162–4.
2. Calabrese LH, Calabrese C, Cappelli LC. Rheumatic immune-related adverse events from cancer immunotherapy. Nat Rev Rheumatol. 2018;14:569–79.

3. Kostine M, Rouxel L, Barnetche T, et al. Rheumatic disorders associated with immune checkpoint inhibitors in patients with cancer-clinical aspects and relationship with tumour response: a single-centre prospective cohort study. Ann Rheum Dis. 2018;77:393–8.
4. Brahmer JR, Lacchetti C, Schneider BJ, et al. Management of immune-related adverse events in patients treated with immune checkpoint inhibitor therapy: American society of clinical oncology clinical practice guideline. J Clin Oncol. 2018;36(17): 1714–68.
5. Naidoo J, Zhang J, Lipson EJ, et al. Multidisciplinary toxicity team for cancer immunotherapy–related adverse events. J Natl Compr Canc Netw. 2019;7(16):712–20.
6. Puzanov I, Diab A, Abdallah K, et al. Managing toxicities associated with immune checkpoint inhibitors: consensus recommendations from the Society for Immunotherapy of Cancer (SITC) Toxicity Management Working Group. J Immunother Cancer. 2017;5(1):95.
7. Thompson JA. New NCCN guidelines: recognition and management of immunotherapy-related toxicity. J Natl Compr Canc Netw. 2018;16:594–6.
8. Das S, Johnson DB. Immune-related adverse events and anti-tumor efficacy of immune checkpoint inhibitors. J Immunother Cancer. 2019;7(1):306.
9. McGonagle D, Bragazzi NL, Amital H, Watad A. Mechanistic classification of immune checkpoint inhibitor toxicity as a pointer to minimal treatment strategies of selected emergent autoimmune diseases to further improve survival. Autoimmun Rev. 2020;19(2):102456.
10. Martins F, Sykiotis GP, Maillard M, et al. New therapeutic perspectives to manage refractory immune checkpoint-related toxicities. Lancet Oncol. 2019;20:e54–64.
11. Horvat TZ, Adel NG, Dang TO, et al. Immune-related adverse events, need for systemic immunosuppression, and effects on survival and time to treatment failure in patients with melanoma treated with ipilimumab at memorial sloan kettering cancer center. J Clin Oncol. 2015;33(28):3193–8.
12. Vokes NI, Liu D, Ricciuti B, et al. Harmonization of tumor mutational burden quantification and association with response to immune checkpoint blockade in non-small-cell lung cancer. JCO Precis Oncol. 2019;3:1–12.

13. Braaten TJ, Brahmer JR, Forde PM, et al. Immune checkpoint inhibitor-induced inflammatory arthritis persists after immunotherapy cessation. Ann Rheum Dis. 2019;79(3):332–8.
14. Perez-Ruiz E, Minute L, Otano I, et al. Prophylactic TNF blockade uncouples efficacy and toxicity in dual CTLA-4 and PD-1 immunotherapy. Nature. 2019;569:428–32.
15. Verheijden RJ, May AM, Blank CU, et al. Association of Anti-TNF with decreased survival in steroid refractory ipilimumab and anti-PD1-treated patients in the Dutch melanoma treatment registry. Clin Cancer Res. 2020;26:2268–74.
16. Kim ST, Tayar J, Trinh VA, et al. Successful treatment of arthritis induced by checkpoint inhibitors with tocilizumab: a case series. Ann Rheum Dis. 2017;76:2061–4.
17. Calabrese C, Cappelli LC, Kostine M, Kirchner E, Braaten T, Calabrese L. Polymyalgia rheumatica-like syndrome from checkpoint inhibitor therapy: case series and systematic review of the literature. RMD Open. 2019;5(1):e000906.
18. Stroud CR, Hegde A, Cherry C, et al. Tocilizumab for the management of immune mediated adverse events secondary to PD-1 blockade. J Oncol Pharm Pract. 2019;25(3):551–7.
19. Noseda R, Bertoli R, Muller L, Ceschi A. Haemophagocytic lymphohistiocytosis in patients treated with immune checkpoint inhibitors: analysis of WHO global database of individual case safety reports. J Immunother Cancer. 2019;7(1):117.
20. Vitiello GA, Miller G. Targeting the interleukin-17 immune axis for cancer immunotherapy. J Exp Med. 2020;217(1)
21. Ruiz de Morales JMG, Puig L, Dauden E, et al. Critical role of interleukin (IL)-17 in inflammatory and immune disorders: an updated review of the evidence focusing in controversies. Autoimmun Rev. 2020;19:102429.
22. Brahmer JR, Lacchetti C, Thompson JA. Management of immune-related adverse events in patients treated with immune checkpoint inhibitor therapy: American society of clinical oncology clinical practice guideline summary. J Oncol Pract. 2018;14(4):247–9.
23. Lu C, Talukder A, Savage NM, Singh N, Liu K. JAK-STAT-mediated chronic inflammation impairs cytotoxic T lymphocyte activation to decrease anti-PD-1 immunotherapy efficacy in pancreatic cancer. Onco Targets Ther. 2017;6(3):e1291106.
24. Winthrop KL. The emerging safety profile of JAK inhibitors in rheumatic disease. Nat Rev Rheumatol. 2017;13:234–43.

25. Salem JE, Allenbach Y, Vozy A, et al. Abatacept for severe immune checkpoint inhibitor-associated myocarditis. N Engl J Med. 2019;380(24):2377–9.
26. Cappelli LC, Gutierrez AK, Baer AN, et al. Inflammatory arthritis and sicca syndrome induced by nivolumab and ipilimumab. Ann Rheum Dis. 2017;76(1):43–50.
27. Cappelli LC, Shah AA, Bingham CO. Cancer immunotherapy-induced rheumatic diseases emerge as new clinical entities. RMD Open. 2016;2(2):e000321.
28. Pollack MH, Betof A, Dearden H, et al. Safety of resuming anti-PD-1 in patients with immune-related adverse events (irAEs) during combined anti-CTLA-4 and anti-PD1 in metastatic melanoma. Ann Oncol. 2018;29(1):250–5.
29. Cappelli LC, Brahmer JR, Forde PM, et al. Clinical presentation of immune checkpoint inhibitor-induced inflammatory arthritis differs by immunotherapy regimen. Semin Arthritis Rheum. 2018;48(3):553–7.
30. Esfahani K, Buhlaiga N, Thebault P, Lapointe R, Johnson NA, Miller WH Jr. Alemtuzumab for immune-related myocarditis due to PD-1 therapy. N Engl J Med. 2019;380(24):2375–6.
31. Ma YF, Chen C, Li D, et al. Targeting of interleukin (IL)-17A inhibits PDL1 expression in tumor cells and induces anticancer immunity in an estrogen receptor-negative murine model of breast cancer. Oncotarget. 2017;8(5):7614–24.
32. Cutolo M, Sulli A, Paolino S, Pizzorni C. CTLA-4 blockade in the treatment of rheumatoid arthritis: an update. Expert Rev Clin Immunol. 2016;12(4):417–25.
33. Lo B, Abdel-Motal UM. Lessons from CTLA-4 deficiency and checkpoint inhibition. Curr Opin Immunol. 2017;49:14–9.
34. Esfahani K, Elkrief A, Calabrese C, et al. Moving towards personalized treatments of immune-related adverse events. Nat Rev Clin Oncol. 2020;3:1–2.

Chapter 15
Benefit-Risk Considerations

Maria E. Suarez-Almazor

Immunotherapy and more specifically immune checkpoint inhibitors (ICI) have revolutionized the treatment of cancer, extending life expectancy in patients with advanced disease who in the past had few therapeutic options for survival. Moreover, in order to improve cancer outcomes, ICI are increasingly being used in combination with other immune therapies or other cancer treatment modalities such as chemotherapy, targeted agents, or radiation. While combination therapies may improve survival, they also can increase the frequency and spectrum of related adverse events. Immunotherapy was initially approved exclusively for patients with metastatic cancer but is now increasingly being proposed for use at earlier cancer stages. Immune checkpoint inhibitors have been approved as adjuvant therapy in patients with locally advanced melanoma after they have undergone potentially curative surgical resection [1]. Currently, there are several trials evaluating ICI in the adjuvant setting for other cancers. This expanded use of ICI in combination therapy or at earlier cancer stages raises

M. E. Suarez-Almazor (✉)
Department of Health Services Research, University of Texas MD Anderson Cancer Center, Houston, TX, USA
e-mail: msalmazor@mdanderson.org

M. E. Suarez-Almazor, L. H. Calabrese (eds.), *Rheumatic Diseases and Syndromes Induced by Cancer Immunotherapy*,
https://doi.org/10.1007/978-3-030-56824-5_15

new considerations with respect to the risk-benefit profile of these agents. In addition, as the use of ICI expands to cancer patients in the community at large, potential differences in risks may become evident as patients not initially represented in clinical trials are treated. Of special interest are those with preexisting autoimmune diseases who may be predisposed to flares of their disease or to increased rates of immune-related adverse events (irAE).

Clinicians and their patients often face complex decisions that require careful considerations of potential benefits and risks which need to be considered within the broad context of patient preferences and values. This is of particular relevance in situations that require thoughtful balance of "quality vs. quantity" of life as can be the case for patients with cancer and concomitant comorbidities such as rheumatic diseases or as a consequence of developing rheumatic irAE, which result in significant symptom burden and impairment. This chapter describes a conceptual framework for the discussion of risks and benefits in cancer patients who have concomitant rheumatic diseases or have experienced irAE and are facing decisions about immunotherapy. These discussions require a multidisciplinary approach including rheumatologists, oncologists, and other specialists, as patients often present with multiple organ irAE.

Evaluating the Potential Benefits and Risks of Therapies

From a practical perspective, it is important to define the potential benefits of immunotherapy with respect to various cancer outcomes that matter to patients. The Food and Drug Administration (FDA) provides a comprehensive framework for the evaluation of benefit-risk considerations, which is primarily used as guidance for device approval but can be modified and applied to medical treatments such as immunotherapy [2].

Benefits

Beneficial health outcomes have several dimensions that are relevant for decision-making but are not always clearly framed or explained within patient-doctor interactions or in educational materials.

Types of Benefits

For most cancer treatments, the types of benefits that are important to patients relate to length of survival, cancer recurrence, cancer progression, symptom burden, and quality of life.

Symptom burden is an important component of quality of life, and it applies both to the health effects caused by the cancer (e.g., pain) and cancer treatment (i.e., adverse events). Health-related quality of life encompasses the individual's sense of well-being and ability to carry out activities of daily living [3]. The World Health Organization defines health as a state of complete physical, mental, and social well-being, not merely the absence of disease. Cancer has a major impact on all domains of well-being, physical, mental, and social. Cancer treatment can increase the quality of life by improving symptoms and function, but it can also result in harms that impact well-being.

The type of benefit will vary according to tumor type and the extent of disease at the time of treatment. Therefore, the expectations for patients with metastatic or locally advanced disease will be different than the expectations for those receiving ICI in the adjuvant setting, once their primary treatment is completed and there is no evidence of disease.

Magnitude of Effect

What most patients want to know with respect to cancer prognosis is the probability they have of dying from the cancer. With respect to specific cancer outcomes, patients want to know whether the given therapies can result in complete remission and, if so, for how long can it be sustained. If complete remission is not likely, can the therapy result in partial remission, with regression in the size and extent of the cancer? When complete or partial regression is not possible, patients want to know whether the cancer therapy can arrest progression and for how long.

Duration

Many cancer outcomes are best measured in terms of duration, as patients and providers care about survival and length of time until cancer recurs or progresses. There are several quantitative duration measures that can be used in the context of therapeutic decision-making [2]:

(i) *Overall survival* is the length of time from the date of cancer diagnosis until death from any cause.
(ii) *Cancer-specific survival* is measured from the time of diagnosis until death from cancer. Patients dying from other non-cancer causes are censored, namely, considered alive until death from the other causes.
(iii) *Disease-free survival* (or relapse-free survival) is the length of time after a treatment ends that a patient survives before having a cancer recurrence.
(iv) *Progression-free survival* is measured from the time a treatment is completed until the cancer gets worse, usually determined by imaging in solid tumors and other biomarkers in hematological malignancies.

Likelihood of Patients Experiencing a Benefit

Some of the measures used in clinical trials and observational studies of cancer therapies can be difficult to conceptualize as they are expressed in terms of relative benefit. Measures such as relative risk or hazard ratios give information on the likelihood of having of one outcome in one group of patients receiving a therapy compared to another group not receiving that therapy (odds). However, they do not provide an absolute estimate of benefit. It is more intuitive for patients and providers to conceptualize the probability of survival or any other outcome in terms of percentage of patients with that outcome within a period of time. Time interval survival rates have often been used to compare treatments with respect to probability of death and to provide information to patients about alternatives. As an example, a 5-year survival rate is the percentage of people alive after 5 years from the cancer diagnosis or from completion of a specific treatment.

Another important aspect is whether there are some groups of patients that may benefit more than others. In addition to specific tumor characteristics, including the extent and presence of biomarkers, patient characteristics such as age and coexisting comorbidities may influence therapeutic response.

Medical Need

A major component of therapeutic decision-making is the consideration of possible alternatives. In some cases, the magnitude of effect of a given therapy is small, but there may not be other options for treatment.

Patient Values and Preferences

In all therapeutic decisions, patient values and preferences need to be ascertained and considered, and also include caregivers if this is the patient's choice. Patients can have diverse preferences as they may value differently survival vs. quality of life and may also consider other attributes in the decision that relate to social aspects such as finances or important life events.

Harms

Various domains should be considered in the assessment of potential risks.

Types of Harms

Immunotherapy can cause a myriad of irAEs, which vary according to the class of ICI used. In addition, patients with cancer and preexisting autoimmune disease can also experience flares of their disease after treatment with ICI. Although the available data are still not robust, there is increasing indication that patients who develop irAE may develop better immune responses against their tumor, with improvement in survival. On the other hand, it is conceivable that some of the immunomodulating agents used to treat irAE may have a deleterious effect on cancer outcomes, hampering tumoral immune responses. There is some evidence that patients receiving steroids at the initiation of ICI therapy have worse responses than those not receiving steroids [4]. A recent study also reported worse outcomes in patients with ICI-induced irAE who received tumor necrosis factor inhibitors (TNFi) compared to those who did not, a finding that has not been corroborated by others yet [5].

Severity and Impact

Common rheumatic irAE, such as arthralgia, may be mild and not require treatment discontinuation or preclude rechallenging with ICI. However, other less frequent irAE such as pneumonitis or myositis associated with myocarditis can be fatal.

Duration

The duration and potential sequelae of adverse events are important to patients. For some irAE such as diabetes or other endocrine toxicities, organ damage can be permanent, but patients can be treated with hormonal replacement and can continue to receive ICI. Rheumatic irAE such as arthritis can be more prolonged, requiring therapy with disease-modifying antirheumatic drugs (DMARDs) including biologic agents for months; therefore, some patients may be less inclined to continue therapy with ICI.

Likelihood of Risk

The risk of developing specific rheumatic (and non-rheumatic) irAE with different ICI is well known. However, there are many uncertainties regarding specific situations. There are challenging decisions regarding rheumatic irAE for which the evidence is still scarce. What is the likelihood that a patient with a preexisting rheumatic disease will flare? Has the risk for de novo irAE increased in patients with concomitant autoimmune disease? If a patient develops a rheumatic irAE, how likely is it that it will get better if the ICI is continued? If treatment is initially withheld, will the adverse event relapse if a patient is rechallenged with the same agent or with a different ICI? What will be the effects of treatment with corticosteroids or DMARDs on cancer outcomes?

Patient Tolerance of Risk and Uncertainty

Patients will vary with respect to their level of concern for a specific harm, given its likelihood, severity, and potential consequences. Furthermore, tolerance of uncertainty also varies among people [6]. There are many unanswered questions with respect to the risk for harms in patients with rheumatic adverse events or preexisting conditions. Moreover, perfect certainty about health outcomes is almost never attainable. People with high tolerance of uncertainty are more likely to have less decisional conflict and better emotional well-being than those with poor tolerance. Patients who are anxious about unknown risks may prefer to defer to physicians' recommendations [7]. Discussions on risks and benefits need to consider the level of tolerance of individual patients in order to make decisions than balance health outcomes with patient preferences.

Multidisciplinary Approach

A team approach to decision-making is advisable given the complexities of balancing benefits, harms, and uncertainties in patients with cancer receiving ICI who develop rheumatic complications or have concomitant diseases. In addition to oncologists and rheumatologists, some decisions may require input from other subspecialties, as these patients often develop multiple adverse events involving different organs. Many institutions are implementing immune toxicity clinical work groups, resembling tumor boards, to provide timely input, multidisciplinary expertise, and comprehensive management for patients with complicated irAE, or those who face complex multifaceted decisions [8]. Finally, for patients who develop anxiety in the face of uncertainty about alternative decisions, psychological evaluation and counseling might be helpful in reducing anxiety and assisting patients in making decisions that are congruent with their values and preferences.

Case Studies

1. Ms. A is a 68-year-old female with a 15-year history of seropositive rheumatoid arthritis that has been difficult to control. The patient initially received oral weekly methotrexate, with partial benefit. She was then treated with TNFi, initially adalimumab, with an inadequate response, followed by infliximab, which was also not effective. The next line of therapy was abatacept, which initially showed some benefit but was discontinued after 18 months when her rheumatoid arthritis flared once again. Two years ago,

Ms. A started treatment with tofacitinib, added on to methotrexate, with an excellent response and no adverse events.

Three months ago, Ms. A was diagnosed with stage III melanoma of her right arm with metastases to axillary lymph nodes. Upon diagnosis, tofacitinib and methotrexate were discontinued, and the patient underwent resection of her tumor and regional lymph nodes. Within 6 weeks of discontinuing therapy, her rheumatoid arthritis flared significantly, and the patient, after discussion with her oncologist and rheumatologist, decided to restart treatment with tofacitinib, with awareness that there is uncertainty about the effects of tofacitinib on cancer progression. Ms. A was offered by her oncologist adjuvant therapy with nivolumab for her melanoma. After careful consideration of the potential benefits and risks, and discussion with her healthcare providers, Ms. A. decided not to undergo adjuvant therapy, as she feels that the potential gains in survival at her age, given that her tumor has been resected, are not important enough to sacrifice her quality of life by risking another rheumatoid arthritis flare that may be difficult to control.

2. Mr. B is a 54-year-old male who was diagnosed with stage I non-small cell lung cancer 4 years ago. The patient underwent surgery and remained without disease until a year ago when he experienced a recurrence in his lung cancer, with metastases to local lymph nodes. The tumor recurrence was not deemed suitable for surgery, and the patient underwent therapy with radiation and chemotherapy, with little response. The patient started treatment with an ICI, pembrolizumab, shortly thereafter, with good tumoral response showing tumor shrinkage after 3 months. After a few infusions of immunotherapy, Mr. B developed severe acute polyarthritis involving his shoulders, wrists, metacarpophalangeal and proximal interphalangeal joints, and knees, with marked morning stiffness and difficulty in performing activities of daily living such as dressing or grooming. His rheumatoid factor and anti-cytric citrullinated peptide antibodies were negative. Erythrocyte sedi-

mentation rate (ESR) was 84. Pembrolizumab was put on hold, and the patient was started on prednisone 40 mg daily, and oral weekly methotrexate was added to his therapeutic regimen, with progressive improvement in pain, swelling, and functional status over the following weeks which allowed tapering of the prednisone to 15 mg daily. Mr. B was offered to be rechallenged with pembrolizumab. After considering his options, he decided to be treated again, as his lung cancer had responded to immunotherapy, and there are no other alternatives for him at this time. He is willing to risk a flare of his arthritis irAE in order to increase his probability of survival.

Conclusions and Future Directions

Decision-making in cancer patients with rheumatic comorbidities with regard to immunotherapy requires thoughtful multidisciplinary discussions with patients considering individual benefits and harms, and patient values and preferences. Prior clinical trials have not included patients with preexisting autoimmune conditions, and there are no trials to evaluate strategies for the management of rheumatic irAE. Therefore, patients need to be presented with the available data and be told about uncertainties. Patients' tolerance for risk and their preferences in decision-making need to be carefully considered. While some patients may feel comfortable making decisions, others may prefer more direct advice from their providers, and these preferences should be considered in the discussions. Future research quantifying risks and benefits of immunotherapy in special populations, such as those with preexisting autoimmune diseases, will aid in counseling patients. Furthermore, clinical trials should also be conducted to determine what the best approaches might be in treating rheumatic irAE without sacrificing tumor responses.

References

1. Weber J, Mandala M, Del Vecchio M, et al. Adjuvant nivolumab versus ipilimumab in resected stage III or IV melanoma. N Engl J Med. 2017;377(19):1824–35. https://doi.org/10.1056/NEJMoa1709030.
2. Food and Drug Administration, U.S. Department of health and human services, 2016. factors to consider when making benefit-risk determinations in medical device premarket approval and de novo classifications guidance for industry and food and drug administration staff. https://www.fda.gov/media/98657/download.
3. World Health Organization. https://www.who.int/about/who-we-are/constitution.
4. Fucà G, Galli G, Poggi M, et al. Modulation of peripheral blood immune cells by early use of steroids and its association with clinical outcomes in patients with metastatic non-small cell lung cancer treated with immune checkpoint inhibitors. ESMO Open. 2019;4:e000457. https://doi.org/10.1136/esmoopen-2018-000457.
5. Verheijden RJ, May AM, Blank CU, et al. Association of anti-tnf with decreased survival in steroid refractory ipilimumab and anti-pd1-treated patients in the dutch melanoma treatment registry. Clin Cancer Res. 2020;26(9):2268–74. https://doi.org/10.1158/1078-0432.CCR-19-3322.
6. Strout TD, Hillen M, Gutheil C, et al. Tolerance of uncertainty: A systematic review of health and healthcare-related outcomes. Patient Educ Couns. 2018;101(9):1518–37. https://doi.org/10.1016/j.pec.2018.03.030.
7. Steginga SK, Occhipinti S. The application of the heuristic-systematic processing model to treatment decision making about prostate cancer. Med Decis Mak. 2004;24(6):573–83. https://doi.org/10.1177/0272989X04271044.
8. Naidoo J, Zhang J, Lipson EJ, et al. A multidisciplinary toxicity team for cancer immunotherapy-related adverse events. J Natl Compr Cancer Netw. 2019;17(6):712–20. https://doi.org/10.6004/jnccn.2018.7268.

Chapter 16
Patient Education and Shared Decision-Making

Maria A. Lopez-Olivo

Patients receiving cancer immunotherapy must be informed so they can understand the therapy they are receiving, understand the potential for adverse events, and make appropriate related decisions. They may face a myriad of learning barriers, including complexity of information, inadequacy of timing and methods of knowledge delivery, avoidance (as a way of coping), and, in some instances, inability to read [1]. The strategies used for cancer education and decision-making can be adapted and implemented by rheumatologists and other specialists, incorporating the aspects that relate to rheumatic immune-related adverse events or preexisting rheumatic diseases.

Patient Education

Patient education is offered to patients to understand their health problem with the purpose of enabling people to take control of their illness and improve their well-being [2]. In

M. A. Lopez-Olivo (✉)
Department of Health Services Research, The University of Texas, MD Anderson Cancer Center, Houston, TX, USA
e-mail: amlopezo@mdanderson.org

M. E. Suarez-Almazor, L. H. Calabrese (eds.), *Rheumatic Diseases and Syndromes Induced by Cancer Immunotherapy*,
https://doi.org/10.1007/978-3-030-56824-5_16

patients with induced rheumatic diseases and syndromes due to cancer immunotherapy, patient education requires a multidisciplinary approach involving oncologists, rheumatologists, and other health professionals to deliver well-coordinated and relevant information. The benefits of using education strategies in patients receiving (or considering) cancer immunotherapy can be extrapolated from experience in cancer patients in general. Evidence suggests that patient education may result in a greater ability to cope with potential immune-related adverse events, reduced hospitalizations, adherence to treatment recommendations, and improved satisfaction, among others [3].

Patient education can be processed, communicated, and applied in different formats, such as text, images, videos, and in-person presentations. The selection of the best format is influenced by the audience who will receive the information (e.g., age-specific, cultural competencies, and health literacy), how the information will be used, the purpose of receiving the information, and the formats already in existence. A study surveying 625 patients regarding the preferred method of education delivery for patients with cancer reported that direct discussion with the treating physician was favored by more than two thirds of the participants over other methods, including printed material, discussion with nurses, media, or talking with peers [4].

To be successful, patient education needs to go over an evidence-based process with four vital components: assessment, planning, implementation, and evaluation [5]. During a learning needs assessment, patient preferences are evaluated regarding content, style, reading level, and delivery timing and methods [5, 6]. The Joint Commission on Accreditation of Healthcare Organizations and the National Cancer Institute – Cancer Patient Education Network recommend to assess the patient's needs before proceeding with any other component of the patient education process [3, 7]. For the planning stage, factors that can influence patient engagement need to be considered such as patient's motivation, willingness to learn, ability to engage across different levels of the healthcare system, and practices of the organization and community.

Educational strategies with specific goals should be developed to address the patients, learning needs and potential determinants of engagement. The implementation phase of the process is the actionable component. Patients and health professionals (including doctors, nurses, dietitians, social workers, psychologists, pharmacists, occupational and physical therapists, and health educators) work together to perform the plan. The evaluation phase is the part where the success of the process is measured and reassessed to identify any adjustments needed. Multiple health education models and frameworks exist as useful resources to tackle the challenges of assessing needs, education planning, implementation, and evaluation [3].

Learning Needs

In the context of cancer immunotherapy, and resulting immune-related adverse events, the patients' learning needs include (i) knowledge about the frequency and characteristics of immune-related adverse events and (ii) understanding that decisions about the treatment of immune-related adverse events can affect cancer outcomes. Therefore, before making healthcare decisions, these patients need to know the benefits and risks of receiving immune checkpoint inhibitors in the context of a preexisting rheumatic disease or the implications of discontinuing or restarting immune checkpoint inhibitors after they have had an immune-related adverse event.

Other areas that require specific attention have been highlighted in a qualitative study exploring the experience of patients with inflammatory arthritis due to immune checkpoint inhibitors [8]. The study reported five common themes among the participants. Patients expressed the need to be aware of (i) the complexities and time that may be needed for diagnosis, (ii) the difference between immune-related adverse events and other adverse events, (iii) the potential impact to quality of life due to the cancer immunotherapy-induced rheumatic diseases and syndromes, (iv) the difference between social support needed for cancer and the specific support needed for the rheumatic disease or syndrome, and (v) the complexity in the decision-making process for treatment and continuation of the immunotherapy taking into account the potential impact in cancer outcomes such as survival or recurrence [8].

Education Strategies

Several strategies have been proposed to be used in clinical settings for cancer care, which can be adapted to health discussions and education on cancer immunotherapy and related risks and benefits. The National Cancer Policy Forum (NCPF) has listed 11 strategies to facilitate health communication [9]. Figure 16.1 shows the strategies proposed. The strategies that can be addressed by health professionals and will be expanded in this chapter include checking the patients' health literacy and cultural values, involving patients in the decision-making process, using all possible health communication channels including social media, being proactive about discrediting misinformation, and initiating discussions to help them understand care plans. Patients receiving cancer immunotherapy can benefit of these strategies to better understand their disease, potential immune-related adverse events, and treatment choices. In the context of cancer immunotherapy-induced rheumatic diseases and syndromes,

Educational Strategies					
Evaluate patients' health literacy	Check patients' values	Shared decision-making	Use all forms of health communication	Discredit false information	Discuss care plans

Figure 16.1 Education strategies listed by the National Cancer Policy Forum (NCPF) to facilitate health communication [9] and adapted in the context of management of cancer immunotherapy-induced rheumatic diseases and syndromes

patients need to know the benefits and risks of (i) receiving immune checkpoint inhibitors in the context of a preexisting rheumatic disease or (ii) discontinuing or restarting immune checkpoint inhibitors after they have had an immune-related adverse event. In addition, patients need to be clear about their options and what is more important to them.

Assessment of Health Literacy

Patients with cancer who receive immunotherapy and develop immune-related adverse events can be overwhelmed by the health information provided even when they are able to read, write, and speak and are highly functional in society. These overwhelming feelings are exacerbated for patients with limited health literacy in whom is unlikely that the provided health information will be retained or processed as intended. For example, patients may have difficulty comprehending terms related to immune-related adverse events, understanding the role of the immune system, and grasping probabilities of benefits and harms with different treatment options for adverse events and with the withholding or discontinuation of immunotherapy. These issues need to be explained in lay terms that are understandable to patients.

Health literacy has been defined as "the degree to which individuals have the capacity to obtain, process and understand basic health information and services needed to make appropriated health decisions" [10]. According to the National Assessment of Adult Literacy, approximately 80 million adults have limited health literacy [11, 12]. Health literacy can be influenced by the individual's culture, communication skills, numeracy skills, and knowledge of health topics. Poor health literacy disproportionately impacts individuals with lower education or income levels, ethnic minority groups, elderly individuals, and non-native speakers of English [13]. Patients who have limited health literacy may have problems understanding their health condition or their treatment options. With this lack of knowledge, patients may not be informed and able to participate in decisions about their healthcare options. Furthermore, limited health literacy has been associated with increased rates of hospitalization and decreased use of preventative services [14, 15].

There are multiple validated tools to evaluate health literacy. The tools most commonly used in the research studies, which are considered gold standards for measuring health literacy, may be lengthy and not optimal for clinical settings [16–18]. Two brief instruments that might be more appropriate in busy clinical settings are the Newest Vital Sign and the Chew et al. [19, 20]. These instruments can be further simplified in one item: "How confident are you filling out medical forms by yourself?" Respondents who frequently or "all the time" have difficulty in filling medical forms can be categorized in those with limited health literacy. Using this question during the clinical encounter can help health professionals to avoid technical terms and provide information that is concise and simple. Also, health professionals should corroborate that the health information to be delivered to patients and caregivers can be understood by using their preferred language and addressing their communication needs [7].

Patients' Values

One key component in patient education and shared decision-making is to take into account what matters most to patients. The terms values and preferences are often used interchangeably; however, several authors differentiate both terms as values expressing what is desirable and preferences being connected to attitudes [21]. The understanding of patients' values and preferences is an important feature of patient-centered care, which has been linked to better prediction of health behaviors, acceptance of patients' expectations and needs, and more effective communication [22, 23].

Patients with cancer on immune checkpoint inhibitors who develop adverse events need to be clear about the goals of their treatment (e.g., increasing survival time versus quality of life) and the importance they place on different treatment consequences and health outcomes. Patients who develop adverse events from treatment are vulnerable and may become anxious failing to express their needs, expectations, and preferences. Several methods exist in the literature regarding the recording of values and preferences, but as described in the section above, those used in research studies may be lengthy and not optimal for clinical settings [24]. There is scarce evidence regarding tools for eliciting patient values and preferences in clinical settings.

A more appropriate approach in busy clinical settings is to explore the role patients want to play in their treatment decisions during the clinical encounter. In patients living with cancer, a study has reported that over 60% prefer to be more involved in their decisions about treatment [25]. Rheumatologists can ask a simple question to ascertain what role patients may want to play in a decision about their treatment. Patients may choose to make the decisions on their own (after receiving the information), make the decision jointly with the health professional, or let the health profession make the decision (after receiving the information) [26]. This can help prevent health providers acting paternalistically and respect their patients' preference for making decisions.

Shared Decision-Making

Patients who experience adverse events with cancer immunotherapy face complex, dynamic, and multidimensional decisional conflicts. Examples of these shared decision-making scenarios include (i) holding or continuing treatment with an immune checkpoint inhibitor after experiencing an adverse event, considering the potential impact discontinuation may have in tumor response and cancer outcomes; (ii) selecting a treatment for adverse events, such as corticosteroids or disease-modifying antirheumatic drugs, which may impact the efficacy of immune checkpoint inhibition; (iii) in patients with preexisting autoimmune disease, deciding on whether to receive or not an immune checkpoint inhibitor given the higher risk of flares; and (iv) in patients with preexisting autoimmune disease who flare after checkpoint blockade, whether to discontinue this treatment.

The consensus statement from the European League Against Rheumatism regarding the points to consider for the diagnosis and management of rheumatic immune-related adverse events due to cancer immunotherapy with checkpoint inhibitors has as one of its overarching principles that the "Management of rheumatic and musculoskeletal immune-related adverse events should be based on a shared decision-making process between patients, oncologists and rheumatologists" [27].

The hallmark of patient-centered care is that health professionals and patients work together to determine the care options that are most aligned with the patients' preferences; this process is called shared decision-making. In fact, the Informed Medical Decisions Foundation defines shared decision-making as "a collaborative process that allows patients (and families) and their providers (and the health care team) to make health care decisions together, taking into account the best scientific evidence available, as well as the patient's values and preferences." This process considers the perspectives of the providers as the entity bringing the evidence-based knowledge and the patients as the entity with the right to be informed of potential harms and benefits of all available options. At the same time that providers feel confident in the care they prescribe, the decision-making process allows patients to receive the support needed to make individualized decisions and reduce their feelings of uncertainty, being uninformed, unclear about values, or unsupported.

Figure 16.2 shows the elements needed for shared decision-making [28] using one of the examples outlined above (considering immune checkpoint inhibitors in patients with a preexisting autoimmune disease). First, an individualized course of action is necessary to address variations in patient

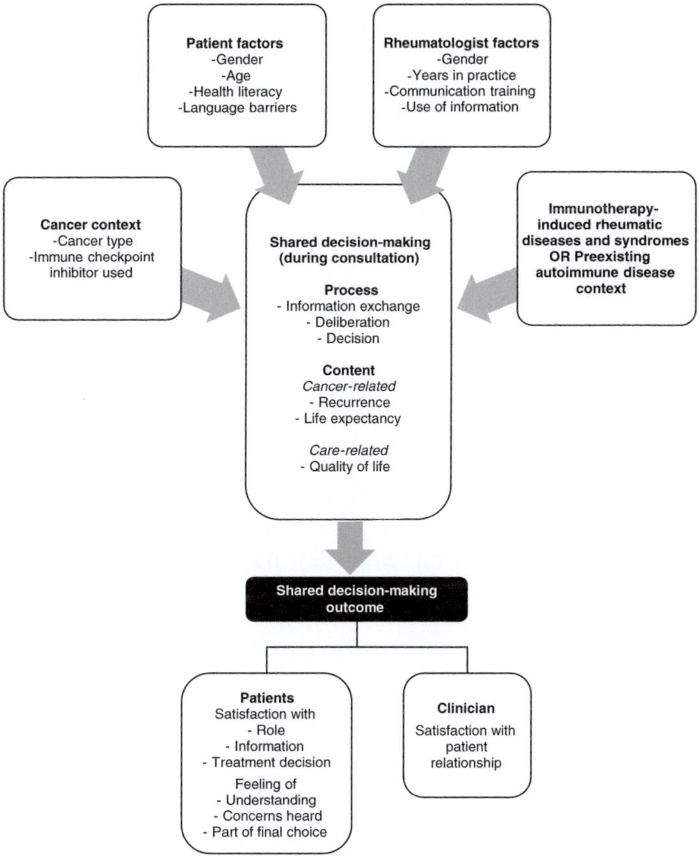

FIGURE 16.2 Elements of shared decision-making. (Adapted from a model described by Leon-Carlyle et al. [28])

(e.g., gender, age, health literacy, and language barriers), rheumatologist (e.g., gender, years in practice, communication training, and use of information), and disease factors (e.g., cancer stage, autoimmune disease, disease activity, and autoimmune disease treatment). Second, collaborative deliberation is needed so that patients and their providers can understand the decision to be made, the options available, and the impact each option will have for the patient's particular circumstance. During the consultation, information is exchanged about the potential impact that the decision to start or not the immune checkpoint inhibitor agent will have in the immune disease and cancer outcomes (e.g., treatment options, immune disease flares, adverse events (related or not to the immune checkpoint inhibitors), and the quality of life). Then a deliberation and decision is made. Finally, shared decision-making results in care decisions that safely and effectively consider the needs of each patient given their specific situation [28]. The shared decision-making process results in patients who are satisfied with the role they played regarding healthcare, their decision, and the information provided. In addition, shared decision-making results in patients who feel that have a better understanding of their options as well as feel that their concerns are heard and have a part in the final choice. The process also improves clinician satisfaction with the relationship with their patients.

Forms of Health Communication

The Accreditation Council for Graduate Medical Education expects medical graduates to demonstrate competency in communication [29]. Multiple approaches exist to communicate with patients regarding their informational needs and engage them in managing their own health. Patient-provider interactions can influence patients' behaviors such as self-efficacy or compliance and lead to enhance patient safety, improve outcomes, reduce cost, and increase patient satisfaction [30]. During the encounter, besides showing attentive listening skills, empathy, and using open-ended questions, providers should aim to address the patient's knowledge, beliefs, expectations of benefits, and external influences. Therefore, the delivery of information and the quantity of information need to be individualized to improve the patient's experience. Content may be delivered in paper format or electronically (e.g., sites or applications accessible on mobile devices or computers, digital optical discs, or compact discs) with interactive features and friendly information about different treatment options showing graphs or images of the differences among several options. The development of educational material should involve a systematic and rigorous process where only up-to-date evidence is considered. Information should be balanced, provided in sufficient detail and using plain language [31].

Brochures or other types of educational material can help guide the conversation regarding immunotherapy options with patients. For patients with cancer who are candidates to receive immunotherapy, these tools can help to better understand the uncertainty and the possible immune-related adverse events associated with each agent and the individual preferences such as their tolerance to risks and/or adverse events. Although they are most effective if used during the clinical encounter (i.e., together with the counseling of a provider), they can also be delivered by other health professionals in the waiting room before the encounter to help patients prepare questions to discuss with the provider or after the encounter so patients can review the material at their own pace and be prepared to discuss later. Patients could receive a summary to be used to facilitate interdisciplinary communication with other providers. The Oncology Nursing Society has proposed to provide wallet cards to patients receiving immunotherapy that can be accessed through their website and are publicly available [32]. The goal is to help inform providers who may not be part of the multidisciplinary team the possible impact of immunotherapy agents in the patients' care.

Discredit False Information

Health professionals should ensure that medical information obtained by their patients is accurate, inclusive of known risks and benefits, commensurate with medical expertise, and based on scientific evidence [33]. However, patients may be exposed to false health information given the accessibility to the Internet and the many unregulated sources. Health information can be delivered via social media sites such as social networking sites, blogs, and online forums [34]. According to the Code of Medical Ethics Opinion 8.12, providers and healthcare organizations, along with public health agencies and communications experts, can confront false health beliefs in the clinical setting.

During the encounter, patients should be given the opportunity to express their concerns and any understanding they have regarding the decisions they need to make. This allows providers to correct and redirect the patients to evidence-based information to make an informed decision about their care. The simple AskShareKnow questions have been used in clinical settings to quickly assess patients' understanding of their options [35]. For example, for patients contemplating the decision to hold or to continue the immune checkpoint inhibitor, the rheumatologist could ask patients to consider the following questions: "what are my options? (i.e., withhold or discontinue), what are the possible benefits and harms of those options? (i.e., impact discontinuation may have in tumor response or other cancer outcomes), what will happen if I do nothing? (i.e., not making the decision)." Explaining the potential impact of these decisions on cancer outcomes and quality of life in lay terms can help patients appraise the severity of the problem, understand what to expect from their decisions, and feel more confident about their decisions. Providing this information during decision-making motivates patients to better process their fears and feel a heightened perception of control [36]. As mentioned above, health messages need to be culturally specific and tailored to the beliefs, values, and preferences of the targeted individual or population. Additional items to be implemented in clinic include those reported by patients to value most during the clinical encounter:

(1) to be seen as individuals rather than a disease, (2) compassion, (3) professional knowledge and/or skills, (4) partnership, and (5) empowerment [37].

Discussing Immune-Related Adverse Events Management Plans

The combination of getting complex information regarding options, prognosis, and costs can cause emotional distress such as anxiety, fear, and depression. The National Cancer Institute states that the goals of an effective and supportive patient–provider communication are to establish trust and rapport, gather information from the patient, deliver information about the decision to make, and address emotions and concerns [38]. Evidence suggests ineffective patient–provider communication may result in increased healthcare utilization and costs [39, 40], and when health professionals are more effective in communicating with their patients, adherence to medical advice and protocols is more likely [41].

Management planning helps providers to communicate with their patients and close care gaps. It promotes more comprehensive discussions of the patients' needs, providing cancer-related and quality of life information, and delineating strategies that better fit ongoing health needs [42]. One method commonly used is the SPIKES method. This approach is easy to implement in busy clinical settings: rapport should be established and patient's perception of the medical situation should be assessed; then the patient's permission is requested to explain, information is provided, and emotions are addressed; finally a management plan is structured and summarized [43].

Conclusions and Future Directions

Imparting information to patients can improve patient's sense of control, reduce emotional distress, improve adherence, create realistic expectations, encourage self-efficacy and participation, and develop feelings of safety. It is important to assess the learning needs of each patient and characterize the information (active information seekers versus avoiders) and participation style (active versus passive engagement in the decision-making process). Research about how individual styles affect patient–provider interactions and the informational strategies that can be implemented according to these styles is still undergoing. Nonetheless, because many patients are often not prepared to ask important questions, rheumatologists should always establish a structured and ongoing dialogue with patients with cancer immunotherapy-induced rheumatic diseases and syndromes regarding plans of care and expectation regarding outcomes.

In summary, different alternatives exist to deliver education and ensure patient engagement and understanding and address the concerns and emotions of patients who develop toxicity with cancer immunotherapy. Information delivered to these patients need to be presented according to individual patient characteristics, such as reading levels, preferred learning methods, and the desire of being informed. Shared decision-making is increasingly used in clinical practice as a way to empower patients who are facing complex decisions for conditions where many uncertainties and preference-sensitive treatment options exist. Rheumatologists should work with other members of the multidisciplinary team to help patients in their decisions regarding the management of immune-related adverse events and in restarting immunotherapy. These decisions should align with patient values and preferences.

Future studies are needed to identify the specific learning needs of these patients to develop educational tools and materials that can facilitate decision-making. Tools such as decision aids can better help deliver health information about the disease, treatments, outcomes, and the prognosis of the condition and help clarify individual preferences and understand the importance of the benefits and harms of all available options.

References

1. Foltz A, Sullivan J. Reading level, learning presentation preference, and desire for information among cancer patients. J Cancer Educ. 1996;11(1):32–8.
2. Zangi HA, Ndosi M, Adams J, Andersen L, Bode C, Bostrom C, et al. EULAR recommendations for patient education for people with inflammatory arthritis. Ann Rheum Dis. 2015;74(6):954–62.
3. Cancer Patient Education Network. Establishing comprehensive cancer patient education programs: standards of practice. 2013. Available at https://www.cancerpatienteducation.org/docs/CPEN/Educator%20Resources/CPENStandardsofPractice.Nov14.pdf. Accessed 24 Jan 2020.
4. Chelf JH, Deshler AM, Thiemann KM, Dose AM, Quella SK, Hillman S. Learning and support preferences of adult patients with cancer at a comprehensive cancer center. Oncol Nurs Forum. 2002;29(5):863–7.
5. Butow P, Brindle E, McConnell D, Boakes R, Tattersall M. Information booklets about cancer: factors influencing patient satisfaction and utilization. Patient Educ Couns. 1998;33(2):129–41.
6. Wyatt JC, Sullivan F. What is health information? BMJ. 2005;331(7516):566–8.
7. The Joint Commission. Advancing effective communication, cultural competence, and patient- and family-centered care: a roadmap for hospitals. Oakbrook Terrace. 2010.
8. Cappelli LC, Grieb S, Orbai AM, Shah AA, Bingham IIICO. "I was prepared for the other side effects; I wasn't prepared for this one": a qualitative study of the patients' experience of inflammatory arthritis due to immune checkpoint inhibitor therapy for cancer [abstract]. Arthritis Rheumatol. 2018;70(suppl 10):5774. https://acrabstracts.org/abstract/i-was-prepared-for-the-other-side-effects-i-wasnt-prepared-for-this-one-a-qualitative-study-of-the-patients-experience-of-inflammatory-arthritis-due-to-immune-ch/. Accessed 10 June 2020.
9. Eastman P. The link between health literacy and Cancer communication. Oncol Times. 2019;41(16):1–5.
10. Services USDoHaH. Healthy people 2010. Washington, DC: US Government Printing Office Originally developed for Ratzan

SC, Parker RM 2000 Introduction In National library of medicine current bibliographies in medicine: health literacy Selden CR, Zorn M, Ratzan SC, Parker RM, Editors NLM Pub No CBM 2000-1 Bethesda, MD: National Institutes of Health, US Department of Health and Human Services. 2000.
11. Kirsch IS, Jungeblut A, Jenkins L, Kolstad A. Adult literacy in America: a first look at the results of the National Adult Literacy Survey (NALS). Washington, DC: National Center for Education Statistics, US Department of Education; 1993.
12. Ylitalo KR, Meyer MRU, Lanning BA, During C, Laschober R, Griggs JO. Simple screening tools to identify limited health literacy in a low-income patient population. Medicine (Baltimore). 2018;97(10):e0110.
13. Paasche-Orlow MK, Parker RM, Gazmararian JA, Nielsen-Bohlman LT, Rudd RR. The prevalence of limited health literacy. J Gen Intern Med. 2005;20(2):175–84.
14. Baker DW, Parker RM, Williams MV, Clark WS. Health literacy and the risk of hospital admission. J Gen Intern Med. 1998;13(12):791–8.
15. Baker DW, Gazmararian JA, Williams MV, Scott T, Parker RM, Green D, et al. Functional health literacy and the risk of hospital admission among Medicare managed care enrollees. Am J Public Health. 2002;92(8):1278–83.
16. Parker RM, Baker DW, Williams MV, Nurss JR. The test of functional health literacy in adults: a new instrument for measuring patients' literacy skills. J Gen Intern Med. 1995;10(10):537–41.
17. Davis TC, Long SW, Jackson RH, Mayeaux EJ, George RB, Murphy PW, et al. Rapid estimate of adult literacy in medicine: a shortened screening instrument. Fam Med. 1993;25(6):391–5.
18. Nguyen TH, Park H, Han HR, Chan KS, Paasche-Orlow MK, Haun J, et al. State of the science of health literacy measures: validity implications for minority populations. Patient Educ Couns. 2015;98(12):1492–512.
19. Weiss BD, Mays MZ, Martz W, Castro KM, DeWalt DA, Pignone MP, et al. Quick assessment of literacy in primary care: the newest vital sign. Ann Fam Med. 2005;3(6):514–22.
20. Chew LD, Bradley KA, Boyko EJ. Brief questions to identify patients with inadequate health literacy. Fam Med. 2004;36(8):588–94.
21. Warren C, McGraw AP, VB L. Values and preferences: defining preference construction. Rev Cognit Sci. 2011;2:193–205.

22. Street RL Jr, Haidet P. How well do doctors know their patients? Factors affecting physician understanding of patients' health beliefs. J Gen Intern Med. 2011;26(1):21–7.
23. Kennedy BM, Rehman M, Johnson WD, Magee MB, Leonard R, Katzmarzyk PT. Healthcare providers versus patients' understanding of health beliefs and values. Patient Exp J. 2017;4(3):29–37.
24. Mangin D, Stephen G, Bismah V, Risdon C. Making patient values visible in healthcare: a systematic review of tools to assess patient treatment priorities and preferences in the context of multimorbidity. BMJ Open. 2016;6(6):e010903.
25. Singh JA, Sloan JA, Atherton PJ, Smith T, Hack TF, Huschka MM, et al. Preferred roles in treatment decision making among patients with cancer: a pooled analysis of studies using the control preferences scale. Am J Manag Care. 2010;16(9):688–96.
26. Degner LF, Sloan JA, Venkatesh P. The control preferences scale. Can J Nurs Res. 1997;29(3):21–43.
27. Kostine M, Finckh A, Bingham CO, Visser K, Leipe J, Schulze-Koops H, et al. EULAR points to consider for the diagnosis and management of rheumatic immune-related adverse events due to cancer immunotherapy with checkpoint inhibitors. Ann Rheum Dis. 2020 https://doi.org/10.1136/annrheumdis-2020-217139.
28. Leon-Carlyle M, Spiegle G, Schmocker S, Gagliardi A, Urbach D, Kennedy E. Using patient and physician perspectives to develop a shared decision-making framework for colorectal cancer. Implement Sci. 2009;4(1):1–5.
29. Accreditation Council for Graduate Medical Education. Educational program 2008. Available at: http://wwwacgmeorg/acgmeweb/Portals/0/PDFs/commonguide/IVA5d_EducationalProgram_ACGMECompetencies_IPCS_Documentationpdf.
30. Ha JF, Longnecker N. Doctor-patient communication: a review. Ochsner J. 2010;10(1):38–43.
31. International Patient Decision Aid Standards (IPDAS) Collaboration. International patient decision aid standards. http://ipdasohrica/.
32. Oncology Nursing Society. Immunotherapy wallet cards. 2020. Available at https://www.ons.org/clinical-practice-resources/immunotherapy-patient-wallet-card. Accessed 11 June 2020.
33. American Medical Association. Code of medical ethics. Opinion 812. 2016. Available at: https://www.ama-assn.org/sites/ama-assn.

org/files/corp/media-browser/code-of-medical-ethics-chapter-8.pdf. Accessed 14 Feb 2020.
34. Centers for Disease Control and Prevention. The health communicator's social media toolkit. Atlanta, GA. 2010. Available at: http://www.cdc.gov/socialmedia/tools/guidelines/pdf/socialmediatoolkit_bm.pdf. Accessed 02 Feb 2020.
35. Shepherd HL, Barratt A, Jones A, Bateson D, Carey K, Trevena LJ, et al. Can consumers learn to ask three questions to improve shared decision making? A feasibility study of the ASK (AskShareKnow) Patient-Clinician Communication Model((R)) intervention in a primary health-care setting. Health Expect. 2016;19(5):1160–8.
36. White K, Meyer G, Martell D. Effective health risk messages: a step-by-step guide. Thousand Oaks: Sage Publications; 2001. p. 16–7, 26-7, 53.
37. Bastemeijer CM, Voogt L, van Ewijk JP, Hazelzet JA. What do patient values and preferences mean? A taxonomy based on a systematic review of qualitative papers. Patient Educ Couns. 2017;100(5):871–81.
38. Communication in Cancer Care (PDQ(R)): health professional version. PDQ cancer information summaries. Bethesda. 2002.
39. Rai A, Han X, Zheng Z, Yabroff KR, Jemal A. Determinants and outcomes of satisfaction with healthcare provider communication among cancer survivors. J Natl Compr Cancer Netw. 2018;16(8):975–84.
40. Walling AM, Keating NL, Kahn KL, Dy S, Mack JW, Malin J, et al. Lower patient ratings of physician communication are associated with unmet need for symptom management in patients with lung and colorectal cancer. J Oncol Pract. 2016;12(6):e654–69.
41. Lin JJ, Lake J, Wall MM, Berman AR, Salazar-Schicchi J, Powell C, et al. Association of patient-provider communication domains with lung cancer treatment. J Thorac Oncol. 2014;9(9):1249–54.
42. Hewitt M, Greenfield S, Stovall E. From cancer patient to cancer survivor: lost in transition. Washington, DC: National Academies Press; 2005.
43. Baile WF, Buckman R, Lenzi R, Glober G, Beale EA, Kudelka AP. SPIKES-A six-step protocol for delivering bad news: application to the patient with cancer. Oncologist. 2000;5(4):302–11.

Index

M. E. Suarez-Almazor, L. H. Calabrese (eds.), *Rheumatic Diseases and Syndromes Induced by Cancer Immunotherapy*, https://doi.org/10.1007/978-3-030-56824-5

J

K

L

M

N

MIX
Papier aus verantwortungsvollen Quellen
Paper from responsible sources
FSC® C105338

If you have any concerns about our products,
you can contact us on
ProductSafety@springernature.com

In case Publisher is established outside the EU,
the EU authorized representative is:
Springer Nature Customer Service Center GmbH
Europaplatz 3, 69115 Heidelberg, Germany

Printed by Libri Plureos GmbH
in Hamburg, Germany